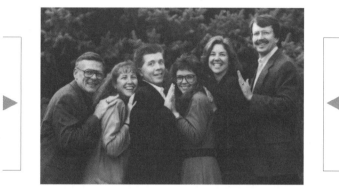

Our "Compacted" Compact Clinicals Team

Dear Valued Customer,

WELCOME to Compact Clinicals. We are committed to bringing mental health professionals up-to-date diagnostic and treatment information in a compact, timesaving, and easy-to-read format. Our line of books provides current, thorough reviews of assessment and treatment strategies for mental disorders.

We've "compacted" complete information for diagnosing each disorder and comparing how different theoretical orientations approach treatment. Our books use nonacademic language, real-world examples, and well-defined terminology.

Enjoy this and other timesaving books from Compact Clinicals.

Sincerely,

Melanie A. Dean

Melanie Dean, Ph.D.
President

Compact Clinicals Line of Books

Compact Clinicals currently offers these condensed reviews for professionals:

For Clinicians

Attention Deficit Hyperactivity Disorder
The latest assessment and treatment strategies
> C. Keith Conners, Ph.D.

Bipolar Disorder
The latest assessment and treatment strategies
> Trisha Suppes M.D., Ph.D., and Ellen B. Dennehy, Ph.D.

Borderline Personality Disorder
The latest assessment and treatment strategies
> Melanie Dean, Ph.D.

Conduct Disorders
The latest assessment and treatment strategies
> J. Mark Eddy, Ph.D.

Depression in Adults
The latest assessment and treatment strategies
> Anton Tolman, Ph.D.

Obsessive Compulsive Disorder
The latest assessment and treatment strategies
> Gail Steketee, Ph.D., and Teresa Pigott, M.D.

Post-Traumatic and Acute Stress Disorders
The latest assessment and treatment strategies
> Matthew Friedman, M.D., Ph.D.

For Physicians

Bipolar Disorder: Treatment and Management
Trisha Suppes, M.D., Ph.D., and Paul E. Keck, Jr., M.D.

Conduct Disorders

The latest assessment and treatment strategies

Fourth Edition

J. Mark Eddy, Ph.D.

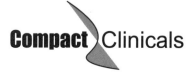

This book is intended for use by properly trained and licensed mental health professionals, who already possess a solid education in psychological theory, research, and treatment. This book is in no way intended to replace or supplement such training and education, nor is it to be used as the sole basis for any decision regarding treatment. It is merely intended to be used by such trained and educated professionals as a review and resource guide when considering how to best treat children and adolescents with conduct disorders.

Conduct Disorders
The latest assessment and treatment strategies
Fourth Edition

by

J. Mark Eddy, Ph.D.

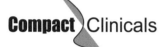

Published by: Compact Clinicals
7205 NW Waukomis Dr., Suite A
Kansas City, MO 64151
816-587-0044

©2006 Dean Psych Press Corp. d/b/a Compact Clinicals

Medical Editing: Kathi Whitman, In Credible English, Inc.,®
Kansas City, Missouri

Book Design: Coleridge Design, Kansas City, Missouri

Library of Congress Cataloging in Publication data:

Eddy, J. Mark
Conduct disorders : the latest assessment and treatment strategies / by
J. Mark Eddy — 4th ed.
        p.   ;   cm.
    Includes bibliographical references and index.
    ISBN-13: 978-1-887537-27-8
    ISBN-10: 1-887537-27-9
    1. Conduct disorders in children. 2. Conduct disorders in adolescence.
3. Conduct disorders in children—Treatment. 4. Conduct disorders in
adolescence—Treatment.
    [DNLM: 1. Conduct Disorder—diagnosis—Adolescent—Handbooks. 2. Conduct
Disorder—diagnosis—Child—Handbooks. 3. Aggression—Adolescent—Handbooks.
4. Aggression—Child—Handbooks. 5. Conduct Disorder—therapy—Adolescent—
Handbooks. 6. Conduct Disorder—therapy—Child—Handbooks.   WS 39 E21c 2006]
I. Title.

    RJ506.C65E33 2006
    618.92'89–dc22
            2005029079

10 9 8 7 6 5 4 3 2 1

Read Me First

As a mental health professional, often the information you need can only be obtained after countless hours of reading or library research. If your schedule precludes this time commitment, Compact Clinicals is the answer.

Our books are practitioner oriented with easy-to-read treatment descriptions and examples. Compact Clinicals books are written in a nonacademic style. Our books are formatted to make the first reading, as well as ongoing reference, quick and easy. You will find:

► *Anecdotes* — Each chapter contains a fictionalized account that personalizes the disorder entitled, "From the Patient's Perspective."

► *Sidebars* — Narrow columns on the outside of each page highlight important information, preview upcoming sections or concepts, and define terms used in the text.

► *Definitions* — Terms are defined in the sidebars where they originally appear in the text and in an alphabetical glossary on pages 79 through 81.

► *References* — Numbered references appear in the text following information from that source. Full references appear on pages 83 through 94.

► *Case Examples* — Our examples illustrate typical adult client comments or conversational exchanges that help clarify different treatment approaches. Identifying information in the examples (e.g., the individual's real name, profession, age, and/or location) has been changed to protect the confidentiality of those clients discussed in case examples.

► *Key Concepts* — At the end of each chapter, we include a review list of key concepts from that chapter. Use these lists for ongoing quick reference as well as for reviewing what you learned from reading the chapter.

Contents

Chapter Three:
Psychological Treatments for the Conduct Disorders   29

Chapter Four:
Biological Influences and Treatments for the Conduct Disorders 63

Appendix: References for the Clinician's Bookshelf 73

Glossary 79

References 83

Index 95

Chapter One:
Overview of the Conduct Disorders

This chapter answers the following:

- ▶ **What are the Conduct Disorders?** — This section presents the six different diagnoses used to categorize child antisocial behaviors.
- ▶ **How Common are the Conduct Disorders?** — This section presents prevalence rates among children and adolescents.
- ▶ **What is the Prognosis for those with a Conduct Disorder?** — This section highlights research on whether or not children with conduct disorders will continue experiencing symptoms through adolescence and into adulthood.

FOR decades, children and adolescents displaying chronic and serious antisocial or "conduct disordered" behavior have accounted for almost half of all referrals to child mental health clinics.[1-3] Youth with a conduct disorder (CD) typically present with a history of persistent disobedience, aggression, temper tantrums, lying, and stealing. Their victims may have suffered physical abuse, injury, disability, or death; emotional abuse and injury; and property damage and/or other financial losses. Prior to referral, a wide array of professionals may have interacted with these youth and their parent(s), including school counselors, principals, police officers, emergency medical technicians, paramedics, nurses, physicians, judges, and juvenile justice system staff.[1, 4] Because of the high emotional, social, and financial costs associated with each of the above consequences, the conduct disorders are considered some of the most expensive child mental health problems in the U.S.

Effective treatment can help mitigate the myriad problems related to the conduct disorders for the youth, his or her victims, their families, and society. However, treatment can be extremely difficult, particularly when complicated by factors such as:

- ▶ How long the conduct problems have been exhibited
- ▶ The youth's ongoing access to peer networks dominated by antisocial friends
- ▶ Demoralized and disengaged parents

This book is a succinct guide to today's "best practices" for assessing and treating CD, complete with ample references and resources for more extensive study.

1

What Are the Conduct Disorders?

Clinicians use the term "conduct disorder" to describe a persistent pattern of youth antisocial behaviors that violates fundamental social rules and/or the basic rights of others. Conduct-disordered behaviors include:

- ▶ Aggression to people or animals
- ▶ Destruction of property
- ▶ Deceitfulness or theft
- ▶ Serious violations of rules
- ▶ Negativistic, hostile, or defiant behavior

Each of these problems can disrupt the ability of parents to consistently and effectively supervise, encourage, and discipline their children.[5] Disruption in the parenting of a child increases the likelihood that the child will exhibit antisocial behaviors.[6, 7]

Most children exhibit some antisocial behaviors during their development. For example, disobedience and temper tantrums are normal behaviors at certain stages. To warrant a conduct disorder diagnosis, a youth must display a variety of *antisocial behaviors* to a *clinically significant* degree.

In this book, "conduct disorders" will refer to the six different diagnoses given for ongoing patterns of child antisocial behaviors by the ***Diagnostic and Statistical Manual of Mental Disorders — Fourth Edition, Text Revision [DSM-IV(TR)]***.[8] These diagnoses are:

- ▶ Conduct Disorder (CD)
- ▶ Oppositional Defiant Disorder (ODD)
- ▶ Disruptive Behavior Disorder Not Otherwise Specified (DBD-NOS)
- ▶ Adjustment Disorder: With Mixed Disturbance of Emotions and Conduct
- ▶ Adjustment Disorder: With Disturbance of Conduct
- ▶ Child or Adolescent Antisocial Behavior

antisocial behavior — behavior that violates fundamental social rules and/or the basic rights of others

clinically significant — a pattern of behavioral and/or psychological symptoms that has become established enough, severe enough, and impairing enough to interfere with a child's day-to-day functioning in the home, the school, and/or the community

From The Patient's Perspective

Shawn M.

Mom just got a call from my school counselor. He said I've been skipping school, failing some classes, and getting into trouble. So what. It's not like I'm the only one. He also told her who some of my friends are. Now I'm really in trouble.

How Common are the Conduct Disorders?

At any point, from two to six percent of American youth exhibit a conduct disorder.[4] Prevalence rates for conduct disorders vary depending on age, sex, and geographical location.[9-13]

Age — Prevalence rates vary across childhood as follows:

- ▶ Elementary school: two percent of girls and seven percent of boys[9]
- ▶ Middle school: two to 10 percent of girls and three to 16 percent of boys[10-12]
- ▶ High school: four to 15 percent of boys and girls[9, 12, 13]

In studies directly comparing rates across age groups, the prevalence of conduct disorders increases as children reach adolescence.[11, 12]

Gender — Studies that compare boys and girls across age groups indicate that prevalence rates are more equal between the sexes during middle to late adolescence than during early childhood.[11-13]

Geographical Location — Rates are higher for younger children from urban areas than from rural areas. However, rates are similar for adolescents in urban and rural areas.[9, 14]

From The Parent's Perspective

Jeannie M.

Just got a call from school. I'm so mad at Shawn. He hasn't been going to all of his classes. He's failing some required classes. He's even been hanging out with some kids who stand outside and smoke and get in trouble a lot. I can't believe this is happening right now. I am so tired, and Dan isn't around enough lately. I think that's what the real problem is. The school counselor says we should go to see a therapist. I don't see how that's going to help. The last time I saw a therapist was a waste of time. Shawn just needs to shape up.

What is the Prognosis for those with a Conduct Disorder?

Risk factors are interrelated across development. For example, children who exhibit hyperactive behaviors are more likely to have an early onset of antisocial behaviors.[25, 26] Youth with an early onset of antisocial behaviors tend to commit more frequent antisocial behaviors.[27] Individuals who commit more frequent antisocial behaviors are more likely to commit violent acts.[28]

One of the strongest predictors of current youth antisocial behavior is previous child antisocial behavior.[15-18] However, this prediction is not as strong as was previously thought. Only 50 percent of children who display antisocial behaviors during elementary school continue to do so during adolescence, and only 40 to 75 percent of adolescents who display antisocial behavior continue such behaviors as adults.[19-21]

Several risk factors increase the chance that an elementary school-aged child displaying conduct-disordered behaviors will continue to do so during adolescence and adulthood.[22-24] These factors include:

▶ Displaying hyperactive, impulsive, and/or inattentive behaviors (e.g., difficulty paying attention and sitting still in the classroom)

▶ Having an early onset of antisocial behaviors (i.e., before or during early adolescence)

▶ Committing many different types of antisocial behaviors (e.g., lies, cheats, steals, and fights)

▶ Exhibiting a high frequency of antisocial behaviors (e.g., gets in many fights)

▶ Displaying antisocial behaviors in multiple settings (e.g., fights at home, during school, and on the neighborhood playground)

▶ Associating with peers who display antisocial behavior

Of all the risk factors, an early history of antisocial behavior and an ongoing association with antisocial peers appear to be most important in terms of long-term outcomes (see figure 1.1).

During early adolescence, it is common for child and peer antisocial behavior to be quite intertwined, with many youth antisocial behaviors committed with, in front of, or against peers.[24, 29]

Key research findings on age of onset indicate that:

▶ Those who first display extensive antisocial behaviors in elementary school versus later have a significantly higher risk of displaying adult antisocial behavior.[30, 31]

▶ The average age of antisocial behavior onset for adults diagnosed with antisocial personality disorder (the adult equivalent of the conduct disorders) is age eight or nine.[32]

▶ Only about 10 percent of those who did not exhibit antisocial behaviors during childhood and adolescence begin to do so during adulthood.[33]

▶ There is a greater likelihood that "early starters" will commit multiple, serious offenses, and are more likely to be incarcerated as adults.[20, 23, 34, 35]

Figure 1.1   Key Predictors of Subsequent Violent, Serious Delinquent, or Criminal Behavior

<table>
<tr><td rowspan="4">Age Predictor Measured</td><td colspan="2">Middle Childhood (age 6 to 11 years)</td><td colspan="2">Early Adolescence (age 12 to 14 years)</td></tr>
<tr><td>Child antisocial behavior</td><td>.38</td><td>Child social ties</td><td>.39</td></tr>
<tr><td>Child substance use</td><td>.30</td><td>Peer antisocial behavior</td><td>.37</td></tr>
<tr><td>Male gender</td><td>.26</td><td>Child antisocial behavior</td><td>.26</td></tr>
</table>

Average correlation across studies listed.
Adapted from a meta-analysis by Lipsey & Derzon (1998).

Most of the information on the predictors of future antisocial behavior come from long-term studies of boys. In the few such studies of girls, the strongest predictors of subsequent antisocial behaviors are the same as for boys: a prior history of antisocial behavior and association with antisocial peers.[37] An additional key risk factor that appears more important for girls than for boys is a history of physical and/or sexual abuse.[24, 37]

Although many adults who displayed frequent antisocial behaviors as children do not commit criminal acts as adults, they often suffer other significant impairments.[38] Studies have linked a history of childhood antisocial behavior to adult alcoholism, psychiatric problems, romantic relationship problems, poor work performance, and poor physical health.[6, 18, 20, 34, 35, 39-41]

Adolescent girls with conduct problems are more likely to become mothers at a very young age, to be single parents, and to have children that display early signs of psychosocial problems, including conduct problems.[36]

Key Concepts for Chapter One:

1. The conduct disorders are some of the most costly child mental health problems in the U.S.

2. Although some antisocial behaviors occur in most children as they develop, those with conduct disorders display a variety of antisocial behaviors that are clinically significant.

3. The conduct disorders comprise six different DSM-IV(TR) diagnoses for ongoing patterns of child or adolescent antisocial behavior.

4. Although prevalence rates for the conduct disorders vary depending on age, sex, and geography, prevalence tends to increase as children reach adolescence.

5. Young boys from urban areas appear to have a higher incidence of CD; however, rate differences between boys and girls as well as between youth in urban and rural settings tend to decrease as children enter adolescence.

6. Those children with an early history of antisocial behavior and an ongoing relationship with antisocial peers appear to be most at risk for continued conduct problems as adolescents and adults.

Chapter Two:
Diagnosing the Conduct Disorders

This chapter answers the following:

▶ **What Criteria are Used to Diagnose the Conduct Disorders?** — This section presents DSM-IV (TR) criteria for the six diagnoses that relate to child antisocial behaviors.

▶ **How Can Clinicians Develop an Effective Assessment Strategy?** — This section presents a process for developing an assessment strategy and implementation plan.

▶ **What Other Disorders Commonly Occur with Conduct Disorders?** — This section discusses disorders comorbid with the conduct disorders and offers guidance for making a differential diagnosis.

D IAGNOSING conduct disorders can be challenging, often because how children present themselves in the clinician's office can vary dramatically. Some children may be withdrawn, hostile, and minimally cooperative (e.g., giving one-word answers to questions). Others may act shy, cling to a parent, speak minimally, and refuse to engage in activities with the clinician. Still, others may be quite restless and inattentive. Much to the consternation of their exasperated parents, some children who are quite non-compliant at home may comply quite readily with the demands placed on them by the clinician.

Just as children who display conduct-disordered behaviors can behave differently during an interview than they do during their everyday activities, their behavioral repertoires at home, at school, and in the community may be strikingly different.

Whatever behaviors clinicians observe during intake, there is no evidence that the information gained from such observations reliably assists in diagnosing a conduct disorder. Although some children with a conduct disorder exhibit challenging behaviors during interviews, many do not misbehave during office evaluations. [42, 43]

What Criteria are Used to Diagnose the Conduct Disorders?

In *DSM-IV (TR)*, child antisocial behaviors are categorized into six diagnoses (five of which are considered mental disorders). Only one diagnosis of the following can be made at a time:

▶ **Conduct Disorder** — Conduct disorder (CD) categorizes an ongoing pattern of behaviors that clearly violates the rights of others or disregards the accepted rules of home, school, and/or community. Major CD symptoms are aggression towards people or animals, destruction of property, lying and stealing, and rule breaking. For example, during the past six months, Jake frequently bullied and threatened others, initiated physical fights, and used a knife during several of those fights.

DSM-IV (TR) — the Diagnostic and Statistical Manual of Mental Disorders, Fourth Edition, Text Revision, published by the American Psychiatric Association

7

Figure 2.1 DSM-IV(TR) Criteria for Conduct Disorders

I. *312.8 Conduct Disorder*

A. A repetitive and persistent pattern of behavior in which the basic rights of others or major age-appropriate societal norms or rules are violated, as manifested by the presence of three (or more) of the following criteria in the past 12 months, with at least one criterion present in the past six months:

Aggression to people and animals

(1) often bullies, threatens, or intimidates others
(2) often initiates physical fights
(3) has used a weapon that can cause serious physical harm to others (e.g., a bat, brick, broken bottle, knife, gun)
(4) has been physically cruel to people
(5) has been physically cruel to animals
(6) has stolen while confronting a victim (e.g., mugging, purse snatching, extortion, armed robbery)
(7) has forced someone into sexual activity

Destruction of Property

(8) has deliberately engaged in fire setting with the intention of causing serious damage
(9) has deliberately destroyed other's property (other than by fire setting)

Deceitfulness or theft

(10) has broken into someone else's house, building, or car
(11) often lies to obtain goods or favors or to avoid obligations (i.e., "cons" others)
(12) has stolen items of nontrivial value without confronting a victim (e.g., shoplifting, but without breaking and entering; forgery)

Serious violations of rules

(13) often stays out at night despite parental prohibitions, beginning before age 13 years
(14) has run away from home overnight at least twice while living in parental or parental surrogate home (or once without returning for a lengthy period)
(15) is often truant from school, beginning before age 13 years

B. The disturbance in behavior causes clinically significant impairment in social, academic, or occupational functioning.

C. If the individual is age 18 years or older, criteria are not met for Antisocial Personality Disorder.

Code based on age at onset:

Childhood-Onset Type: onset of at least one criterion characteristic of Conduct Disorder prior to age 10 years

Adolescent-Onset Type: absence of any criteria characteristic of Conduct Disorder prior to age 10 years

Unspecified Onset: age at onset is not known

Specify severity:

Mild: few if any conduct problems in excess of those required to make the diagnosis **and** conduct problems cause only minor harm to others

Moderate: number of conduct problems and effect on others intermediate between "mild" and "severe"

Severe: many conduct problems in excess of those required to make the diagnosis **or** conduct problems cause considerable harm to others

II. *313.81 Oppositional Defiant Disorder*

A. A pattern of negativistic, hostile, and defiant behavior lasting at least six months, during which four (or more) of the following are present:

(1) often loses temper
(2) often argues with adults

Figure 2.1 (continued)

 (3) often actively defies or refuses to comply with adults' requests or rules

 (4) often deliberately annoys people

 (5) often blames others for his or her mistakes or misbehavior

 (6) is often touchy or easily annoyed by others

 (7) is often angry and resentful

 (8) is often spiteful or vindictive

Note: Consider a criterion met only if the behavior occurs more frequently than is typically observed in individuals of comparable age and developmental level.

B. The disturbance in behavior causes clinically significant impairment in social, academic, or occupational functioning.

C. The behaviors do not occur exclusively during the course of a Psychotic or Mood Disorder.

D. Criteria are not met for Conduct Disorder, and, if the individual is age 18 years or older, criteria are not met for Antisocial Personality Disorder.

III. 312.9 Disruptive Behavior Disorder Not Otherwise Specified

This category is for disorders characterized by conduct or oppositional defiant behaviors that do not meet the criteria for Conduct Disorder or Oppositional Defiant Disorder. For example, include clinical presentations that do not meet full criteria either for Oppositional Defiant Disorder or Conduct Disorder, but in which there is clinically significant impairment.

IV. 309.4 Adjustment Disorder: With Mixed Disturbance of Emotions and Conduct

A. The development of emotional or behavioral symptoms in response to an identifiable stressor(s) occurring within 3 months of the onset of the stressor(s).

B. These symptoms or behaviors are clinically significant as evidenced by either of the following:

 (1) marked distress that is in excess of what would be expected from exposure to the stressor

 (2) significant impairment in social or occupational (academic) functioning

C. The stress-related disturbance does not meet the criteria for another specific Axis I disorder and is not merely an exacerbation of a preexisting Axis I or Axis II disorder.

D. The symptoms do not represent bereavement.

E. Once the stressor (or its consequences) has terminated, the symptoms do not persist for more than an additional six months.

Specify if:

Acute: if the disturbance lasts less than six months

Chronic: if the disturbance lasts for six months or longer

Adjustment Disorders are coded based on the subtype, which is selected according to the predominant symptoms. The specific stressor(s) can be specified on Axis IV.

V. 309.3 Adjustment Disorder: With Disturbance of Conduct

Criteria A through E above and:

This subtype should be used when the predominant manifestation is a disturbance in conduct in which there is violation of the rights of others or of major age-appropriate societal norms and rules (e.g., truancy, vandalism, reckless driving, fighting, defaulting on legal responsibilities).

VI. V71.02 Child or Adolescent Antisocial Behavior

This category can be used when the focus of clinical attention is antisocial behavior in a child or adolescent that is not due to a mental disorder (e.g., Conduct Disorder or an Impulse-Control Disorder). Examples include isolated antisocial acts of children or adolescents (not a pattern of antisocial behavior).

Only one of these six diagnoses (presented in descending order of severity) can be made at any given time.

1. CD

2. ODD

3. DBD-NOS

4. Adjustment Disorder (mixed)

5. Adjustment Disorder (conduct)

6. Child or Adolescent Antisocial Behavior

▶ **Oppositional Defiant Disorder** — Oppositional defiant disorder (ODD) categorizes an ongoing pattern of child behaviors that are defiant and hostile toward others, particularly toward authority figures. For example, over the past year, a child may have frequently lost her temper, became angry, argued, and refused to cooperate with her parents and teachers.

▶ **Disruptive Behavior Disorder-Not Otherwise Specified** — Disruptive behavior disorder-not otherwise specified (DBD-NOS) categorizes an ongoing pattern of CD and/or ODD behaviors that fail to meet the criteria for a CD or ODD diagnosis. For example, during the past six months, a child may have frequently initiated fights, argued with adults, and defied adult requests, but he reportedly demonstrated no other CD or ODD symptoms.

▶ **Adjustment Disorder with Mixed Disturbance of Emotions and Conduct** — This adjustment disorder categorizes antisocial behaviors and emotional symptoms that begin within three months of an identifiable psychosocial stressor (e.g., moving into a high-crime neighborhood, parental conflict). Further, the symptoms do not meet criteria for one of the previously mentioned disorders. For example, Joey has intense mood swings and fights frequently with schoolmates, with the mood swings and fighting commencing within a month following his father's death.

▶ **Adjustment Disorder with Disturbance of Conduct** — An adjustment disorder characterized by antisocial behaviors only.

▶ **Child or Adolescent Antisocial Behavior** — Child or adolescent antisocial behavior categorizes isolated antisocial behaviors that are not considered indicative of a *mental disorder*. For example, Chris shoplifted three times during the past six months, but apparently exhibited no other CD or ODD symptoms.

mental disorder — a clinically significant pattern of behavioral or psychological symptoms associated with one or more major negative outcomes (e.g., distress, pain, injury, disability, confinement)

According to DSM-IV(TR), CD can be diagnosed if the specified criteria are met whether or not other psychiatric diagnoses exist.[2] The same is true of ODD except when the symptoms occur exclusively in the presence of a diagnosed mood disorder or a psychotic disorder. When this occurs, the clinician should assume that the oppositional behaviors are part of the constellation of symptoms of the mood or psychotic disorders, rather than representative of ODD.

Diagnostic Clarifying Information

Clarifying information involves determining clinical significance and specific criteria that serve as predictors of antisocial behavior. Making any psychiatric diagnosis is a subjective process: the clinician must decide that a child, relative to his or her peers, is behaving in ways that are deviant enough to warrant a psychiatric label.

Clinical Significance

When diagnosing a child with a conduct disorder, the clinician must decide whether a pattern of antisocial behaviors has become established enough, severe enough, and impairing enough to be labeled clinically significant. Impairment is probably most crucial to the idea of clinical significance; the maladaptive behaviors that qualify the child for a conduct disorder diagnosis should significantly interfere with the child's day-to-day functioning in one or more settings (i.e., home, school, and/or community).

Specific Criteria

The symptom, "often stays out at night despite parental prohibitions, beginning before age 13," is an example of a cluster of behaviors dubbed *"wandering."*[44] Wandering (or conversely, a lack of parental *monitoring*) is strongly predictive of child antisocial behavior.[16,44,45] In DSM-IV (TR), wandering in spite of parental rules is no longer considered a predictor of antisocial behavior, but rather a conduct-disordered behavior in its own right.

The symptom, "often bullies, threatens, or intimidates others," might better describe how girls may present when exhibiting CD. Researchers have hypothesized that girls tend to use *"relational aggression,"* such as intimidation and threatening, more than boys.[46-48] However, at present, there exists scant data to support this hypothesis.

Early and Late Subtypes

Diagnostic criteria focus on two subtypes based on age of onset of symptoms:

▶ "Early" — defined as onset before age 10

▶ "Late" — defined as onset at age 10 or older

These subtypes are based on findings that children who first exhibit antisocial behaviors during elementary school are at high risk for continuing to behave antisocially as adults.[23]

Researchers hypothesize that "early starters" learn their behavioral repertoires first through social interactions in the home, then through their social interactions at school, and finally through association with antisocial peers. In contrast,

wandering — spending time in unstructured settings without adult supervision

monitoring — hour-to-hour each day, a parent knows whom their son or daughter is with, where he or she is, and what he or she is doing

relational aggression — harm perpetrated against others using indirect, non-physical means, such as manipulation, threats, and exclusion

Although DSM-IV (TR) uses age 10 to divide "early" and "late" subtypes, some researchers consider age 13 or 14 (i.e., the end of middle school) as a more appropriate "cut" point.[49]

researchers hypothesize that "late starters" tend to learn their behavioral repertoires predominately through antisocial peer association. Late starters are more likely to discontinue their antisocial behaviors prior to adulthood.[30, 31] Some research findings support both the early- and late-starter hypotheses.[49, 50]

deviant peer groups — groups of youths who behave outside of socially accepted norms

As discussed in the behavioral therapy section of chapter three, groups of antisocial peers, or *deviant peer groups,* appear to play a central role in the development and maintenance of child antisocial behavior.

How Can Clinicians Develop an Effective Assessment Strategy?

The optimum way to conduct an effective assessment would be to observe the child over time in each setting. This is usually not possible, except in university training clinics where student clinicians are available.

To adequately assess conduct-disorder symptoms, clinicians must investigate how children behave in each key setting. The most common way to conduct this type of cross-setting assessment is to survey adults who spend significant time in each setting. However, adult reports of child behaviors are affected by factors other than true behavioral variation.[51, 52] The current emotional state or the past experiences of adults may bias their perceptions of the child's behavior. For example, some adults may see behaviors as aversive or deviant when other adults would rate the same behaviors as neutral. In a series of studies on bias, parents with children who either did or did not exhibit antisocial behaviors viewed videotapes of other parent/child interactions and rated specific child behaviors as *prosocial,* neutral, or deviant. Those parents of children with problem behaviors tended to classify a greater number of child behaviors as "deviant" than parents of children without problem behaviors or independent observers.[53, 54]

prosocial — responsible, socially considerate behavior

Assessment does not end when treatment begins; it is used to monitor ongoing treatment progress.

The most effective way to overcome the specific biases of various raters and to reliably map out a child's behavioral repertoire is to simultaneously consider multiple points of view as well as

From The Patient's Perspective

Shawn M.

We've been seeing a therapist. I just want to be left alone. I know I should start going to school more, but nothing else is wrong. At least the therapist is not blaming me for everything, at least not yet. She's talking to Mom a lot, and Mom doesn't seem too happy about that. The therapist even wants Dad to come in. That will be interesting.

how children behave in multiple settings. Thus, the clinician will need to develop a carefully planned assessment strategy that evaluates these aspects versus DSM-IV (TR) criteria.

The DSM-IV (TR) criteria for CD are listed on pages 8 through 9.

Assessing a child from multiple vantage points provides clinicians with a more reliable, valid picture of a child's current functioning and environment. At the end of data collection, the clinician integrates the information in a way that will inform and guide the course of treatment. A reliable and valid assessment strategy includes:[15]

- ► Multiple modes of measurement (e.g., observations, interviews, self-report scales)
- ► Multiple informants (e.g., parents, teachers, child, observers)
- ► Observation of behavior within multiple settings (e.g., home, school, community)
- ► Data collected at multiple time points

Each procedure used should yield unique information for constructing a treatment plan.[55] Given these parameters, a reasonable assessment strategy might include the following implementation methods:

1. Global rating scales completed by parents, children, and teachers
2. Clinical interviews with parents, children, and teachers
3. Observations of family interactions in the clinic and in the school or home

From The Parent's Perspective

Jeannie M.

Shawn got caught shoplifting, and he is on probation for a year. Now we are required to see a therapist. Why does everything have to be so hard right now? I guess there is a real problem with Shawn. I don't see how this is all my fault, but the therapist keeps talking to me about changes I need to make at home. She does say that it seems more difficult to make families work these days. No kidding. She does have a few ideas that seem like they might make things better. I talked with Dan tonight, and he might be able to come to an appointment. It would really help if he were more involved.

4. Repeated brief telephone interviews with parents

5. Examination of historical records

The clinician uses the information collected during each of these procedures to specify both positive and problem behaviors that the child currently displays. Further, the clinician identifies the strengths and problems present in the various settings in which the child interacts. This information is then used to construct a tailored treatment plan.

Handling the Initial Call

The first call parents make to a clinic should lay the groundwork for the first face-to-face interview between the family and the clinician.[56] Clinic staff that handle such calls can press for specific information, including the types and frequency of the child's problem behaviors, the dates of specific major problem incidents, and the general reactions of the parents to the problem. Parents can also be queried about previous treatment history as well as about how the child functions in major settings (e.g., home, school, and community). The staff member should also briefly describe the intake and treatment process and answer any questions.

The objective of the initial call is to infuse structure and improve the efficiency of the first, face-to-face interview between the family and the clinician.

At the end of the 10 to 15 minute call, the staff member should request that parents do the following:

▶ Complete behavior rating scales (mailed the same day as the call).

▶ Have the child (if age 10 years or older) complete appropriate behavior rating scales.

▶ Ask the child's school teacher(s) to complete behavior rating scales.

▶ Return all completed behavior rating scales several days prior to the intake interview.

Parents can be told that if forms are not returned prior to the day of the interview, their appointment will be postponed. Setting up this contingency screens out parents who are probably not yet ready to pursue treatment. Further, a critical factor in treatment success is the ability of parents to promote consistent, structured activities. If parents cannot return questionnaires by a predetermined date, they probably will have difficulty fulfilling the requirements of a treatment program. On the other hand, a major portion of the clinician's caseload may involve parents who have trouble with such requirements. These parents may be distrustful of authority and may not be willing to comply during the early phases of treatment. Thus, using such a screening approach might result in unjustly eliminating parents from a helpful treatment program that they might have completed.

Collecting Behavioral Rating Scales

Two useful questionnaires for diagnosing a conduct disorder are the Child Behavior Checklist (CBC-L) and the Disruptive Behavior Disorders Checklist (DBD).[57, 58] Used together, these questionnaires yield estimates of both the type and severity of a child's antisocial behaviors.

CBC-L

The CBC-L is widely used in both clinical and research settings. However, the CBC-L questions do not directly address all the DSM-IV(TR) conduct disorder behaviors. The CBC-L comprises both a lengthy list of problem behaviors and numerous questions on academic and social functioning. It can be completed by parents, teachers, and youth (ages 11 to 18 years).[57, 61, 62] Scales of interest in terms of the conduct disorders (i.e., Delinquent Behavior, Aggressive Behavior, Attention Problems, and Anxious/ Depressed) as well as prosocial functioning (e.g., Activities and Academic Performance) are computed by combining specific CBC-L items. The most recent version of the CBC-L family of measures is named the Achenbach System of Empirically Based Assessment. Each measure (e.g., parent version, teacher version) has subscales that map directly on to the DSM-IV. Normative data allows the clinician to compare scores a child receives to those of a general population sample of children and adolescents.[59, 60]

For the parent CBC-L, the following are moderate to strong for the conduct disorder-related scales:

- ▶ *Internal reliability*
- ▶ *Test-retest reliability*
- ▶ *Inter-parental agreement*
- ▶ *Across-time correlations*

Values for the youth CBC-L are similar, except for across-time correlations, which tend to be low.

The teacher CBC-L (called the Teacher Rating Form, or TRF) has similar psychometric properties, except that agreement between teachers tends to be moderate, especially on the Delinquent Behavior subscale.

In terms of validity, the CBC-L questionnaire items are *face valid*. Further, both the parent and teacher conduct disorder-related scales correlate moderately to strongly with similar scales from other self-report measures completed by parents or teachers. Finally, the parent, teacher, and youth CBC-L scores discriminate between clinic-referred and non-referred samples.[57, 61, 62]

Collecting behavioral rating scales facilitates having parents, teachers, and the child estimate the type and severity of antisocial behaviors.

The CBC-L norms may not be universally applicable, even within the U.S.[59, 60]

internal reliability — the extent to which the various items on a test are related to one another

test-retest reliability — the extent to which those tested obtain similar scores relative to each other on each administration of the test

inter-parental agreement — the degree of agreement on test scores between parents

across-time correlations — the extent to which a person's test scores remain in a similar rank compared to others across time (e.g., a highly stable test might have Suzy score high on three separate testings, Sam moderate, and Jean low)

face valid — the content of test items directly assesses a self-evident psychological construct

DBD

Although less psychometric information is available on the DBD, the items relate directly to each of the symptoms in the DSM-IV(TR) for ADHD, CD, and ODD. Total symptom counts can be computed for each disorder. In a large sample of boys in regular education classes as well as in a smaller sample of boys in special education classes, the internal reliabilities of the ADHD, CD, and ODD scales were strong.[58, 63] Although empirical validity information is currently unavailable, the main advantage of the DBD is its face validity.

Scores on the DBD and/or the CBC-L can indicate that completion of further questionnaires might be useful. For example, if there are concerns about child depression, the Child Depression Inventory might be used to further assess child perceptions.[64] Thorough information about a variety of such "specialty" self-report scales are available from multiple sources listed in the appendix.

Many questionnaires have been developed that assess both child and family functioning.[65–67]

Conducting Intake Interviews

Once the behavior rating forms have been returned, the clinician reviews all the information collected and notes issues to pursue during the first intake meeting. Using these notes to guide content, the clinician structures the interview as follows:

1. Greeting the family and attempting to set a comfortable tone for the intake
2. Educating the family about the assessment process
3. Questioning the parent(s) and child separately about the presenting problem and related issues
4. Arranging with the parents to collect further baseline assessment data

Prior to parent, child, and teacher interviews, the clinician integrates responses from the behavior rating scales (see pages 15–16) into a diagnostic framework by making a checklist that compares possible diagnoses and their symptoms. This framework can be used to guide further questioning.

Parent Interviews

In the parent interview, the clinician should:

1. Begin to establish a working alliance with the parents.
2. Gather specific information about the child's current problem behaviors and prosocial functioning.
3. Specify how parents, teachers, and other pertinent adults currently deal with problems.
4. Gather the child's *developmental history* and a *psychosocial history.*

developmental history — significant events and milestones during childhood such as age the child first walked or talked

psychosocial history — history of significant social developments such as family and peer interaction and adjustment at school

5. Query the parents regarding what they want to happen as a result of their contact with the clinician.

6. Make plans regarding follow up appointments.

At the session beginning, the clinician should describe the intake process and inform the parents of the various intake and treatment details and time lines. Parents should be informed of any laws that dictate clinician behavior in certain situations, such as what the clinician must do if information is obtained about child abuse and neglect or about a potential suicide or homicide. Prior to continuing, parents should be given a written informed consent form, which should be signed prior to moving forward with the interview.

During the initial interview, the clinician should query parents about:

▶ Onset of the presenting complaint and other behavior problems

▶ Development of symptoms across time

▶ Previous attempts to deal with the problem in professional and lay settings

▶ Family history of the problem

After clarifying the child's specific symptoms, the clinician can ask the parents about their specific reactions to each problematic child behavior at home as well as the reactions of teachers and other adults in settings outside the home. This information provides the clinician with some knowledge of the rewards and punishments children receive for their antisocial behaviors as well as a sense of how difficult the child's problems have been to deal with in the past.

The clinician should ask about the state of current family relationships, parental friendships, and parent-teacher relationships. Family participation in community and neighborhood life should also be queried. For example, knowing that a family closely identifies with or practices certain religious or cultural traditions is important information that can be incorporated into the intervention process. During therapy, strengths present in each of these areas can help support changes in child behavior.

Parents should be asked what absolutely needs to change for them to feel that treatment is successful. This gives the clinician some idea about what the patient really wants from their visit to the clinic.

The parent intake interview ends with the clinician getting releases from the parents for all pertinent records (e.g., school records, juvenile court records) as well as permission to directly communicate with key adults involved with the child (e.g.,

Some parents may have difficulty with the suggested parent interview. Being flexible and varying the content, structure, and pacing of interventions is important throughout assessment and treatment, particularly with parents who have had negative experiences with previous mental health professionals or agencies.

pediatrician, teachers, previous clinicians). Arrangements are also made for other baseline assessments, such as multiple telephone calls with the Parent Daily Report (see telephone interview on page 20) and clinic, home, or school observations.

Child Interviews

In the child intake interview, the clinician should:

1. Begin to establish a working alliance with the child.
2. Learn about the child's perspective on the presenting problems.
3. Gain knowledge about the child's friendship network and relationships with significant adults.
4. Determine the child's general intellectual and emotional functioning.

In therapeutic interventions for the conduct disorders, the clinician-child relationship is an important one, and a concerted effort needs to be made to develop a positive relationship.

To achieve the primary goal of establishing a working relationship with the child, the clinician should keep the tone of the interview light, questioning in a matter-of-fact manner that does not push or threaten the child. The actual interview questions often yield little new information, but may provide some insights on specific problem areas.

The use of a brief mental status exam and/or neuropsychological screen is also quite helpful in deciding whether further testing is necessary.[65, 66]

Besides informal questioning, a more formal structure can be imposed by administering several subscales from a standardized achievement test (e.g., the Woodcock-Johnson) and an intelligence test (e.g., the vocabulary section from the Wechsler Intelligence Scale for Children).[65, 68] These measures provide the clinician with basic information on the child's current intellectual functioning and allow the clinician to observe the child under academic conditions. With this information, the clinician can decide whether or not to recommend further psychological testing.

Teacher Interviews

During the teacher intake interview (usually done over the telephone), the clinician should:

1. Begin to establish a working alliance with the teacher (to facilitate possible school interventions during treatment).
2. Gather specific information about how the child's current problem behaviors impact academic and social functioning in the school setting.
3. Learn how problem behaviors are currently being dealt with at school.
4. Determine teacher perceptions about the relationship between the parents and the school.

The clinician should query the teacher about each of the above areas. Specific questions should seek to clarify or expand the teacher's responses to the behavior rating scale.

Using Other Assessment Methods

Following the intake interviews, the clinician should determine which standard assessment methods best fit the assessment strategy. These methods include:

- ▶ Standardized clinical interviews
- ▶ Common psychometric instruments
- ▶ Telephone interviews
- ▶ Observations
- ▶ Historical records

At present, there is no evidence that medical laboratory tests provide the clinician with information that would aid in diagnosing or treating any of the conduct disorders.

Standardized Clinical Interviews

Standardized diagnostic interviews may help clinicians diagnose conduct disorders more efficiently and reliably. One popular interview is the Diagnostic Interview for Children (DISC).[66, 67] The DISC takes from 50 to 70 minutes for a trained person to administer and covers the major forms of child and adolescent psychopathology, including the mood, anxiety, disruptive-behavior, and substance-use disorders. Two versions of the DISC are available:

- ▶ DISC-C: for children ages six through 18
- ▶ DISC-P: for parents

With adolescents, test-retest reliabilities for the conduct disorder scales on the DISC-C are moderate to strong. However, with elementary school-aged children, the reliabilities of the DISC-C scales are quite low. In contrast, test-retest reliabilities for the DISC-P conduct-disorder scales are strong for children of all ages.[71] Agreement between parent and child on DISC diagnoses tends to be low.[72] In terms of validity, both DISC instruments discriminate between clinic-referred and non-referred samples.[73]

Common Psychometric Instruments

For the conduct disorders, there is currently no evidence that frequently used psychometric instruments, such as the Rorschach Inkblot Test, the Thematic Aptitude Test, the Minnesota Multiphasic Personality Inventory-Adolescent (MMPI-A), or the Weschler Intelligence Scale for Children-Third Edition (WISC-III), reveal information that leads to a more accurate conduct disorder diagnosis.[68,74,75] However, administering **portions** of intelligence and achievement tests can be quite useful during the preliminary clinical interview with the child. Complete evaluations can be done in the clinic if parents request such a service.

The DISC was developed for use within highly supervised research situations. When the DISC has been used under regular clinic conditions, lower reliability values have been noted.[69, 70]

baseline — the period of time prior to the beginning of a therapeutic intervention

inter-interviewer reliability — degree of agreement among the ratings of various interviewers

Clinicians may want to investigate options available through the child's school. Free, school-sponsored evaluations of intelligence, achievement, speech and language, and motor development are mandated by Federal law.[55] Obtaining such evaluations from the school may take some time, but in conduct disorder cases, the presenting problems (e.g., disobedience, aggression, stealing) are usually problematic enough that they need to be addressed prior to academic interventions.

Parent Daily Report (PDR) Telephone Interviews

The PDR is a brief behavioral checklist administered over the telephone for roughly five minutes by a trained staff member.[53, 56] The PDR addresses child antisocial behaviors (including the symptoms of the conduct disorders) and can be customized to include parent-identified problem behaviors (e.g., child behaviors identified by the parents as particularly problematic at *baseline*). During the interview, parents report on the occurrence/non-occurrence of each behavior.

The PDR can be used to:

1. Establish the baseline level of child antisocial behavior (e.g., one to two weeks of daily PDR data can be collected to yield estimates of children's average performance as well as their day-to-day variability).

2. Monitor changes in antisocial behavior throughout treatment.

PDR scores collected during treatment (typically one to five calls per week) can be plotted and compared to the data collected during baseline to visually track how a child's antisocial behaviors change during the course of treatment.

In several samples, the PDR has been a reliable and valid measure of problem behavior.[78] *Inter-interviewer reliability* for the PDR is generally quite high.[79] Test-retest reliability for scores from one day to the next is moderate. However, data summarized from several PDRs (i.e., the average of several scores) is more reliable. In terms of validity, total scores for targeted problem behaviors on the PDR correlate significantly with both home observational data and global self-reports of the same behaviors.[79]

Observations

Through observation, the clinician can assess the frequency, intensity, and quality of a child's antisocial and prosocial behaviors on a moment-by-moment basis. Responses of parents, siblings, peers, and teachers can also be assessed, giving the clinician clues about the types of rewards and punishments children receive for the negative and positive behaviors they display.

If observations are done in the home or at school, the clinician can also assess the broader social and physical characteristics of the environments in which children spend most of their time.[80]

The most common observation tasks are detailed in figure 2.2.

Figure 2.2   Common Observation Tasks

Observation Task	How Performed	Advantages
Play Task (used with younger children and parents)	Child and a parent play together with toys/games of their choice, clean-up, and then participate in several structured, goal-directed activities (e.g., parent directs child in a parent-chosen activity, completing a maze, child teaches parent a game, working on an art project together).[84]	• Can be done in the clinic in 10 to 15 minutes • Can be easily videotaped for later viewing by the clinician and the parents • Present families with a standard "testing" situation
Problem-solving Task (used with older children and adolescents)	Child and parents attempt to discuss and generate solutions to a current family problem.[85]	
Unstructured Home Observations	Independent rater or the clinician observes the child and family in their home during the dinner hour or early evening.[86]	• Take place in the child's natural environ-ments (but require more staff time to complete)
Observations Outside the Home	Independent rater or the clinician observes the child in the class-room and on the playground.[80, 84]	

To code family interactions, independent observers or clinicians can use a simple behavioral coding system. The Parent-Child Interaction Coding System (PCIS) and Family Observation Schedule (FOS) are relatively easy to learn and use.[55, 80] Both systems include codes for parent commands, parent negative statements, child compliance, and child noncompliance. Since these behaviors are often at the center of conflict in families with a child diagnosed with a conduct disorder, the PCIS and FOS are ideal for capturing clinically relevant information as well as for monitoring changes during treatment.

To code the behavior of a child during school, a simple coding system should be used. One possible system is the Direct Observation Form (DOF) comprising similar items to the afore-mentioned parent and teacher CBC-L forms.[86] To code the DOF, the independent observer or clinician watches the child in a school setting for a 10-minute period (e.g., classroom, recess, lunch time) and then completes and scores the form. Subscales

Observations are often used as part of a formal "functional analysis," during which a clinician attempts to experimentally identify the variables that influence child problem behaviors. Once these variables are known, a treatment program is designed that attempts to change these variables in order to change child behaviors.[81–83]

When coders receive training and consistent monitoring, evidence supports the reliability and validity of these coding systems. Unfortunately, the reliability and validity of the systems in the general clinical context are unknown.

Although there are numerous reliable coding systems available, (some of which also have validity data) many are difficult to use outside a research group setting.[84, 87]

on the DOF that are of particular relevance to the conduct disorders include:

- ▶ Aggressive Behavior
- ▶ On Task
- ▶ Hyperactive
- ▶ Attention Demanding
- ▶ Depressed

The clinician should repeat the 10-minute observation procedure within the same setting on different days (e.g., a total of four times in the classroom) and average the DOF scores for the child's final score.

Several randomly-selected children (or several children identified by the teacher as "average") in the class can also be observed and rated, giving the clinician information on how the child compares to his or her classmates. The DOF has good *inter-observer reliability* and *correlates* with other measures of behavioral problems.[86, 88] Further, scores on the DOF discriminate between referred and non-referred samples.[88]

Besides the use of formal coding systems during observations, clinicians or observers should write narrative descriptions or complete questionnaires that document their general impressions of the child and his or her surroundings.[89] Several observer impression questionnaires have been developed to index a variety of child prosocial and antisocial behaviors as well as parenting behaviors and styles. These questionnaires tend to have good reliability and to correlate significantly with other measures of conduct disorder and parenting behaviors.[89, 90]

Historical Records

If parents consent, official records afford a low-cost, potentially high-yield assessment opportunity.[91] Treatment records will provide the clinician with session notes from previous intervention experiences, behavioral observations recorded during inpatient or residential stays, and/or testing data from previous psychological assessments. Academic records document standardized testing, grades, discipline contacts, and developmental problems. Medical records may document changes in the child's behavior over time, providing a different point of view on the child's developmental history. Juvenile court records document formal police contacts with the child (e.g., detainment for suspected criminal activity). Child protective services division contacts due to reported child abuse or neglect may be incorporated into juvenile court records as well as documented in separate agency records. However, information gained from historical records should be interpreted with caution, for it may be quite incomplete and/or inaccurate. For

inter-observer reliability — degree of agreement among the ratings of various observers

correlates — the extent to which two scores are linearly related to each other (e.g., as one score goes up, the other tends to go up or down)

example, less than five percent of juvenile-reported crimes result in police arrest and official documentation.[92]

Presenting Assessment Results

Once baseline assessment has been completed, the clinician integrates the collected information in a manner that will facilitate treatment planning and treatment process. Simply tallying up whether or not to diagnose a conduct disorder is not very helpful for treatment planning. Such a tally will undoubtedly reveal that the various people that were queried do not agree on the nature and/or extent of the problem. It may even reveal that they do not agree on whether or not a problem exists. For example, in several studies where parents, teachers, and/or children were asked about the child's antisocial behavior, 55 to 95 percent of the children given a conduct disorder diagnosis were identified by only one respondent.[9, 93] Some raters tend to rate a child as having conduct problems more than others. Elementary school teachers are three times more likely to identify a child as displaying a conduct disorder than are parents, and adolescents are two to three times more likely to identify themselves as meeting diagnostic criteria than their parents.[9] This high rate of reporting by adolescents has been found in several large surveys, with greater than 50 percent of adolescents admitting to committing more than one kind of antisocial behavior.[94, 95]

A more practical and useful way to integrate information is through the use of a descriptive analysis framework.[80, 96] During a descriptive analysis, the clinician considers how specific problem behaviors might be related to what happens in the surrounding environment. The clinician uses the complete set of data to specify the following for each problem behavior (e.g., hitting a sibling):

1. **Antecedents —**
   a. **External:** conditions that exist external to the child prior to the occurrence of a problem behavior (e.g., child and sibling are playing together)
   b. **Internal:** conditions that exist within the child that may be related to the problem behavior (e.g., hitting is more likely when a child is tired after a long day at school and daycare)
2. **Behavior** — the problem behavior itself (e.g., hitting a sibling)
3. **Consequences** — conditions that exist immediately after the problem behaviors occur (e.g., parent yells at child to stop hitting and return toy to sibling, child yells back at parent, parent and child argue, parent backs off)

The clinician then hypothesizes about how the antecedents, problem behavior, and consequences relate to each other (e.g.,

> *A descriptive analysis specifies:*
> *1. Antecedents (External and Internal)*
> *2. Behavior*
> *3. Consequences*

See chapter three for more discussion on the development of the conduct disorders.

repeated occurrences of such situations that teach children to use aversive behavior to get what they want). Such hypotheses are then used to guide and focus the treatment plan. Decisions can be made about what is appropriate for the clinician to deal with during treatment, and what issues should be immediately referred elsewhere (e.g., individual therapy for parents, marital therapy, psychiatric consult for possible medication assessment).

Once the clinician compiles the relevant information and makes tentative plans for treatment, decisions must be made on how best to present this information to the family. The cornerstone of successful treatment is for parents and clinician to arrive at a common perception of the problem and potential solutions.[78]

Assessment results are usually presented to parents and children during separate meetings. "Guided Participation" is a useful framework for such a presentation.[80] The clinician alternates summarizing the results and implications of the assessment with time for parents to think about, discuss, and question the clinician's reasoning. After presenting the data and listening to parental feedback, the clinician introduces the treatment model that seems most appropriate for the child's problem, specifies goals for the proposed intervention, and discusses treatment duration and costs.

What Other Disorders Commonly Occur with Conduct Disorders?

Conduct problem behavior is commonly present in youth who are diagnosed with other psychiatric disorders. Not surprisingly then, the conduct disorders frequently co-occur with other types of psychiatric disorders, and the clinician should probe a wide range of symptomatology during the assessment phase of treatment so that an adequate treatment plan can be developed.

In most cases, the presence of other disorders is not likely to change the basic treatment plan for addressing the conduct disorder, but is likely to necessitate the addition of other types of treatment approaches (e.g., individual therapy, medication) and perhaps involve other clinicians so that *comorbid* problems are adequately addressed.

comorbid — the simultaneous presence of two or more disorders

The most common comorbid disorders with CD are:

- ▶ Attention deficit hyperactivity disorder (ADHD)
- ▶ Anxiety disorders
- ▶ Major depressive disorder
- ▶ Substance abuse/dependence

In a study that combined data from several population studies, of the 13 percent of children who received a diagnosis of CD or ODD:[97]

- ▶ Thirty-one percent were also diagnosed with ADHD.
- ▶ Twenty-four percent were also diagnosed with an anxiety disorder.
- ▶ Twenty-one percent were also diagnosed with a mood disorder, such as major depressive disorder or bipolar I disorder.

An additional disorder that includes conduct problem behaviors and that has received some recent attention in the research literature is intermittent explosive disorder (IED).[98, 99] IED is characterized by serious, unexpected acts of aggressive behavior that either appear to be unprovoked or are clearly extreme responses to any provocation that is present. These incidents are unrelated to substance use or medical status. Besides these incidents, a youth does not exhibit other signs of a conduct disorders.

Attention Deficit Hyperactivity Disorder

In samples of children diagnosed with an attention deficit disorder, as many as 65 percent may display significant levels of defiance.[100] Across a variety of studies, up to 40 percent of children and 65 percent of adolescents diagnosed with ADHD meet full diagnostic criteria for ODD, and 20 to 50 percent of these children and adolescents also meet full diagnostic criteria for CD.[55, 101] A recent longitudinal study of a representative sample of the U.S. population found that children diagnosed with ADHD were more likely to develop ODD.[102]

Several or all of the key symptoms of ADHD (inattention, impulsivity, and hyperactivity) may occur for a variety of reasons besides the presence of ADHD. For example, children who have experienced trauma, such as abuse, may display several ADHD-like symptoms.

According to DSM-IV (TR), CD can be diagnosed if the specified criteria are met, whether or not other psychiatric diagnoses exist.[8] However, a diagnosis of ODD is given only if the symptoms occur independently of a mood or psychotic disorder and if the symptoms are distinguishable from those of ADHD. For example, children displaying attention-deficit-disordered symptoms, such as inattention, impulsivity, and hyperactivity, often exhibit associated symptoms of ODD, such as noncompliance. To diagnose co-occurring ODD and ADHD, the clinician must decide that in addition to ADHD symptoms, the child is truly exhibiting hostile, angry, and defiant behavior.

The co-occurrence of ADHD and the conduct disorders is high enough that there is some debate about whether they are actually distinct behavioral syndromes, or rather parts of the same syndrome.[103] Results from a recent, systematic literature review indicate that ADHD and the conduct disorders are conceptualized best as different syndromes.[26] However, their co-occurrence does have important future implications. For example, compared to boys with only one or neither syndrome, boys with both ADHD and conduct problems are much more likely to exhibit either type of problem at long-term follow-up.[26, 101] Unfortunately, insufficient data exist on long-term outcomes for girls.

Because of the link between ADHD and the conduct disorders, a thorough assessment of current and past ADHD symptoms is important when diagnosing a conduct disorder.

Major Depressive Disorder/Dysthymia/ Anxiety Disorders

Acting out behaviors that are common in the conduct disorders often occur in the presence of depressive disorders.

In a comprehensive review of studies of childhood psychiatric disorder comorbidity, those youth diagnosed with conduct disorder were more likely than others to be diagnosed with a depressive disorder, and to a significantly lesser degree, with an anxiety disorder.[101] However, other research found that depression and conduct disorder tended to be more comorbid in girls than boys.[102]

Bipolar I Disorder

Some research indicates that approximately 20 percent of children and adolescents with bipolar I disorder also exhibit a conduct disorder.[104] In younger children, conduct problems are usually related to poor judgement and grandiosity, and in adolescents often to issues such as running away, stealing, and driving under the influence of substances.[105, 106]

Substance Abuse/Dependence

The conduct disorders and substance use disorders have been linked in a variety of studies.[107] For both boys and girls, substance use disorders co-occur at a significant level with conduct disorder, but not with ODD.[107] Some researchers argue that conduct problems and substance use problems are linked through early use: the earlier someone with conduct problems begins to use substances, the more likely he or she will abuse substances during adulthood.[108] This popular hypothesis has yet to be tested directly. There is evidence that youth with a conduct disorder (other than ODD) are significantly likely to have a later substance abuse or dependence disorder. However, this relationship becomes insignificant (for boys, but not girls) when controlling for other possible comorbidities.[102]

Heavy use of substances is often preceded and followed by conduct problem behavior and association with peers with similar problems.[109] Abuse and dependence may lead to an exacerbation of conduct problems and the initiation of a conduct disorder.

Outcomes for youth with multiple psychiatric disorders tend to be poorer. For example, in a study of adolescents with substance use disorders, those with CD and/or ADHD were more likely to use substances again more quickly following treatment, despite having received more follow-up treatment services.[110]

Differential Diagnosis

Before making a CD diagnosis, a wide variety of psychopathology and background stressors should be considered in relation to the presenting problems to differentiate between CD and ADHD, substance abuse or dependence disorders, depressive disorders, or bipolar I disorder. Those with other types of psychological problems, including post-traumatic stress disorder or mental retardation, may also exhibit conduct problems.

The presence of both a conduct disorder and one of these other disorders requires the clinician to decide whether the conduct problems are a manifestation of a conduct disorder or rather just one aspect of one of these other disorders. The following provides an overview of factors to consider in differentiating other disorders most commonly associated with CD symptoms from a conduct disorder:

▶ **Attention deficit hyperactivity disorder** — Behavioral problems associated with ADHD are primarily due to inattention, hyperactivity, and impulsivity, NOT the oppositionality and defiance characteristic of ODD. Direct observation of the child in the home and school setting as well as interviews with parents and teachers can help differentiate ADHD from the conduct disorders.

▶ **Bipolar I disorder** — Those with bipolar I disorder will have a history of cycling depression and mania or intense, frequently recurring periods of emotion and irritability not typical of CD. Additionally, in bipolar disorder, defiant behaviors are precipitated by a mood shift rather than a behavioral pattern (without a prominent mood problem) as in CD. Those with bipolar disorder may also report psychotic symptoms not present with CD.

▶ **Major depressive disorder/dysthymic disorder** — Those with depressive disorders exhibit significant changes in energy and activity levels as well as sleep and appetite disturbances uncharacteristic of CD.

▶ **Substance abuse/dependence** — Current and past substance use should be carefully examined in terms of links to conduct problem behavior. Symptoms are typically related to onset, duration, or cessation of substance use.

Key Concepts for Chapter Two:

1. Only one of the six CD diagnoses can be made at any given time.

2. Age of onset (before or after age 10) is key to DSM-IV(TR) diagnostic subtypes. "Late starters" (those who begin to display antisocial behaviors after age 10 to 13) typically discontinue such behavior before adulthood.

3. Adequately assessing CD requires gathering information on behavior patterns from various sources (e.g., parents, teachers, peers) and in multiple settings (e.g., school, home, community).

4. Using results of behavior rating scales, clinicians can structure effective parent, child, and teacher interviews.

5. Standard assessment measures used for diagnosing CD include standardized clinical interviews, questionnaires, telephone interviews, observation, and historical records.

6. Assessment results are more helpful in terms of treatment when presented in terms of antecedents and consequences for each problem behavior.

7. The most common disorders comorbid with the conduct disorders are ADHD, anxiety disorders, and major depressive disorder.

8. Youth with a conduct disorder (other than ODD) also may suffer from substance abuse/dependence.

Chapter Three:
Psychological Treatments for the Conduct Disorders

This chapter answers the following:

- ▶ **What is the Behavioral Therapy Approach to Treating CD?** — This section explains social learning theory and behavioral interventions for treating CD: parent training, school-based programs, and multidimensional treatment foster care. For each intervention, information addresses treatment process, follow up, and effectiveness.

- ▶ **What is the Cognitive Therapy Approach to Treating CD?** — This section explains cognitive theory, treatment methods, and effectiveness.

- ▶ **What is the Family Therapy Approach to Treating CD?** — This section covers both functional family therapy and multisystemic treatment as well as effectiveness of these approaches.

- ▶ **How is Group Therapy Used to Treat CD?** — This section focuses on group therapy conducted in community centers or day camps as well as group therapy effectiveness.

- ▶ **How is the Psychodynamic Approach Used to Treat CD?** — This section discusses attachment theory and presents treatment and efficacy information on a dyadic skills training program.

W HEN treating children and adolescents diagnosed with a conduct disorder, clinicians must consider four key issues:

1. **Basis of the diagnosis** — Conduct disorders are diagnosed solely on the basis of child behaviors. The most effective treatment programs focus on changing specific problematic behaviors.

2. **Focus of the treatment program** — Regardless of what factors initiate conduct problems, the conduct disorders are developed and maintained through a child's social interactions with parents, teachers, and peers. The most effective treatment programs focus first on changing the characteristics of these interactions.

3. **Scientific support for psychotherapy** — Research studies, including randomized controlled trials, support the use of some treatment programs, most notably parent training, school-based behavior management programs, and child problem-solving skills programs. The most effective treatment programs use parent training in combination with other programs.

Of the over 250 different types of psychological therapies practiced with children and adolescents, parent training has emerged as the clear treatment of choice for those exhibiting conduct-disordered behavior.[111–115] However, notable limitations exist in the evidence base for youth psychotherapy research, and many interventions studied may not have received fair tests of their efficacy.[116–118]

29

Chapter four presents the biological foundations of the conduct disorders as well as medications used.

4. **Use of medications as a secondary treatment** — For some children, medications may decrease the intensity or frequency of certain conduct-disordered behaviors, which in turn may improve the child's response to ongoing psychosocial interventions.[119] Typically, physicians prescribe medications when the conduct disorder co-occurs with an attention deficit hyperactivity disorder (ADHD), and/or the conduct disorder includes displays of severe and extreme aggression.

The most effective treatment programs use medication, if indicated, as an adjunct to psychological therapy, rather than as the sole treatment method.

The following sections present each therapy type (behavioral, cognitive, family, group, and psychodynamic) in terms of the process of treatment sessions and follow-up methods after termination as well as research findings on treatment efficacy.

What is the Behavior Therapy Approach to Treating CD?

Behavior therapy attempts to strengthen the child's prosocial behavior repertoire, thereby changing the social interactions between parents, teachers, peers, and the child that may promote negative behavior. There are several different versions of behavior therapy. "Social Learning" behavioral theorists hypothesize that the day-to-day interactions between children with a conduct disorder and their parents, teachers, and peers inadvertently teach and maintain aggressive and other antisocial child behaviors.[83][120] According to these theorists, this process occurs through the unintended *negative reinforcement* of aversive behaviors. For example, consider the following sequence of events:

negative reinforcement — the discontinuation of an undesired event (e.g., parents fighting) following a behavior (e.g., child hits sibling) rewards the occurrence of that behavior (i.e., the hit)

▶ A parent tells a child to put a candy bar back on the shelf at the grocery store checkout line.

▶ The child complains and whines.

▶ The parent repeats the request more sternly.

▶ The child says "no."

▶ The parent threatens to punish the child.

▶ The child yells.

▶ The parent threatens, and the child yells louder.

Interaction sequences such as these are called "coercive interactions."

The sequence ends when the parent backs down; the child stops yelling; and the parent purchases the candy bar. Unfortunately, the discontinuation of the parent's threat increases the likelihood that the child will yell again when in a similar demand situation. Further, the discontinuation of the child's yelling increases the likelihood that the parent will back down again in a similar situation.

When negative reinforcement sequences occur again and again within a relationship, the participants are "taught" that aversive behaviors are effective at "shutting off" the negativity of others. Unfortunately, when such behavior sequences predominate in a family, *positive reinforcement* sequences are usually quite scarce. Over time, one result of a high rate of negative reinforcement and a low rate of positive reinforcement within a family is a child who is deficient in positive social skills and extremely proficient in deviant behaviors. Another result is the withdrawal of parents from parent-child interaction, which provides the child with more adult-unsupervised time both inside and outside the home.

Children who are skilled in deviant behaviors and who have low levels of adult supervision tend to have difficulties in conventional situations, such as school and on the playground. A common outcome of conflict in these situations is rejection by peers and adults. In concert, difficulties in school and with peers can lead to a cascading set of problems for the child, the family, and the community.[15, 83] If a child then begins to associate with peers involved in delinquent activities (e.g., deviant peers), the child will likely be exposed to and begin to participate in more serious antisocial behaviors (e.g., violent acts) as well as other problem behaviors, such as early sexual behavior and substance use.

This section covers the three recommended behavioral treatment programs for the conduct disorders:

- ▶ Parent Training (pages 31–41)
- ▶ School-Based Programs — CLASS and RECESS (pages 41–43)
- ▶ Multidimensional Treatment Foster Care (pages 43–45)

For each program, information presented includes treatment process, follow-up after termination, and program efficacy.

Parent Training

Ample evidence exists that parent behaviors, such as inconsistent discipline and inadequate supervision, are related to child conduct problems.[15, 83] On the basis of these findings, clinicians have designed parent training programs to help redirect parents' efforts from inadvertently shaping problem behaviors to systematically teaching prosocial behaviors. Parent training helps parents become effective "behavior modifiers," who accurately

Coercive family processes provide the means and the opportunity for a child to learn and practice aversive behaviors across multiple settings, behaviors that ultimately lead to the CD diagnosis.

positive reinforcement — the delivery of a desired event (e.g., parent says, "Great job, Joe!" and gives Joe a hug) following a behavior (e.g., child playing nicely with sibling), which results in an increase of that behavior

A variety of group and individual parent training treatment programs are available. See **Appendix: Recommended Resources** for a list of these programs.

monitor what problems exist within their family, make plans to resolve such problems, and implement these plans.

Although many versions of parent training exist for treating the conduct disorders, one of the earliest and most influential programs was developed by Gerald R. Patterson and John B. Reid and their colleagues at the Oregon Social Learning Center (OSLC).[56, 121] This program has been adapted to a variety of treatment settings and embodies many of the primary elements of current parent training programs.[15, 83] These primary elements include:

► An assessment phase in which the clinician attempts to build a well-defined and positive working relationship with the parents

► Treatment sessions with parents (the child with CD and siblings may attend certain sessions) typically held weekly for 60–90 minutes

For more information on using the PDR in telephone interviews, see page 20.

► The Parent Daily Report (PDR), which records data for monitoring treatment effectivenss that is collected by a clinical staff member over the phone

► Troubleshooting phone calls between the clinician and the parents (typically once or twice a week)

The average length of treatment is three to four months; however, termination should be a joint decision between clinician and family.[55] Average clinician contact time during treatment is 20 to 40 hours, approximately one-third of which is spent on the telephone.[119]

Content adaptations for parent training can be made for older or younger children than those for whom the program was designed.

Designed for children in elementary school or for those in early- to mid-adolescence, parent training involves both an assessment and a treatment phase.

From The Patient's Perspective

Shawn M.

I haven't been able to see my friends like I used to, and that makes me mad. But, Mom isn't angry with me and things seem to be better at home, even between Mom and Dad. Dad even went to see the therapist with us. I couldn't believe it. I guess things aren't so bad; I'm doing better at school. But now I have to make sure I get all of my homework done before I can watch TV at night. It seems that there are all kinds of new rules just to get to do what I want. Mostly it works out okay.

Assessment Phase

To establish an effective parent training relationship, the clinician should:

- ▶ **Build a trusting relationship with the parents —** Make frequent phone contacts and home visits to gather the information needed to remove potential barriers. Spend time listening to parents, validating their feelings, and empathizing with their situation.

- ▶ **Treat the parents as expert colleagues —** Instruct, advise, and support parents in a respectful fashion. Build on the strengths of a family.

- ▶ **Actively model the techniques that are being taught —** Illustrate the use of appropriate skills at every opportunity. Invite all family members to selected family problem-solving sessions, and show parents how to appropriately involve children in family decisions.

- ▶ **Teach parents to more accurately observe their own and their child's behavior —** Learning to make observations in the home or clinician's office gives the family direct information about family functioning on a moment-by-moment basis.

The assessment process begins in earnest during the PDR phone calls that occur in the two-week baseline period following the face-to-face intake meeting. During these calls, clinicians guide parents to focus on observable child behaviors and succinctly report on what they observe.

Following the initial, two-week baseline assessment, the clinician asks parents to read a book on the principles of social learning

From The Parent's Perspective

Jeannie M.

Well, things are going better. After a couple of months of working on talking with each other better and keeping better track of Shawn, things seem more in control. I know that Dan and I tend to back off when we're tired or problems start. Now, I realize that to get some amount of control, we need to do just the opposite. We are paying better attention to Shawn's activities and making sure he gets his homework done. He gets to do the fun things he likes if he does his chores and homework. It seems to be working out.

theory and treatment (see *Appendix: Recommended Resources*). Once parents have read this material, the clinician tests the parents on their newly learned knowledge.

The process of making a baseline assessment, asking parents to read, and testing knowledge prior to treatment screens those families where:

▶ Either one or both parents are not ready to enter treatment.

▶ The parents do not want to pursue a parent-type of therapy.

▶ The parents need more time to think about what they really want to do about their current situation.

During the next visit, the clinician presents and discusses baseline PDR information and the results of the book test and highlights family and child concerns and strengths.

After this presentation, if the parents remain interested in continuing treatment, the child joins the parents, and the clinician teaches the family observational skills by having them track and record simple, well-defined behaviors during the session.

rate-per-minute — the average number of specific behaviors of interest occurring in one minute

For example, the clinician asks family members to observe how many times the clinician blinks during a five-minute period. The clinician then takes all the data collected and calculates *rate-per-minute* summaries (e.g., 10 blinks in five-minutes is equivalent to a rate of two behaviors per minute).

Often, various family members' ratings do not match. This provides the opportunity for the clinician to discuss how difficult it is to accurately track even simple behaviors and then to present ideas for improving parental tracking. The clinician then helps parents pinpoint two problematic and two desired child behaviors and asks the parents to track these four behaviors over the next three days for two pre-specified hours each day (i.e., each parent tracks for one hour).

After training the parents in the presence of the child, the clinician engages the child in the discussion, and fully explains what will be happening at home and why. The clinician asks the child to develop a list of desired changes for the family and to bring the list back to the next session.

At the end of the session, the clinician asks the parents to pay a "breakage fee" (with the actual amount adjusted for family income). The full "breakage fee" amount is refunded if parents meet all treatment program expectations. Although this fee can be used to cover the cost of materials (e.g., the social learning book), it functions primarily as a penalty fund. For example, if parents arrive late or miss scheduled appointments, money can be deducted from the fund. Additional fees can be collected if the fund becomes exhausted.

On each of the next three days following this appointment, the clinician calls the parents at a prearranged time. During these calls, the clinician asks for the rate per minute of the four target behaviors and the length of time each parent observed the target behaviors. If the original behavioral definitions have proven to be difficult to use, the clinician helps refine them. Each call generally lasts no longer than five minutes per parent. During the third call, the clinician schedules the first treatment phase appointment.

Treatment Phase

During the treatment phase, parent training focuses on:

> ▶ Delivering effective positive reinforcements to family members

> ▶ Setting up, maintaining, and modifying a "contingency contract"

> ▶ Correctly utilizing "time outs" as a consequence for child misbehavior

> ▶ Controling anger during frustrating and conflicting parent-child interactions

> ▶ Effectively monitoring a child's whereabouts and behaviors

> ▶ Using family conferences to solve and to prevent problems

The main tasks for the clinician during treatment are:

▶ Teaching the family new skills

▶ Helping the family apply new skills

▶ Creating and maintaining an effective follow-up process

PDR calls continue throughout the entire treatment phase.

Depending on the needs of a particular family, training also addresses:[56, 80, 122]

> ▶ Communicating and working together more effectively with teachers and school administrators

> ▶ Tutoring children in academic skills

> ▶ Working out marital problems that interfere with parenting

> ▶ Dealing with other personal issues that can interfere with parenting, such as feelings of depression[123]

During the first treatment sessions, the clinician teaches the basic parenting skills of positive reinforcement, *contingency contracting*, and time out using the methods of discussion, modeling, and role-playing. For example, positive reinforcement skills include:

contingency contracting — a plan for the positive and negative consequences that follow specific child behaviors

> ▶ Establishing eye contact

> ▶ Labeling the behavior being supported

> ▶ Using an enthusiastic tone of voice (e.g., looking at the child, the parent says, "John, I really appreciate that you took out the trash. Thanks so much!")

"Yes, but..." statements are cloaked as reinforcers, but are really punishing statements.

The clinician helps parents deliver unqualified reinforcers (e.g., "Yes, you did a good job!"), rather than using "Yes, but ..." statements. For parents who have trouble expressing warmth, the clinician can work with the parent on various ways to express positive emotion. Role plays between clinician and parent, parent and parent, and parent and child can also be particularly helpful.

The content and process of parent training must be adapted to the needs, problems, and strengths of each family.

Parents learn a variety of techniques to increase the chances that their child will display positive behaviors. These techniques include:

- ▶ Modeling the desired positive behaviors
- ▶ Actively using positive reinforcement skills with all the children in the family, particularly during times when siblings are being cooperative with each other
- ▶ Practicing ways to clearly describe to the child those behaviors desired by the parents as well as the positive consequences they will receive for such behaviors

Contingency Contracts

To facilitate the use of positive reinforcement, parents learn to write and use a contingency contract — a written document agreed upon by family members that specifies both desired and undesired behaviors as well as positive or negative consequences for displaying these behaviors.

token economy system — a program of earning points or other currency that can be traded in for specific rewards

The contract outlines a simple *token economy system* in which children earn points for displaying specific behaviors. Earned points can be exchanged for rewards from a pre-selected menu (e.g., playing a game with a parent or watching a favorite TV show).

The first contract parents use focuses solely on a few positive behaviors (e.g., doing what is asked, playing nicely with siblings). Parents give rewards frequently as the child displays these positive behaviors. Once this type of contract works well at home, parents develop a new contract using the PDR data that has been collected since the parent first began the assessment phase. The new contract:

- ▶ Specifies one desired behavior (e.g., doing chores) and one undesired behavior (e.g., noncompliance)
- ▶ Lists how many points can be earned or lost whenever the child displays each of these behaviors
- ▶ Lists rewards for earning a specific number of positive points as well as consequences for having zero or negative points at the end of the day (e.g., going to bed 30 minutes early)

More advanced contracts include more behaviors.

Time Out

Once parents are proficient in positive reinforcement and contingency contracting, the clinician introduces nonviolent discipline techniques, such as time out. Time out is an alternative punishment to yelling, spanking, or grounding. Clinicians model for and role-play with parents how to give effective time outs using the following process:

> ► Parents give the child one warning following the occurrence of the problem behavior.

> ► If the behavior continues, parents tell their child to go to a predetermined, out-of-the-way place that the child perceives as boring (e.g., the bathroom) for a specified timeframe.

> ► If the time out reaches a predetermined maximum, such as 10 minutes, parents withdraw a privilege for a small period of time (e.g., watching television for the rest of the afternoon).

Parents are warned that using time out on a consistent basis into a family is often quite challenging, and that the clinician will try to assist during this difficult adjustment period by calling and consulting with the parents on a daily basis. Finally, the clinician explains time out to the child and engages the child in role-playing to demonstrate how this technique works. Parents are instructed not to physically take their child to time out, and not to engage their child in a discussion or argument during time out.

Clinicians may find it helpful to review simple anger control techniques with the parents. Sometimes, teaching parents how to accurately recognize when they are becoming angry can help circumvent problems. Encouraging parents to give themselves five-minute time outs or to count to 10 prior to speaking to their child can help diffuse volatile situations. In extreme circumstances, parents may be asked to sign a contract specifying that instead of expressing their anger verbally or physically against family members, they will call the clinician the first moment they are beginning to feel angry. For some parents, this type of contract can help disrupt angry outbursts and can assist the parent in beginning to use more constructive communication techniques.

The clinician informs parents that correct, consistent use of the contingency contract and of time outs typically results in predetermined, target problem behaviors coming under some parental control in seven to 14 days.

In between treatment sessions, the clinician continues to call the parents once or twice a week so that issues are dealt with immediately that could disrupt the positive teaching

For older children, substitute work consequences for "time out."

Time outs are brief, and usually begin at three to five minutes in length. If the child refuses to go, their time in time out is slowly increased in one-minute increments (up to 10 minutes) until they do go.

Because parent-training techniques serve to reduce the intensity and modify the quality of discipline confrontations, effective parent training should ultimately reduce parent distress and anger.

As the child's behavior gets under control, the number of time outs parents need to give should drop. If this does not occur within seven to 14 days, parents are likely misusing the techniques.

relationship established between the parents and the child. As noted earlier, the clinician or another staff member also continues to make separate data-collection PDR calls to monitor child behavior changes.

Structured Weekly Sessions

Once parents begin to use contingency contracting and time out in the home, the clinician can use the following week's session to refine the family's basic skills by:

▶ Detailing what happened at home with the contract during the previous week, and provide the family ample praise for positive results and efforts

▶ Reviewing PDR data

▶ Reviewing data collected by the parents on any new problem behaviors they would like to address

▶ Expanding the contract by specifying new behaviors and/or changing rewards and/or delaying rewards

▶ Spending the last 10 to 15 minutes of the sessions dealing with family crises or other topics, as necessary

Ask parents to collect data on new problem behaviors they would like to change.

During these weekly sessions, one of the primary teaching formats used is the role-playing of reinforcement and discipline scenarios. Parents practice together or with the clinician, and the clinician then provides feedback on their performance.

One particularly useful role-playing technique is the "wrong way–right way" method.[95] Parents are instructed to role-play a parent-child interaction the wrong way, and the clinician praises their "good" acting abilities. This gives the clinician the opportunity to comment on ineffective or problematic parenting in a nonthreatening and disengaged context. It also allows parents to discuss and acknowledge how miserable it feels to be a parent in a "wrong way" situation. Next, the clinician instructs the parent how to act the "right way." The clinician actively, but gently, shapes the role-play as necessary. This can be done by whispering in the ear of one or both participants. This technique can be particularly useful when parents act out difficult interactions they experienced with their child during the previous week.

After parents master these basic skills, the clinician presents more advanced parenting skills, such as monitoring and holding family problem-solving conferences.

Monitoring

As children reach adolescence, monitoring youth activities when they are away from home is crucial to limiting the extent and growth of conduct problems. Youth who spend unsupervised time with deviant friends are particularly likely to commit antisocial acts.[16, 44] During treatment, the clinician teaches parents to be specific about their adolescents' whereabouts and schedules throughout the day. Parents learn to ensure compliance with the planned schedule. Behaviors related to staying on schedule are written into the contingency contract and appropriate consequences are detailed.

Clinicians need to encourage parents to get to know and to keep in regular contact with their child's friends and the friends' parents.

Family Problem-Solving Conferences

During the final stage of treatment, siblings join the parents and child in treatment sessions. Family members learn how to plan and conduct family conferences and to construct, modify, and change contracts to help solve family problems. A fundamental message of parent training is that all family members have an equal stake in the functioning of the family.

During treatment sessions, the clinician helps families follow the conference structure appropriately. At first, parents lead the conference; later, the child and siblings take turns leading. Family members take turns documenting decisions made during the meeting. Members also make formal contracts specifying what is to happen as a result of the decisions and when the contract will be re-negotiated.

Families generate a set of rules to govern the way family members communicate with each other during conferences. For example:

1. Each person's opinion is of equal worth during a conference.
2. Those who perceive themselves as "victims" in a particular situation are always right. Family members are encouraged to help the victim pinpoint the problem, and members paraphrase the problem. The "victim" provides feedback about the accuracy of their paraphrasing.

Frequently, clinicians videotape the structured family conferences. When reviewing the tape, the clinician can discuss ways for the family to improve the process of the family conference. For family members who are having trouble accepting that positive changes are actually happening, videotaping can also highlight the positive behaviors of certain family members (e.g., the positive behaviors of the child).

The basic family conference structure involves:

▶ *Discussing the pleasant high points for the family during the week*

▶ *Reviewing problems that arose during the week*

▶ *Conducting problem solving, if necessary (e.g., pinpointing the problem, brain-storming possible solutions, choosing the best solution)*

▶ *Documenting the problem-solving results*

▶ *Planning a family activity that promotes family prosocial interaction.*

As the family improves their ability to conduct family conferences, the clinician should expand the purpose of family meetings to deal with the family crises that likely arose during the previous week. The clinician encourages families to conduct and to tape record additional weekly conferences at home. These recordings help the clinician provide targeted feedback on family progress and monitor the generalization of skills to the home setting.

Intensive Interventions

At least 20 percent of parents respond poorly to clinic visits and phone calls, and require more intensive intervention.[56] For these parents, home visits can be conducted during which the clinician assesses family interaction, role plays appropriate behaviors, and supervises the correct performance of skills. Home visits should be used if clear changes in child behavior are not observed within three weeks after contingency contracting begins. During a home visit, the clinician can point out problems as they naturally occur and follow this up with immediate role-playing and modeling of what can be done to improve parent effectiveness.

One or two such visits may be sufficient for some families, but more intensive work in the home may be required for others.[56]

Follow-up After Program Termination

Families are encouraged to call for "booster shot" meetings with the clinician as needed. Approximately 50 percent of families request such a service. In one study, 12 of 28 families requested additional intervention for an average of seven hours during the first year after treatment termination. The average decreased to four hours during the second year and one hour during the third year.[124]

Effectiveness of Parent Training Programs

The impact of parent training on child antisocial behavior has been studied extensively, and the research literature has been reviewed myriad times.[23, 121, 125–128] Most researchers have focused on immediate or short-term outcomes, and many have found positive treatment effects. With the Oregon Social Learning Center (OSLC) program, approximately one in three families benefits from parent training standard techniques. With more extensive outpatient interventions (such as school interventions), the initial success rate can probably approach two out of three families.[56]

Parent training is one of the few empirically supported treatments for both the conduct disorders and associated problems, such as ADHD.[125, 129] The most rigorously investigated program is that of Carolyn Webster-Stratton. This video-based program has been found effective for children with conduct problems within a variety of different samples.[130-133]

Four factors appear to improve treatment success:

1. Offering parents as many sessions as needed
2. Using experienced clinicians[23, 134]
3. Teaching parents general principles of behavior management[23]
4. Addressing other factors besides parenting during treatment[56, 134-136]

Unfortunately, studies of long-term treatment effects are few. However, several studies have found that some child behaviors learned through parent training continue over time.[137-139]

School-Based Programs (CLASS and RECESS)

Many clinicians conduct treatment programs within the schools in an attempt to modify problematic behaviors that occur in the classroom or at recess. Two of the most well-developed and well-researched treatment packages for school-based behavior management are:

1. CLASS (Contingencies for Learning Academic and Social Skills)[140, 141]
2. RECESS (Reprogramming Environmental Contingencies for Effective Social Skills)[140, 142]

Clinicians conduct initial treatment sessions with an individual child in the classroom and on the playground. This serves a dual purpose. First, clinicians can model how to deliver the program for teachers and playground supervisors in the natural environment. Second, clinicians can demonstrate how well the program works when delivered correctly. During the later stages of the program, clinicians serve as consultants to teachers and/or playground supervisors as they administer the program.

CLASS Treatment Process

During the first five days, the clinician provides the child with continuous feedback about their behavior for several school periods each day. Using green and red cards to signal whether the child is behaving appropriately (green) or inappropriately (red), the clinician monitors the child's behavior throughout two, 20- to 30-minute periods. If the green card is displayed, the child receives a point and verbal praise every one to two minutes. If the red card is displayed, the child loses a point. If the child earns 80 percent of the possible points in a period, then the class earns a group-activity reward (e.g., the class is given five minutes of extra recess, the class gets to play a special game)

These programs build children's prosocial behavioral repertoires by:

► *Providing immediate and clear consequences for appropriate and inappropriate behaviors during school*

► *Linking school behavior to home consequences via school-home cards*

Although originally designed for children ages five through eight, aspects of each program can be easily adapted for use with older, elementary-school-aged children.

Both CLASS and RECESS last six to eight weeks, and each takes approximately 40 hours of direct contact time by the clinician.

immediately following the end of the period. The clinician documents the child's performance during both periods on a school-home behavior card.

Parents and teachers learn to communicate effectively using a simple system such as a school-home card.

The school-home card lists the biggest problems identified by the teacher. At the end of each class period, the clinician (and later the teacher) marks those problems that occurred. The child brings the card home at the end of the day, and the parents provide a consequence for appropriate (e.g., points and verbal reinforcement) or inappropriate (e.g., early bedtime) behavior. Parents also determine a consequence (e.g., no television) if the child fails to bring the contract home.

Both parents and teachers should use brief time outs to deal with negative behaviors.

During days six through 20, the teacher administers the treatment program, using the red and green signaling cards intermittently, and fading them out completely by day 15. Parents and teachers gradually increase the magnitude of rewards at home and school as well as the interval required to earn each reward. For example, by day 16, the child must perform successfully for five days to earn a reward. During days 21 to 30, teachers and parents only give verbal praise or similar naturally occurring consequences as rewards.

RECESS Treatment Process

After reviewing playground rules, the clinician tells the children that the entire class will earn rewards for the child's appropriate behavior.

During the first few school days of the RECESS program, the clinician meets with parents, teachers, recess monitors, and the child to orient them to the program and explain each person's role. The clinician defines and models for the child exactly what differentiates positive social behaviors (e.g., maintaining eye contact, smiling, sharing) from negative ones (e.g., hitting, noncompliance). With the help of the child, the clinician then teaches these concepts to the entire class.

The clinician provides ample verbal praise for the child's positive behaviors.

At this point, the clinician implements the behavioral program with the child during each recess period. At the beginning of each recess period, the child receives one point for each five-minute interval in the recess period (e.g., three points for a 15-minute period). The child is told to try to keep these points by interacting positively with others throughout the period and by following all playground rules.

If the child retains a specific number of points across all recess periods in an entire day, the entire class participates in a fun group activity at the end of the school day.

During this time, the child loses one point each time they act negatively toward another child or adult or each time they break a playground rule. The clinician tells the child each time a point is lost. If the child loses all points, they receive a time out for the remainder of recess. If the child behaves in an especially good manner or handles a difficult situation appropriately, a bonus point is awarded, which cannot be lost.

During days 8 through 10, the recess supervisor administers the program under the direct supervision of the clinician and continues the program for three more weeks (days 11 through 25). The program also begins to operate in the classroom. In the classroom, the child receives regular praise for good behavior and earns access to recess by following classroom rules and interacting positively during academic periods immediately before recess. The child earns points at the beginning of class and must retain them. Children who lose all points are not allowed to go to recess, and thus, lose the chance to earn points during recess for that period.

During the final phase (days 26 through 40), external controls, such as points and time outs, gradually fade to be replaced by verbal praise and other naturally occurring rewards both at home and at school.

Follow-up After Program Termination

These programs may be continued indefinitely, and the school-home behavior card can be an ongoing mechanism both to reinforce appropriate behavior at school and to keep communication open between teachers and parents.

Effectiveness of School-Based Programs

Empirical support exists for behavioral, school-based programs for childhood externalizing disorders, most notably for ADHD.[129, 143, 144] Both the CLASS and RECESS packages have been tested extensively using a variety of research designs.[140] Results indicate that while these programs are in effect, both reduce the negative social behaviors of children exhibiting conduct-disordered behaviors. There is some evidence that the CLASS program has long-lasting effects. In two studies, children who received CLASS were utilizing significantly less special education services 18 to 36 months after program termination.[145]

Multidimensional Treatment Foster Care

When the juvenile court or a clinician and the family determine that an adolescent diagnosed with a conduct disorder needs an out-of-home placement, a promising program is multidimensional treatment foster care (MTFC).[78] The goals of MTFC are to:

> ▶ Minimize the display of conduct-disordered behaviors
> ▶ Minimize the influence of deviant peers
> ▶ Encourage prosocial behaviors
> ▶ Promote the development of academic skills

Adolescents diagnosed with a conduct disorder are individually placed with foster parents who have been carefully screened and then trained to deliver the MTFC program. An adolescent spends an average of four to six months in foster care, during

The school-home report card along with a home reward system is used to support the class program.

A naturally occurring reward might be allowing a child to accompany his or her parents to the grocery store as a reward for good behavior during the afternoon.

To monitor the progress of the child during treatment, clinicians encourage teachers to complete rating scales of child behaviors at frequent points and maintain a daily-record form summarizing the child's behavioral performance.

case manager — a person, typically a social worker, who oversees all aspects of the patient's treatment program

which time both they and their parents receive ongoing psychological interventions. A *case manager* supervises the entire intervention program, ensures that treatment goals are being met, and acts as the liaison between MTFC staff and external agencies, including the adolescent's school and the juvenile court. Case managers meet regularly with foster parents and clinicians and are on call 24 hours a day for crisis intervention.

During MTFC, the adolescent and the parents have different clinicians. An extremely important part of treatment is the building of supportive and trusting relationships between adolescent and clinician as well as between the parents and their clinician. These relationships form the base from which more difficult aspects of skills acquisition can be accomplished.

Treatment Process

Throughout the four- to six-month period, adolescents participate in individual therapy that focuses on social skills and problem solving skills (see pages 47–48 on child problem-solving skills in this chapter). Additionally, parents participate in parent training (see pages 31–41 on parent training in this chapter). Toward the middle of treatment, adolescents and parents meet together with both clinicians for family meetings. During these meetings, family members learn more positive ways of discussing important issues and solving problems together. These meetings help bridge the transition from foster care back to home.

During the program, foster parents use the following three-level point system to teach prosocial skills, reward appropriate behavior, and provide consequences for inappropriate behavior:

All privileges must be earned, including phone time, free time, and allowance.

▶ **Level one** — a youth receives close supervision across all settings (e.g., home, school) and relatively immediate reinforcement. Points earned during one day lead to privileges received on the following day. Adolescents who do well can reach level two in two to three weeks.

All contacts with friends occur where the adolescent's whereabouts can be confirmed and monitored.

▶ **Level two** — a youth receives more freedom and more delayed reinforcement. Points earned during one week lead to privileges received during the next week. All privileges must be earned, but more are available, including the chance to buy free time with friends.

Adolescents can be demoted to level one for low point days. If this happens, they must earn their way back to level two by gaining a certain number of points. To move to level three, even more points must be earned. For example, an adolescent must earn 12 bonds that cost 25 points each. One bond can be earned (purchased) per week. Adolescents usually stay at level two for three to four months.

▶ **Level three** — a youth receives even more freedom. Rather than points being earned or lost, adolescents are rated globally each day on their performance of several behaviors. The ratings received determine the adolescent's allowance. Privileges do not have to be earned, but extra rewards can be earned for sustained appropriate behavior. Two or more low ratings for the same behavior on two consecutive days may result in a demotion to level two of up to one week. Official violations (e.g., police contacts) result in a demotion to level one as well as other consequences.

All activities need to be approved, and the adolescent's whereabouts in the community continue to be followed closely.

Follow-up After Termination

MTFC "aftercare" services vary, depending on the needs of the adolescent and family. Clinicians hold parent group and individual sessions with parents to provide further information, assistance, and support in their efforts to manage their adolescent's behavior. Clinicians make frequent telephone contacts with parents to closely monitor the transition from MTFC to home. Clinicians may also hold individual sessions with adolescents to "coach" them in social and community relationship skills. *Respite care* services are provided for families if the parents and their adolescent need "a break" from each other. Other services, such as academic tutoring, can be provided or arranged as needed.

One of the most important jobs of the clinician is to thoroughly convince the parents that they themselves must and can become experts at managing the behavior of their adolescent, often despite a long history of failed attempts.

respite care — short-term out-of-home placements (e.g., a weekend)

Effectiveness of Multidimensional Treatment Foster Care

Researchers have examined MTFC efficacy in several samples of adolescents with conduct disorders referred by the juvenile courts. In the first study, male youth randomly assigned to participate in MTFC had significantly fewer criminal referrals in the one-year period following treatment exit (59 percent) than those assigned to participate in services-as-usual group home programs (93 percent).[146, 147] As predicted, the positive effect of MTFC over group homes on arrests was mediated by lower levels of deviant peer association and higher levels of monitoring, consistent discipline, and positive adult-youth relationships.[148]

Researchers are conducting a similar study at the Oregon Social Learning Center (OSLC) with adolescent girls, and initial impacts on delinquency appear promising.[149, 150] A version of MTFC has also been developed for preschool age children, and positive effects on conduct problems have been found in the first randomized trial.[151]

What is the Cognitive Therapy Approach to Treating CD?

Cognitive therapy attempts to change the thought processes, or cognitions, of a child diagnosed with conduct disorder. Theorists hypothesize that certain cognitions lead to child aggressive behaviors and interpersonal conflict, while others may be conducive to positive social interactions.

The primary goal of treatment is to provide children with a cognitive framework that will help them better solve interpersonal problems.

Children who have developed a repertoire of conduct-disordered behaviors also may have developed cognitive (thought) processes that are ineffective in prosocial situations.[152] For example, children who display aggressive behaviors tend to attribute hostile intentions to their peers even during neutral or ambiguous social interactions.[120] These tendencies have been labeled "social processing deficits," and clinicians have observed that a variety of social processing deficits coincide with child aggressive behavior.[121] Unfortunately for the child, such "deficits" may be adaptive in some social settings in which they interact. However, they may be maladaptive in relatively benign situations.

Cognitive theorists believe that some children unconsciously and rapidly process social behaviors in a way that leads to aggressive responses. They believe that a child perceives and reacts to a social stimulus based on how well aspects of that stimulus have predicted certain outcomes in previous encounters. If such stimuli have often been associated with threatening situations, the affective features most useful in determining a current threat will be attended to and other, less-predictive cues will be ignored.

Information (both process and outcome) of each processing sequence is thought to be stored in long-term memory. The cumulative history that a child has with a particular stimulus is hypothesized to influence later processing.

For example, a peer frowns at a child with conduct problems. The peer's frown is interpreted as a threat, and the child feels a mix of fear and anger. Once the frown is interpreted as threatening, the child accesses an array of previously tried behavioral responses, such as: running away, pushing the peer, making a negative comment, frowning back, or making no response.

Social information processing psychologists hypothesize that cognitive processing errors serve as the immediate "cause" for observed aggressive behavior.[153]

The child evaluates and classifies each response as acceptable or unacceptable given the current situation. The sequence ends when the child exhibits the chosen response (e.g., swears at the peer, which likely starts a verbal argument and leads to a physical fight).

In treating the conduct disorders, those who favor the cognitive approach use child problem-solving skills training programs that focus on the development of adaptive ways to think through interpersonal problems.[154, 155] The goal of this treatment is to make problem solving more *conscious*, proactive, and prosocial.

conscious — within the person's awareness

Problem-solving skills can be taught individually or in small groups (e.g., five to 10 children). Many clinicians prefer small groups because:

▶ Children can practice the skills with peers under the supervision of the clinician.

▶ Group process can be used to facilitate change.[156]

Small groups usually include children of approximately the same age and/or developmental level and possibly of the same gender.[157] Groups may be limited to children with a conduct disorder or may include a mix of children exhibiting different types of problems, children with and without a conduct disorder, or a "target" child's entire classroom. Current research provides no clear answers as to which group composition results in the most effective treatment.

Depending on the program, the number of sessions varies between 10 and 30, spread out over 10 to 20 weeks.[156-158] Some clinician/researchers hypothesize that the most ideal approach is to stretch training across an entire school year and then follow-up with periodic booster sessions. The longer time period provides children with more opportunity for skills rehearsal and may improve their ability to generalize their new skills to the natural environment.[157] Session lengths vary, but usually do not exceed 75 minutes.

Treatment Process

Clinicians conduct problem-solving skills training programs in the context of a *contingency management program*. During the first meeting, clinicians present the rules for the group, provide participants with a list of the rules and consequences, post the rules, and role-play what will happen when the rules are broken.[158] They also detail rewards for appropriate behaviors, including tasks to be accomplished outside the session (i.e., "homework"). Subsequent meetings usually begin with a quick reminder of the rules. A well thought-out contingency management program that is properly introduced and consistently applied greatly enhances the productivity of problem-solving skills training sessions. The contingency management program can also serve as a mechanism for providing approval, giving support, and (ultimately) building trust.

Through games, stories, and social interaction, children are taught to carefully analyze social problems using a methodical, step-by-step approach, such as:[156]

▶ What is wrong?

▶ What can I do?

▶ Which choice is best?

Although developed with elementary-school-aged children, child problem-solving skills training can be adapted for older children.

Several researchers have found that bringing groups of children with problem behaviors together into group therapy settings may result in detrimental outcomes for individual group members (e.g., increases in the problem behaviors of group members).[159-161]

contingency management program — a system for rewarding good behaviors and providing costs for misbehaviors

Clinicians model the use of each step, observe children practicing the steps, and give praise and correction as appropriate.

Treatment sessions typically focus on group problem-solving as well as self-instruction training, but can often include other components (e.g., anger management) and basic social skills (e.g., group entry and play skills).[162–164]

Problem-solving treatment sessions often include these steps:[157, 158]

1. Review the group rules.

2. Verbally reinforce the child for the homework activities he or she completed during the past week.

3. Provide a brief, simple, and well-organized lecture on the topic of the day, emphasizing the precise steps needed to accomplish a specific goal. Supplement this talk with information on posters and handouts.

4. Preferably with a co-clinician, model the skills presented in the lecture during a role-play of a problem-solving situation.

5. With a child in front of the group, role-play a problem-solving situation to again demonstrate the skills presented; provide coaching and feedback.

6. In front of the group, provide coaching and feedback, while two children use the target skills during a problem-solving role-play. If there are two clinicians, this can be done by pairing each child with a clinician and having the clinicians whisper corrective feedback as appropriate. Videotape this session, if possible.

7. Review the role-play (using videotape, if available) and provide further feedback.

8. Briefly review the session.

9. Discuss weekly activities that the child can do to earn points towards rewards. To improve compliance, such tasks can be labeled "show that I can" rather than "homework."[165]

10. Provide any earned rewards.

Self-instruction training sessions typically involve the clinician coaching children to talk themselves through problem-solving steps. A basic format for such training involves the clinician role-playing tasks while verbally (out loud) instructing themselves about what to do; then, the children role-play the situation four times as follows:[166]

▶ Listening while the clinician instructs them

▶ Instructing themselves out loud

▶ Whispering instructions to themselves

▶ Silently instructing themselves

> *Modeling occurs throughout treatment sessions: the clinician not only formally demonstrates for the child how to solve problems in hypothetical situations, but uses problem solving skills as real problems arise during treatment.*[158]

Follow-up after Program Termination

Periodic booster sessions following treatment termination may promote the continued use of problem-solving skills as well as the generalization of these skills to new settings.[157] Using booster sessions is conceptually appealing, but the effect of such on child behavior has not been studied.

Effectiveness of the Cognitive Approach

Problem-solving skills treatments appear to have some positive impacts on child aggressive behaviors, at least during and soon after treatment.[167] In several studies, children exhibiting aggressive behaviors were randomly assigned to child problem-solving skills training, some other type of treatment, or a control group. After treatment, children in the problem-solving skills condition demonstrated greater decreases in aggressive behaviors than children in the other conditions.[156, 162, 168, 169] How well these effects persist over time is unclear. Some studies indicate persistence of treatment effects up to one year after termination, while other studies indicate that many children fail to maintain treatment gains.[156, 158, 170]

What is the Family Therapy Approach to Treating CD?

Family therapy attempts to change family communication processes. Proponents believe that problematic interactions between family members create and maintain child conduct problems. Two types of family-based interventions that appear effective are functional family therapy (FFT) and multisystemic treatment (MST). FFT has an exclusive family focus. MST expands its focus to include not only the immediate family but also the child's school, peers, and community — those systems important in maintaining conduct-disordered behavior.

In numerous studies, researchers have found that family factors, such as parent use of discipline, monitoring, and problem-solving skills, significantly correlate with child antisocial behaviors.[15, 83, 171] In the behavior therapy approach discussed previously, clinicians view all members of a child's nuclear family (or family system) as important players in the development of a conduct disorder. Family therapy theorists also ascribe to this idea, and place the etiology, development, and maintenance of the child's problems primarily within the context of the family's verbal and nonverbal communication patterns.[172] According to these theorists, it is the *dysfunctional* family system, rather than the "identified patient" (e.g., the child diagnosed with a conduct disorder), that should be the focus of treatment. Other associated systems relevant to

dysfunctional — patterns of behavior that have distressing and problematic outcomes

child and family behavior (e.g., the child's network of friends, the teachers and counselor at school, extended family) are also considered to be important in the maintenance of problems within the nuclear family, and thus attempts are made to systematically modify these systems as well.

homeostasis — equilibrium or balance

Family theorists view a child's "conduct disorder" as one of a variety of problematic family symptoms that maintain *homeostasis* within a family system. The disorder is seen as a solution to some problem that currently threatens or once threatened to disrupt the accepted status quo of the family.[164] For example, the primary family problem may be conflict between parents that threatens family survival. When the child diagnosed with a conduct disorder is misbehaving, parents may have to divert their focus away from their marital conflict. Thus, the disorder serves to keep the family together. Since curing the conduct disorder would require that the system respond with a "diversion" that might be equally undesirable, the only way to truly create useful change within the family is to change the family system.[173] Changing the family system requires:

family roles — the way that parents and children relate with one another in terms of power, allegiance, and function

▶ Assessing what purposes maladaptive symptoms (e.g., child antisocial behavior) serve in the system

▶ Then, changing *family roles* and communication and relationship patterns so that these purposes can be served in more adaptive ways

Theorists view healthy families as those in which parents share power and decision making with one another and where clear boundaries exist between parents (as a team) and other family members.

Despite the popularity of family therapy theories, sparse research exists on their outcome for CD.[174–176] However, preliminary supportive outcome data is available for functional family therapy (FFT), and numerous studies have been conducted on multisystemic treatment (MST).

Functional Family Therapy

Communication patterns describe the way families verbally and non-verbally interact with each other on a day-to-day basis. Incongruent messages and other types of poor communication are considered both a cause and an effect of dysfunction within the family.[177]

The primary goal of FFT is to improve and optimize communication within a family. Families are taught to convey their thoughts and feelings more clearly and precisely, to negotiate solutions to problems more effectively, and to use behavioral techniques to provide a more consistent home environment for their children.

FFT was designed for children in early to mid-adolescence. All members of the family attend treatment sessions together. Sessions are held on a weekly basis and last for 60 minutes. Treatment continues until both the clinician and the family determine termination to be appropriate.

Treatment Process

During treatment, the clinician models, shapes, and teaches the family communication skills within the context of ongoing family problem-solving discussions. The process typically follows this pattern:

1. The clinician gives family members reading assignments that introduce social learning principles. (See "Parent Training: For Parents" in the appendix.)

2. Through observing and interviewing the family, the clinician learns about family interactions that seem to be related to the child's conduct-disordered behaviors. The clinician uses this knowledge to help shape the family's problematic interactions into more kind and productive encounters.

3. From the first session, the family works on negotiating solutions to those family problems that the clinician hypothesizes are related to the child's conduct-disordered behaviors. The clinician actively models clear, efficient, and adaptive communication skills, and prompts and reinforces these skills with family members during the negotiation. Throughout negotiations, clinicians frequently state their hypotheses about the meaning of and purposes for various verbal and nonverbal communications used by family members. Family members are encouraged to correct and clarify these interpretations.

4. During continued negotiations, the clinician teaches the family a variety of skills to improve the communication clarity between family members.

Follow-up After Program Termination

Booster sessions can be added as needed to fine-tune communication within the family.

Effectiveness of Functional Family Therapy

There is preliminary support for the efficacy of FFT. In a well-cited study, families with children who had been detained by police for several relatively low-level offenses (e.g., running away; being declared "ungovernable"; being habitually truant; shoplifting; or possessing tobacco, drugs, or alcohol) were randomly assigned to several conditions, including FFT. Relative to a no-treatment control group and two "community-standard" treatment groups, children whose families participated in the FFT condition had lower *recidivism* rates for these low-level offenses six to 18 months after treatment.[178] Unfortunately, the average number of serious criminal offenses (e.g., robbery, burglary) committed remained constant for all treatment groups.

Clinicians assist families in developing clearly defined parameters for child and family behavior. They learn to differentiate family rules (limits that must be followed) from family requests (statements that can be responded to either negatively or positively).

If one or more family members are unwilling to address the major problem at first, families negotiate a minor issue (e.g., performing a chore at home) and later progress to major issues.

A secondary focus of treatment is on helping families develop a token economy system to reward desired child and family behaviors (see the parent training and MTFC sections).

recidivism — a tendency to lapse into a previous pattern of behavior, especially a pattern of criminal habits associated with repeat arrests

The most recent revision of FFT includes several additions to the basic communication skills program (e.g., cognitive interventions targeting inappropriate perceptions that family members hold about each other).[180] The effectiveness of this revised treatment package has not yet been tested.

Clinicians view MST as a "family-preservation" intervention since they use this therapy to treat children diagnosed with conduct disorder who are at imminent risk for being institutionalized due to chronic delinquent behavior. Across the course of treatment, clinicians are available 24 hours a day, seven days a week for intervention activities.

In a follow-up study, siblings within the FFT-treated families also had lower rates of police detainment for any offense 30 to 42 months after treatment.[179] In a study of a different sample, youth who received FFT demonstrated lower rates of recidivism two and one-half years later than a comparison group.[181]

Multisystemic Treatment

In contrast to the exclusive family focus in functional family therapy, multisystemic treatment (MST) focuses on modifying any system (e.g., family, school, peer, community) important in maintaining the child's conduct-disordered behaviors.[182] The primary goal of treatment is to provide parents with the skills and resources needed to independently address the challenges presented by their children.

MST was originally designed for adolescents and their families. Nuclear family members, extended family members, peers, teachers, neighbors, community center staff, and other pertinent figures in a child's life all may be involved in treatment. Clinicians meet with families in whatever location and at whatever time is most convenient for the family (often in the evenings at the family's home). Sessions usually last between 15 and 90 minutes and may occur daily. Treatment continues until the child and parents have achieved a reasonable level of functioning. The average duration of treatment is four months, and average contact time for the clinician is 30 hours.

Treatment Process

MST treatment generally proceeds as follows:

1. The clinician schedules the initial meeting in the family's home. During that meeting, each family member discusses the presenting problem and associated issues. The clinician helps the family clarify problems, assesses family strengths that could assist in alleviating problems, and helps the family set reasonable immediate and long-term goals. An action-oriented plan is developed to meet an immediate goal, giving family members and the clinician explicit, reasonable, and daily tasks to accomplish the plan.

2. While family members are working on the initial plan, the clinician contacts the child's school administrator and teachers, the child's peers, and/or extended family members to further assess the problem and search for possible solutions available within the existing systems.

3. After addressing basic needs, the clinician uses parent training (see pages 31–41), child problem-solving skills training (see pages 39–40), community and school inter-

If peers contribute to the child's problem, clinicians may emphasize pursuing new friendships, and follow this by trying to involve children in activities where relationships with prosocial peers can be fostered.

ventions (see pages 41–43), and other psychological interventions as appropriate. These interventions should build skills and effect changes that promote positive, pervasive, and lasting treatment effects. The primary goal is to focus on the family's present problems. However, problems related to past events are acknowledged and dealt with if possible (e.g., by providing restitution).

4. Family sessions are held regularly throughout treatment. During each session, the clinician probes family members on their efforts to accomplish assigned tasks and gives ample praise if the tasks were completed. If tasks were not completed, the clinician attempts to discern why not and develop a new plan. When families fail to accomplish treatment goals in a reasonable amount of time (i.e., two to three weeks), alternative plans should be made and put into place immediately. Sessions conclude with the assignment of tasks to each participant.

5. Across the course of treatment, clinicians develop interventions both within and between each system (e.g., family, school, peers) as appropriate. In addition, clinicians assess and monitor the child's behavior within each system on a continuous basis.

Follow-up After Program Termination

Booster sessions can be conducted to address further issues as needed.

Effectiveness of MST

To date, numerous studies have examined the effectiveness of MST.[183–185] For example, adolescents with "serious" juvenile offense records were randomly assigned to MST or traditional services (i.e., probation with various stipulations). Relative to the traditional services group, adolescents who received MST were detained by police fewer times, reported committing less offenses, and spent less time incarcerated. However, the only highly significant treatment effect was a shorter duration of incarceration (on average, 10 weeks less).[186] In another study, adolescents with extensive offense records were randomly assigned to MST or "eclectic" (psychodynamic, patient-centered, and/or behavioral) individual therapy.[187] Recidivism approximately five years later was 22 percent for those who completed treatment in the MST group and 71 percent for those who completed individual therapy. Ratings on various other measures tended to favor the MST group.

Clinicians address both the basic psychological and seemingly "non-psychological" needs of the family (e.g., food, child care, transportation, medical care). If the family's basic physical needs are not currently being met, the first goal might be to obtain necessary services and materials by helping the family link up with community resources.

The clinician may work with the child during individual therapy on remedying problem-solving skill deficits or may simply provide emotional support for the child during the treatment process.

How is Group Therapy Used to Treat CD?

Group therapy attempts to change various aspects of the social networks children have with their peers. Proponents hypothesize that unsupervised contact with antisocial peers plays a key role in the escalation and maintenance of child conduct problems. Similarly, adult-supervised contact with peers without behavior problems leads to more positive child behaviors.

As previously discussed, theorists hypothesize that peer groups (particularly deviant peer groups) play a prominent role in the "basic training" of antisocial behavior in children (and adolescents in particular) as well as in the long-term maintenance of such behaviors.[15] The most well known group therapy to effect change in conduct-disordered behaviors involves child problem-solving skills training (see pages 47–49).

Other promising group therapy approaches that attempt to use the group setting to leverage change in the child's conduct-disordered behaviors include:

- ▶ Treatment derived from the theories underlying behavior therapy and family therapy in a community center setting
- ▶ Treatment based on the theoretical persuasions of behavior therapy and cognitive therapy in a day-camp setting

Community Center-Based Group Treatment

Deviant peer groups play a prominent role in the display of conduct-disordered behaviors, particularly when parents or other adults do not supervise contact with deviant peers. Based on this finding, researchers have hypothesized that minimizing contact with deviant peers and maximizing contact with prosocial peers in supervised settings likely decreases conduct-disordered behaviors. Further, treatment provided in "unstigmatized" settings, such as a community center, may result in greater success than treatment confined to clinical settings.[188]

Major activities involve planning and participating in various recreational activities at the community center. Staff members teach problem-solving skills and other prosocial behaviors during group activities on both a formal and informal basis.

Community center group treatment was designed for all school-aged children.[94, 188] Children participate in groups of 10 to 15. Groups comprise children without behavior problems who attend after-school activity programs at a community center as part of their regular schedule as well as one or two children who exhibit conduct-disordered behaviors. The groups meet once a week for two to three hours throughout the school year.

Treatment Process

This approach to group treatment utilizes social learning and traditional group therapy. In social learning groups, clinicians systematically apply individual and group contingencies to reward desired behaviors and discourage undesired behaviors. Clinicians use shaping, modeling, role-playing, and coaching to teach prosocial behaviors. In addition, they engage in continuous assessment of individual behaviors to check intervention effectiveness, and make changes in the treatment plan based on these results.

Social learning treatments use the same basic techniques, discussed in the parent training section on pages 31–41.

Traditional groups reflect social psychological and social group work principles similar to the conceptualizations used in family therapy. The clinician focuses on rules, norms, and consequences, helping leaders emerge, and the mechanisms the group uses to solve problems. Traditional groups do not use the contingencies employed by social learning groups.

Follow-up After Program Termination

Groups are conducted throughout each school year, and can be continued during the summer (see the following section).

Effectiveness of Community Center Group Therapy

One of the best examples of a controlled treatment outcome study of group intervention is the St. Louis Experiment. That study contrasted the efficacy of three treatment methods (Social Learning, Traditional, and Control/Minimal).[93] The study also examined two other factors: the clinician's experience level (low and high) and group composition (mixed and unmixed).

Insight-oriented group therapy has been advanced for the conduct disorders, but these types of treatments have not been found effective.[174]

Regardless of the treatment method to which the child was assigned, children who were in mixed groups appeared to fare better than those who were in unmixed groups, especially if the groups were led by experienced leaders. This is an extremely important finding, since it is common for children who display similar problem behaviors to be grouped together away from prosocial peers to receive various interventions.

In mixed groups, one or two randomly chosen children who displayed conduct-disordered behaviors were assigned to a group of nine to 14 children who did not display such problems. Unmixed groups comprised 10 to 15 randomly chosen children who displayed conduct-disordered behaviors.

Other studies also report negative effects when children with problem behaviors are grouped together for "treatment."[160, 161] For example, a recent study of adolescents "at risk" for substance use and other problem behaviors contrasted the effectiveness of a group parent training intervention, a peer-group intervention, and a parent training/peer-group combined intervention. After treatments, those who received the peer-group intervention used more tobacco and were rated by teachers as having more behavior problems than children who received no intervention.[161]

Day Camp Group Treatment

Summer is a time when many children have large amounts of unstructured and unsupervised time. Unfortunately, children diagnosed with a conduct disorder tend to commit problem behaviors when they are in unstructured and unsupervised situations, especially during adolescence. One promising summer-time treatment option that addresses this and other problems is a structured, day camp treatment program. Several versions of these programs have been proposed, and some have been under development for many years.[189] The Summer Treatment Program (STP) was developed for children with ADHD, many of whom had also been diagnosed with a conduct disorder. It's main goal is to improve a child's ability to relate in a prosocial manner with other children and adults in a variety of settings.

The STP is an intense treatment program focusing on minimizing a child's negative behaviors and increasing a child's positive behavioral repertoire. Originally designed for children in elementary school, the program has recently been extended to children in early- to mid-adolescence.

Children participate with a group of 10 to 12 age-matched children from 8:00 a.m. to 5:00 p.m. weekdays for eight weeks during the summer. The STP utilizes the computers, classrooms, gymnasium, and playing fields of an entire elementary school.

In contrast to the other treatment programs discussed (which are often delivered via an individual clinician), the STP utilizes a large staff. Ideally, each 10- to 12-person group of children requires five direct service counselors, including one "lead counselor" at the masters or doctoral-level. A licensed psychologist supervises the direct service team. Elementary and secondary school teachers, a nurse, and a consulting psychiatrist are also on staff. The success of the program depends heavily on a low staff-to-child ratio.

Treatment Process

The STP focuses on developing academic, sports, and social skills as well as children's individual and group problem-solving skills. All aspects of the program, including skills training and time-out procedures, are tailored to be developmentally appropriate for each age-matched group of children (e.g., time outs are longer for older children than younger). Each day, children participate in classroom experiences, including:

Peer relationship skills are also taught within the context of a "buddy system." Children are paired up, and parents are encouraged to get the children together outside of camp.

Children tend to view the STP as an enjoyable experience rather than as a "treatment program." Embedding the treatment within a summer camp context serves to normalize the experience.

- ▶ Computer-assisted education, art instruction, and academic instruction
- ▶ Instruction on sports rules (e.g., soccer, baseball, basketball) and intensive coaching and supervised practice in sports skills
- ▶ Group problem-solving discussions and role-playing
- ▶ Constant instruction, modeling, and practice of appropriate problem-solving and social skills

Children participate with their group in a variety of skill training and field trip activities each day. A camp-wide token reinforcement program, or point system, is used throughout the summer to reward appropriate behaviors and provide consequences for inappropriate behavior. For example, points are given for following rules, sharing, and ignoring provocation. Points are lost for swearing, interrupting, and physical aggression. Points earned in the system can be exchanged for privileges, honors, and/or parent-provided rewards. Besides a loss of points, children receive time outs immediately following misbehaviors. Initially, children receive relatively long time outs (e.g., 30 minutes). However, the length of the time out is reduced if a child behaves appropriately during time out (e.g., from 30 to 10 minutes).

A clinical staff member, whose sole purpose is to tally points, tracks child behaviors on a moment-by-moment basis. Other clinical staff members "call in" points to the point recorder as they are earned or lost.

Parents participate in debriefing sessions at the end of each day, attend group parent training sessions once a week, and receive regular phone calls about treatment progress.

Follow-up After Program Termination

The STP was designed to be part of a comprehensive, year-round, long-term treatment program.[189] During the school year, parent training continues as needed, and children participate in a one-day-per-week version of the STP, called the "Saturday Treatment Program."

Parents learn basic principles of behavior management during an eight-week, one-day-per-week, group parent training program.

Effectiveness of STP

Parents, teachers, and camp counselor ratings of child problem behavior all tend to improve following the STP. Further, treatment dropout tends to be quite low.[189] Neither STP's short- nor long-term impact has been examined in a controlled investigation; however, a variety of other studies suggest that the intervention is promising.[144]

The STP was one of several components in the psychosocial treatment package for the National Institute of Mental Health-sponsored Multimodal Treatment Study. This study examined the effectiveness of various types of intervention conditions (i.e., psychosocial only, medication only, psychosocial and medication combined, and a "services-as-usual" control) for children diagnosed with ADHD.[190-197] Fourteen months of psychosocial treatment produced positive results for 67 percent of participants for symptoms of aggression, anxiety, social skills, inattention, and hyperactive-impulsive behavior.[198-201]

How is the Psychodynamic Approach Used to Treat CD?

Psychodynamic therapy attempts to change parent-child interactions. Theorists believe that children who experienced poor caregiving during early childhood may have difficulty developing and maintaining positive social relationships. Additionally, those children are thought to be particularly vulnerable to exhibiting conduct-disordered behaviors.

In developmental psychology, the word "attachment" refers to a set of contact-seeking behaviors exhibited by all infants during the later part of the first year of life. During this period, infants become wary of strangers, and become distressed and cry when separated from their mothers (or the infants' primary caregivers). When infants are once again in physical contact with their mothers, their distress tends to subside.

Attachment is the psychodynamic theoretical construct most frequently discussed in terms of the development of conduct problems. The fundamental tenet of attachment theory is that feelings of security and control elicited by infant-mother separations and reunions give rise to "cognitive-affective" schema, or "working models," of both the self, others, and the relationship between self and others.[202, 203] For example, an infant who does not experience consistent attention may develop a schema that people are not to be trusted. Once established, theorists hypothesize that these schema influence the growing child's perceptions, cognitions, and motivations. Thus, these schema are viewed as an important determinant on the way an individual interprets and responds to others' behaviors throughout life.[204] According to this theory, nonresponsive, insensitive caregiving during infancy leads to the development of "insecure" attachment schema, which, in turn, makes a child particularly vulnerable to exhibiting conduct-disordered behaviors.[205]

Insecure children tend to use conflictual behaviors as their primary means of regulating caretaking behaviors, which are likely to initiate the parent-child coercive interactions typical of conduct-disordered behaviors. (See the discussion of behavioral theory on page 30.)

Despite the success of parent training, attachment theorists have criticized the approach for ignoring the causal importance of underlying beliefs. Attachment theorists claim that most of what parent training really changes is appearances, or "surface structure." The real problems, they hypothesize, reside in the "deep structure" of cognitions inside the child's mind, and these are not changed as a result of parent training. Furthermore, in parent-child relationships where there are severe problems (such as physical abuse of the child), attachment theorists argue that helping the parent learn ways to gain further control of their child's behavior is probably unwise, even if the new techniques are nonviolent. Rather, theorists contend that, first and foremost, these parents need to learn to relinquish some of their control over their child.

The dyadic skills training program, an enhanced version of a basic parent training program, was designed for parents of noncompliant young children (ages three to eight years) and attempts to remedy the deficiencies attachment theorists ascribe to parent training programs.[205] Like parent training, there is an assessment phase, followed by treatment consisting of hour-long sessions (with parents and children) held in the clinic on a weekly basis for 12 to 18 weeks.

Assessment Phase

The assessment phase (two-three sessions) involves the assessment strategies discussed in chapter two along with the clinician probing the history and status of the parent-child attachment relationship and as well as the attachment history of the parent (usually the mother) with his or her parents. The clinician observes several separation and reunion situations (e.g., mother leaves child alone in room for several minutes, then returns) and notes the behaviors and emotional expressions that occur during the separations and reunions.

> *Parent and child are observed and behaviors noted during child-directed and parent-directed play, particularly behaviors relating to discipline or "control" issues.*

After assessment, dyadic skills training is recommended when:

▶ Attachment issues are clearly a problem for the parent and child (e.g., exerting control is the most prominent parent behavior observed).

▶ Parents clearly have difficulty demonstrating positive, accepting feelings toward the child.

> *Clinicians frame treatment as a process that will help improve the parent-child relationship.*

Treatment Process

During dyadic skills training, the clinician teaches parents about the normative social, cognitive, and emotional development of preschoolers, and explains the tendency for preschoolers to attempt to be independent and autonomous from parents. From this context, clinicians reframe parent difficulties as a problematic juggling act between closeness, autonomy, and limit setting. The child's difficulties are reframed as part of the natural tendencies of growing up.

Next, the clinician attempts to facilitate an elevation in the child's level of control in the parent-child relationship by increasing unstructured, undirected, parent-child play that occurs in the family, and by training the parent how to play in a way that yields control to the child. Parent-child play sessions are usually videotaped. The clinician and parent watch the videotapes together, and the clinician uses instruction, modeling, role-playing, and coaching to teach parents better ways to respond (or not respond) to their child. The videotapes of play can also be used to elicit the parent's cognitive (e.g., "Chris does that on purpose to make me mad") and affective reactions (e.g., "That makes me

> *Elevating the child's level of control provides a more constructive way for parents and children to communicate. This way of relating may be quite a contrast to the negative discipline confrontations that they have likely been enduring for some time.*

feel sad."), to their child's behaviors and to help parents think from their child's perspective.

Clinicians regularly give homework assignments that include parent-reframing exercises, such as "Chris isn't doing that just to make me mad. She likes playing video games more than taking out the trash."

Parents learn limit setting through "standard" parent training with a focus on using the least restraint possible to maintain order. The clinician helps parents sort their child's negative behaviors into low-level, ignorable behaviors (e.g., whining) and harmful behaviors (e.g., hitting). The clinician encourages parents to reduce limit-setting attempts on ignorable behavior and to be firm on limit setting for harmful behavior. Further, parents learn indirect methods for most limit setting. These include:

- ▶ Using natural consequences
- ▶ Using "when/then" contingencies (i.e., "When you do this first, then you can do that.")
- ▶ Providing choices for the child that coincide with the parent's desires
- ▶ Offering specific, labeled praise for positive behaviors

In addition, parents and children receive homework assignments for practicing problem-solving skills while they make minor decisions or negotiate day-to-day departures and reunions. As their skills improve, they are assigned more stressful situations to negotiate.

Follow-up After Program Termination

Clinicians can make a six-month follow-up phone call to check on the child's progress with both parents and teachers. At this point, further treatment can be pursued if indicated.

Effectiveness of the Psychodynamic Approach

Neither the short-term nor the long-term impact of this treatment package has been investigated in terms of impact on the conduct disorders. However, supportive evidence exists regarding the efficacy of the parent-training component of the program (see parent training on page 31).

Although play therapy is a common psychodynamic approach to treating young children diagnosed with a conduct disorder, evidence to date does not indicate that play therapy is effective in reducing antisocial behavior.[207]

A variety of other attachment-focused programs are under development but also have yet to be evaluated.[206] Most of these programs focus on modifying the parent-infant relationship in ways that are hypothesized to be optimal for development of the child's personality and are intended to prevent negative child outcomes such as the development of a conduct disorder.

Key Concepts for Chapter Three:

1. Psychological treatment programs that focus **both** on changing specific problematic child behaviors and on how children interact with parents, teachers, and peers are most effective for treating the conduct disorders.

2. The most effective conduct disorder treatments combine parent training, school-based behavior management programs, and child problem-solving skills training.

3. Parent training programs that teach parents to be "behavior modifiers" have proven successful in a variety of empirical studies.

4. Key aspects of parent training programs involve the use of positive reinforcement, contingency contracting, time out, structured weekly sessions, monitoring, and family problem-solving conferences.

5. School-based programs provide immediate and clear consequences for school behavior.

6. The cognitive therapy approach to treating CD focuses mainly on child problem-solving training that makes problem solving more conscious, proactive, and prosocial.

7. In family therapy, clinicians use either functional family therapy (EFT) or multisystemic treatment (MST) to change how the child with a conduct disorder communicates with family and significant others.

8. The most effective group therapy for CD appears to be situations where the group includes children without behavior problems rather than consisting solely of members with similar problem behaviors.

9. Intense group treatment, such as the Summer Treatment Program (STP), has shown preliminary efficacy for reducing aggression, anxiety, and problematic social skills, common to those with a conduct disorder.

Chapter Four:
Biological Influences and Treatments for the Conduct Disorders

This chapter answers the following:

▶ **Is there a Genetic Component to the Conduct Disorders?** — This section discusses research on the possibility that biological factors related to problems with conduct could be inherited.

▶ **How are Medications used to Treat the Conduct Disorders?** — This section reviews the most common types of medications used to treat severe aggression as well as related problems such as ADHD.

▶ **What is the Effectiveness of Medication Therapy?** — This section presents efficacy research results for antipsychotics, stimulants, mood stabilizers, and other medications used to treat conduct problems.

T HE conduct disorders appear to result from some inter-action of biological , familial, and social factors:

▶ **Biological factors** — Children may inherit tendencies to display inattentive, impusive, and/or hyperactive behaviors, which increase the likelihood that a child will display conduct problems.

▶ **Familial factors** — The risk of CD is higher for children exposed to parents or other caregivers whose lives are characterized by substance abuse, psychiatric illness, marital conflict, child abuse, and/or antisocial behavior. Additionally, inconsistent parental availability and discipline appear to be consistent factors.

▶ **Social factors** — Exposure to deviant peer groups influences antisocial behavior.

There has been extensive biological research on one of the key symptoms of the conduct disorders, aggression. Researchers have identified a variety of *neurotransmitters* (e.g., serotonin, norepinephrine) and brain structures (e.g., *hypothalamus, amygdala*), which appear to be related to the display of aggressive behaviors.[174, 208] Ample evidence exists that aggressive behavior can be biologically induced (e.g., via physical injury, illness, removal of brain tissue, organic syndromes) and modified (e.g., via hormones, food deprivation, electrical stimulation, medications) to varying degrees in animals and humans.[208–210]

A variety of studies have examined the correlation between physiology and conduct problems; most frequently studied have been heart rate (HR) and electrodermal activity (EDA) during

neurotransmitters — chemical agents that carry information between nerve cells in the body and affect behavior, mood, and thoughts

hypothalamus — a brain structure involved in the control of body temperature, heart rate, blood pressure, etc.

amygdala — a brain structure that plays a role in emotional behavior, such as aggression, motivation, and memory functions

Low levels of serotonin are related to impulsive violence as well as normal aggression towards self and others.[211]

laboratory tasks. Conduct problems tend to be related to low resting HR and low resting EDA, although these relationships are weak.[212] There appear to be similarities between the psycho-physiological responses of children/adolescents with conduct problems and adults with aggression problems or antisocial personality disorder, the adult equivalent of conduct disorder.

Is there a Genetic Component to the Conduct Disorders?

Several researchers have investigated whether biological factors related to conduct problems might be inherited. In the most relevant studies, researchers examined the co-occurrence of adult criminal behavior (a legal rather than a clinical designation) among relatives. Some of the variation in criminal behavior among individuals can be attributed to what are presumed to be "genetic" factors.[213-218]

One hypothesis for how genetic factors might influence the development of a conduct disorder early in life focuses on inherited tendencies to display inattentive, impulsive, and hyperactive behaviors.[30, 219-222] Such behaviors probably contribute to difficulties in parent-child interactions, which in turn could lead to the coercive family processes that behavioral theorists believe teach children a repertoire of antisocial behaviors.[83] Regardless of whether genetics play a role, the presence of both biological and social risk factors greatly increases the risk that a child will exhibit antisocial behavior.[210]

From The Patient's Perspective

Shawn M.

Now they want me to go to see a doctor about medications. I am tired of meeting with all of these people to talk about me. It sure is hard to concentrate sometimes. Maybe there is something that could help with that. I would like to do better with things, but no matter how hard I try, I can't seem to get with it sometimes.

How are Medications Used to Treat the Conduct Disorders?

Currently, there are no FDA-approved medications for treating the conduct disorders. However, research studies indicate medications that impact certain target CD symptoms can be important adjunctive therapy, especially for patients with severe and extreme aggressive behavior. These medications include atypical *antipsychotics*, other antipsychotics, stimulants, mood stabilizers (e.g., lithium and divalproex sodium), and others (antidepressants, anticonvulsants, and noradrenergics).[211, 223, 224] Another key role for medication in CD treatment is to improve attentiveness and reduce antisocial behaviors , making some children more able to benefit from psychosocial intervention.[223]

Medications used to treat ADHD, which is highly comorbid with the conduct disorders, appear to reduce symptoms associated with milder forms of aggression.[224] Research indicates that hyperactive-impulsive-attention problems co-occur with conduct problems at a greater than random rate and that some treatments for ADHD may impact aggression or other conduct problems in some children.[26, 225]

Antipsychotics

Newer antipsychotics, called "atypical antipsychotics," have demonstrated effectiveness for controlling severe aggression and rage with fewer side effects than more traditional antipsychotics. Frequently used, especially for acute agitation in emergency situations, antipsychotics affect neurotransmitters in the brain.[211, 224] For example, researchers in two, double-blind, placebo-controlled trials have found risperidone (an atypical antipsychotic) effective for treating severe conduct and disruptive behaviors in children with subaverage IQs.[226, 227]

Overt aggressiveness and rage seem to be symptoms more responsive to pharmacotherapy, while covert CD symptoms (e.g., lying and stealing) are not as responsive.[119, 211]

antipsychotics — (also referred to as neuroleptics) tranquilizing medications, especially those used in treating mental disorders

Most published studies involve the use of medications for treating CD and comorbid disorders rather than for CD alone.[223]

Because of the risk to youth of extrapyramidal side effects, it may be advisable to favor atypical antipsychotics (e.g., risperidone, ziprasidone, and olanzapine) over more traditional medications.[211]

From The Parent's Perspective

Jeannie M.

Even though things seem more under control now, Shawn is still having trouble at school. Our therapist thinks that Shawn might have a mild case of ADHD, and that he should see a physician and try some medications. Seems like we'll never get a handle on Shawn all the way — there is always something new. But maybe this is one of the last pieces to the puzzle. Would sure be nice.

Figure 4.1, on page 70, provides an at-a-glance view of medications used to treat target symptoms of conduct disorders.

psychotropic — broadly, a substance that impacts the behavior, emotions, and/or thoughts of an individual

stimulants — medications that increase the arousal of the central nervous system

synapse — the space between individual nerve cells in the brain

reuptake — reabsorption of a neurotransmitter into the cell that released it

Special concerns for antipsychotics include:

▶ These medications are not recommended for children under three.

▶ Use cautiously if the patient is concurrently taking anti-convulsants and a variety of other drugs; potentiates effects of central nervous system depressants (e.g., alcohol).

▶ For clozapine, weekly blood counts are mandatory; sei-zure prophylaxis should be considered at higher doses.

▶ Use cautiously with other *psychotropic* medications or if patient has a history of cardiovascular problems.

▶ Monitor involuntary movements continually.

▶ Weight gain associated particularly with atypical antipsychotics can be problematic for patients with glucose intolerance.

Stimulants

Stimulants are the most common medications used to control symptoms of impulsivity characteristic in both conduct disorders and ADHD. Considered highly effective, some research cited in a recent literature review indicates that stimulants significantly reduce aggression in patients without the presence of ADHD.[224, 228, 229]

Based on the high co-occurence of ADHD with CD, one meta-analysis of literature published from 1970–2001 examined the effects of stimulants on overt and covert aggression-related behaviors in children diagnosed with ADHD. In this study, researchers found that, while stimulants impacted comorbid conduct disorder, the effects were not as strong for aggression-related behaviors as for other core ADHD symptoms.[225]

The stimulants (methylphenidate and dextroamphetamine) are the most common psychotropic medications prescribed for children in the U.S., accounting for three to seven percent of prescriptions for youth each year.[230-233] These medications improve sustained attention, attentional allocation, motor inhi-bition, and the organization and speed of motor responses.[234] Stimulants, which have a chemical structure that closely resem-bles the structure of the neurotransmitters in the nervous sys-tem, appear to act by:

1. Increasing the release of dopamine and norepinephrine (neurotransmitters in the brain) into the *synapse*

2. Blocking the *reuptake* of dopamine and norepinephrine[235]

Longer-acting formulations offer a two-fold advantage: first, some patients experience fewer "peaks" and "valleys" in medica-tion effect; second, the risk of substance abuse is less since there is not the associated "high" with this preparation.

Special concerns for the stimulants include:

▶ Do not use with children under six years old.

▶ It is not advisable to prescribe concurrently with other psychotropic drugs, which can elevate levels of both drugs; concurrent use with *MAOI medications* can elevate blood pressure to dangerous levels.

▶ Use with oral steroids (for asthma) can result in dizziness, tachycardia, palpitation, weakness, and/or agitation

▶ Use with antihistamines may decrease effectiveness of stimulant.

▶ Use is generally thought to be contraindicated if there is a history of tics and/or family history of Tourette's syndrome. Use with caution if there is a co-occurring seizure disorder or high blood pressure.

Mood Stabilizers

Various studies cited in a recent article indicate the effectiveness of mood stabilizing medications (e.g., divalproex, lithium, carbamazepine) for reducing violent and self-injurious behaviors.[211]

Divalproex Sodium (Valproate)

This anticonvulsant medication has been used to control manic episodes in patients with bipolar disorder. However, recent research suggests a possible role for divalproex in the treatment of conduct disorder.[236] In a randomized, controlled clinical trial with 71 youths with CD, divalproex sodium improved key variables considered predictive of criminal recidivism — self-reported impulse control and self-restraint.[236]

Special concerns for divalproex sodium include:

▶ Severe side effects include serious or even fatal liver damage, especially during the first six months of treatment, requiring monitoring of liver function.

▶ Use is not recommended for children under two years of age, especially when combined with other anticonvulsants, or children with other disorders (e.g., mental retardation).

▶ Use can cause life-threatening damage to the pancreas, requiring monitoring for pancreatitis.

▶ Cessation requires a gradual reduction in dosage.

▶ Prolongs clotting time.

▶ Requires monitoring of thrombocytopenia and policystic ovary syndrome.

MAOI medications — monamine oxidase inhibitors, which are used to treat depression and other psychiatric disorders

Research indicates that hyperactive-impulsive-attention problems co-occur with conduct problems at a greater than random rate and that some treatments for ADHD may impact aggression or other conduct problems.[26, 225]

Because of the medication's potential for damage to the liver and pancreas, more research on side-effect profiles and longer-term impacts of divalproex is warranted.

▶ Medication increases the effect of painkillers and anesthetics and depresses activity of the central nervous system, which may increase effects of alcohol.

▶ Use caution when combining divalproex with amitriptyline (Elavil®), aspirin, and barbiturates as well as blood thinners; other seizure medications; or sleep aids and tranquilizers.

Lithium

Used typically for bipolar disorder and intermittent explosive disorder, lithium carbonate is a mood stabilizer that prevents or diminishes mood intensity. The medication acts by interfering with the synthesis and reuptake of neurotransmitters and affects levels of serotonin, a chemical messenger in the brain, which can alter mood.

Special concerns for lithium include:

▶ Safety has not been established for children below age 12.

▶ Use with caution with other psychotropic medications.

▶ Drugs that interfere with kidney function (e.g., non-steroidal anti-inflammatory agents), drugs that impact hydration (e.g., diuretics, non-prescription diet systems), and illness may disrupt lithium steady state and lead to drug toxicity. Symptoms of toxicity include diarrhea, vomiting, drowsiness, muscular weakness, lack of coordination. Patients must have constant access to water during treatment.

▶ Use requires monitoring of serum blood levels, thyroid, and renal function.

Other Medications

Other medications have been shown to impact favorably on some conduct-disordered symptoms (e.g., aggression, noncompliance).[237, 238]

Antidepressants (Fluoxetine, Bupropion)

According to a recent review of medications used to treat violent youth, both selective serotonin reuptake inhibitors (SSRIs) and bupropion (a nontricyclic antidepressant) decreased aggressive behavior.[211] In one study cited, fluoxetine and citalopram appeared to decrease aggressive behavior in patients without comorbid depression.[211] Of special concern, however, is that the use of antidepressants could precipitate a manic episode in individuals with a previously undiagnosed bipolar disorder. Of the SSRIs, the authors found that fluoxetine appears to be the medication of choice.[211] One study cited in the article found that taking bupropion resulted in significant improvement in children with ADHD who exhibited prominent CD symptoms and violent behavior.[211]

Special concerns for antidepressants include:

▶ All antidepressant medications have the potential to trigger a manic or hypomanic episode in persons with underlying bipolar disorder.

▶ Use of SSRIs as well as bupropion with other drugs may cause "serotonin syndrome" with nausea, diarrhea, chills, palpitations, agitation, muscle twitching, and delirium. SSRIs can be fatal if taken along with MAOIs.

▶ Bupropion should be avoided in patients with anorexia or bulimia due to possible seizures. Drug-induced seizures can occur in doses greater than 6 mg/kg.

Noradrenergics (Clonidine)

Clonidine is an antihypertensive with some demonstrated efficacy for treating children with ADHD and comorbid oppositional defiant or conduct disorder. Additionally, this medication may be preferred over stimulants for children with low IQs.[239]

Special concerns for clonidine include:

▶ Safety has not been established below age 12.

▶ Concurrent use with tricyclic medications may lessen clonidine effect.

▶ Sudden cessation of the medication must be avoided as it may cause nervousness, agitation, tremor, confusion, and rapid rise in blood pressure. Severe reactions, such as disruption of brain functions, stroke, fluid in the lungs, and death, have also been reported. If the patient is also taking a beta blocker (e.g., inderal or tenormin), the beta blocker must be stopped several days before gradual withdrawal of clonidine.

▶ Use may induce rebound hypertension.

▶ Use with caution for patients who have severe heart or kidney disease, are recovering from a heart attack, or have a cerebral vascular disease.

▶ The medication increases the effects of alcohol and other medications with depressive effects on the central nervous system.

▶ Use with caution to prevent interactions for patients also taking barbiturates, beta blockers, calcium blockers, digitalis, sedatives, or tricyclic antidepressants.

Figure 4.1, on the following page, provides an at-a-glance view of these medications, target symptoms, and most common side effects.

Figure 4.1   Medications for Treating Target Symptoms in Conduct Disorders*

Medication Class/Name[211, 223, 224]	Target Symptoms	Most Common Side Effects
Atypical Antipsychotics Risperidone Ziprasidone Olanzapine Clozapine	Explosiveness, paranoia, psychosis, aggression	Sedation, weight gain, dry mouth, constipation, Parkinson-like symptoms (flat facial expression, stiff muscles, and slowed movements), hypotension. **With risperidone**, sexual dysfunction, elevated prolactin. **With ziprasidone**, dizziness, nausea, and vomiting. **With olanzapine,** potential mental confusion. **With clozapine**, an abrupt drop in blood pressure when suddenly changing from lying to sitting or sitting to standing, rapid heart rate, excessive salivation, nausea, and vomiting.
Other Antipsychotics Haloperidol Pimozide	Explosiveness, severe aggression, rage	Sedation, Parkinsonian symptoms, acute dystonic reactions, weight gain, withdrawal, and tardive dyskinesias (all of which are less pronounced with pimozide). Pimozide is contraindicated witih sertraline.
Stimulants** Methylphenidate Hydrochloride Dextroamphetamine Sulfate	Inattention, impulsivity, hyperactivity, mild aggression, noncompliance	Insomnia, decreased appetite, weight loss (may be greater with dextroamphetamine sulfate), stomach aches, irritability. Possible drug withdrawal symptoms (e.g., extreme fatigue, anxiety, depression) late in day after last dose dissipates or if abrupt cessation of treatment.
Mood Stabilizers Lithium Carbonate Divalproex Sodium	Explosiveness, severe aggression, rage	**With lithium,** weight gain, stomach ache, headache, tremor. **With divalproex sodium,** abdominal pain, abnormal thinking, breathing difficulty, bronchitis, bruising, constipation, depression, diarrhea, dizziness, emotional changeability, fever, flu symptoms, hair loss, headache, incoordination, indigestion, infection, insomnia, loss of appetite, memory loss, nasal inflammation, nausea, nervousness, ringing in the ears, sleepiness, sore throat, tremor, vision problems, vomiting, weakness, weight loss or gain.
Other Medications		
Antidepressants Fluoxetine Bupropion	Anxiety	**With fluoxetine,** agitation, respiratory complaints, headache, dry mouth, tremors. **With buproprion**, blurred vision, constipation, sweating, insomnia, headache, dizziness, hypertension, nausea/diarrhea
Antihypertensives Noradrenergic Clonidine	Inattention, impulsivity, hyperactivity, mild aggression, noncompliance; may be best for hyperaroused child with high levels of motor activity and aggression	Sedation, nausea, vomiting, headache, dizziness, rash with skin patch. Variety of other side effects, including dry mouth, vomiting, weight gain, nervousness, agitation, orthostatic hypotension, cardiovascular problems, kidney problems, fatigue, depression, cardiac arrhythmias. **Note:** Sudden termination of treatment may cause nervousness, agitation, headache, rapid rise in blood pressure.

* Medications included are presented in the order recommended in the treatment algorithm for CD presented in the Annals of the New York Academy of Science [Gilligan, J, and Bandy, L. (2004)].[211] **Because there are no medications specifically approved for treating CD,** clinicians should consult available research and use clinical judgment and medication titration results to determine appropriate dosages for individual patients.

** Clinicians should evaluate (through feedback from child, parents, and teachers) whether or not to continue stimulant use every six to 12 months.[55, 231, 240]

What is the Effectiveness of Medication Therapy?

Evidence indicates that a variety of medications — especially atypical antipsychotics, stimulants, mood stabilizers, and clonidine — offer a positive, short-term impact on a few of the conduct-disorder and related symptoms in some children.

Atypical antipsychotics, especially risperidone, are beneficial for treating severely aggressive behaviors in children hospitalized with CD.[119, 224, 241]

For **stimulants**, problem symptoms usually do not respond equally well to the same dose, and children often respond differently to the same dosage level on different days.[242] From 50 to 75 percent of children accurately diagnosed with ADHD benefit from stimulants through decreases in inattention, impulsivity, hyperactivity, non-compliance, and/or verbal and physical aggression.[233, 243-245] In two controlled studies cited in a recent pharmacotherapy research review, researchers found that methylphenidate decreased aggression in patients without symptoms of ADHD.[224] Another study cited in that same review found mixed results.

New intermediate-acting and extended-release versions of the stimulants offer additional options for symptom control.[246]

A few studies of the effect of long-term maintenance of stimulants have shown positive effects.[233]

For mood stabilizers, lithium appears beneficial for the short-term treatment of severe aggression with a strong affective and episodic component, without significant side effects.[119, 247] However, most research fails to clarify what percentage of patients respond well to lithium.[223, 224] In a randomized, controlled clinical trial of 71 adolescent males diagnosed with conduct disorder (and having been convicted of at least one criminal offense), researchers found that divalproex sodium significantly improved self-reported symptoms — impulse control and self restraint — considered highly predictive of recidivism.[236]

Another small, double-blind controlled study found that divalproex decreased explosiveness and mood lability in children with ODD or CD.[248]

Clonidine, an antihypertensive, appears helpful as well. Researchers in a randomized clinical trial found that clonidine-treated patients scored better on the Conduct and Hyperactive Index subscales of the Connors Behavior Checklist (parent-report) and had fewer unwanted side effects.[239]

The likelihood of CD symptoms reappearing is less after discontinuing medication if effective and sustainable environmental interventions are firmly in place. Further, concurrent, intensive psychosocial treatment tends to reduce the amount of stimulant medication needed to show improvement.[249]

Since medication for the conduct disorders is an adjunct, rather than an alternative to psychosocial treatments, there are no studies that explicitly contrast these two types of treatment for the conduct disorders.

Despite the short-term efficacy of using medications to treat certain symptoms of conduct disorder, there is no evidence that treatment with any medication cures the conduct disorders.[119, 250] Instead, medications assist in symptom management and are commonly viewed as only one component of a treatment program.[144]

Key Concepts for Chapter Four:

1. Although unknown, the etiology of the conduct disorders appears to be related to some interaction of genetic/constitutional, familial, and social factors.

2. Research indicates a biological etiology for at least one of the key symptoms of the conduct disorders, aggression, in some children.

3. The primary role of medications in treating conduct disorders is as an adjunct to psychotherapy used specifically to reduce symptoms of aggression.

4. Medications used to treat aggression and impulse control include antipsychotics, stimulants, and mood stabilizers.

5. Although some research supports the use of medications for short-term reduction of symptoms related to CD, no evidence of long-term efficacy exists.

6. Medications appear to be more effective in reducing overt CD symptoms (e.g., aggression, violent outbursts) than covert ones (e.g., lying, stealing).

7. There are no FDA-approved medications for treating the conduct disorders; dosages should be given based on clinical judgment, research outcomes in controlled trials, medication titration results, and the individual needs of the patient/situation.

Appendix:
References for the Clinician's Bookshelf

Research, Theory, and Treatment

Bloomquist, M. L., & Schnell, S. V. (2002). *Helping children with aggression and conduct problems: Best practices for intervention*. New York: Guilford Press.

Conner, D., & Barkley, R. A. (2002). *Aggression and antisocial behavior in children and adolescents: Research and treatment*. New York: Guilford Press.

Dodge, K., Dishion, T., & Lansford, J. (Eds.) (2005). *Deviant by design: Interventions and policies that aggregate deviant youth, and strategies to optimize outcomes*. New York: Guilford Press.

Fishbein, D. H. (Ed.). *The science, treatment, and prevention of antisocial behaviors: Application to the criminal justice system*. Kingston, NJ: Civic Research Institute.

Kazdin, A. E., & Weisz, J. R. (Eds.) (2003). *Evidence-based psychotherapies for children and adolescents*. New York: Guilford Press.

Loeber, R., & Farrington, D. P. (Eds.) (1998). *Serious and violent juvenile offenders: Risk factors and successful interventions*. Thousand Oaks, CA: Sage.

McCord, J. & Tremblay, R. E. (1992). *Preventing antisocial behavior: Interventions from birth to adolescence*. New York: Guilford Press.

Nathan, P. M., & Gorman, J. M. (Eds.) (1998). *A guide to treatments that work*. New York: Oxford University Press.

Patterson, G. R. (1982). *Coercive family process*. Eugene, OR: Castalia Publishing.

Putallaz, M., & Bierman, K. L. (Eds.) (2004). *Aggression, antisocial behavior, and violence among girls*. New York: Guilford Press.

Reid, J. B., Patterson, G. R., & Snyder, J. (Ed.) (2002). *Antisocial behavior in children and adolescents: A developmental analysis and model for intervention*. Washington, D.C.: American Psychological Association.

Stoff, D. M., Breiling, J., & Maser, J. D. (Eds.). (1997). *Handbook of antisocial behavior*. New York: John Wiley and Sons.

Assessment

Mash, E. J., & Terdal, L. G. (1997). *Assessment of childhood disorders, 3rd Edition.* New York: Guilford Press.

O'Neil, R. E., Horner, R. H., Albin, R. W., Storey, K., & Sprague, J. R. (1990). *Functional analysis of problem behavior: A practical assessment guide.* Sycamore, IL: Sycamore.

Salvia, J., & Ysseldyck, J. E. (1991). *Assessment.* Boston: Houghton Mifflin.

Vance, B. H. (Ed.) (1993). *Best practices in assessment for school and clinical settings.* Brandon, VT: Clinical Psychology Publishing.

Parent Training: For Clinicians

Barkley, R. (1997). *Defiant children: A clinician's manual for assessment and parent training, second edition.* New York: Guilford Press.

Cavell, T. A. (2000). *Working with parents of aggressive children: A practitioner's guide.* Washington D.C.: American Psychological Association.

Dishion, T. J., Kavanagh, K., & Soberman, L. (In press). *Adolescent transitions program: Assessment and intervention sourcebook.* New York: Guilford Press.

McMahon, R. J., & Forehand, R. L. (2003). *Helping the noncompliant child: Family-based treatment for oppositional behavior* (2nd ed.). New York: Guilford Press.

Patterson, G. R., Reid, J. B., Jones, R. R., & Conger, R. E. (1975). *Families with aggressive children.* Eugene, OR: Castalia Press.

Ramsey, E., Beland, K., and Miller, T. (1995). *Second step: Parenting strategies for a safer tomorrow.* Seattle, WA: Committee for Children.

Sanders, M. R., & Dadds, M. R. (1993). *Behavioral family intervention.* Boston: Allyn and Bacon.

Sanders, M. R., Markie-Dadds, C., Turner, K. M. T., & Brechman-Toussaint, M. L. (2000). *Triple P-Positive parenting program: A guide to the system.* Brisbane, QLD, Australia: Families Interventional Publishing.

Webster-Stratton, C. & Herbert, M. (1994). *Troubled families, problem children: Working with parents, a collaborative process.* Chichester, England: John Wiley & Sons.

Parent Training: For Parents

Dishion, T. J., & Patterson, G. R. (1995). *Preventive parenting with love, encouragement, and limits: The preschool years.* Eugene, OR: Castalia Press.

Forgatch, M. S., & Patterson, G. R. (1987). *Parents and adolescents living together, part 2: Family problem solving.* Eugene, OR: Castalia Press.

Gottman, J. (1997) *Raising an emotionally intelligent child: The heart of parenting.* New York: Simon and Schuster.

Patterson, G. R. (1976). *Living with children: New methods for parents and teachers* (revised). Champaign, IL: Research Press.

Patterson, G. R. (1977). *Families: Applications of social learning to family life* (revised). Champaign, IL: Research Press.

Patterson, G. R., & Forgatch, M. S. (1987). *Parents and adolescents living together, part 1: The basics.* Eugene, OR: Castalia Press.

Webster-Stratton, C. (1997). *The incredible years: A troubleshooting guide for parents of children aged 3–8.* Toronto, Ontario: Umbrella Press.

School-Based Interventions

Walker, H. M. (1995). *The acting-out child: Coping with classroom disruption* (revised). Longmont, CO: Sopris West.

Walker, H. M., Colvin, G., & Ramsey, E. (1995). *Antisocial behavior in school: Strategies and best practices.* Pacific Grove, CA: Brooks/Cole.

Multidimensional Treatment Foster Care

Chamberlain, P. (1994). *Family connections: A treatment foster care model for adolescents with delinquency.* Eugene, OR: Castalia Publishing.

Chamberlain, P. (1998). *Blueprints for violence prevention, book eight: Treatment foster care.* Boulder, CO: Center for the Study and Prevention of Violence.

Child Problem Solving Skills Training

Camp, B. W., & Bash, M. A. S. (1985). *Think aloud: Increasing social and cognitive skills, a problem-solving program for children.* Champaign, IL: Research Press.

Greenberg, M. T., Kusche, C. & Mihalic, S. F. (1998). *Blueprints for violence prevention, book ten: Promoting alternative thinking strategies (PATHS).* Boulder, CO: Center for the Study and Prevention of Violence.

Kendall, P. C., & Braswell, L. (1985). *Cognitive-behavioral therapy for impulsive children.* New York: Guilford Press.

Functional Family Therapy

Alexander, J., Barton, C., Gordon, D., Grotpeter, J., Hansson, K., Harrison, R., Mears, S., Mihalic, S., Parsons, B., Pugh, C., Schulman, S., Waldron, H., & Sexton, T. (1998). *Blueprints for violence prevention, book three: Functional family therapy*. Boulder, CO: Center for the Study and Prevention of Violence.

Alexander, J. F., & Parsons, B. (1982). *Functional family therapy*. Monterey, CA: Brooks/Cole.

Multisystemic Treatment

Henggeler, S. W. (1990). *Family therapy and beyond: A multisystemic approach to treating the behavior problems of children and adolescents*. Pacific Grove, CA: Brooks/Cole.

Henggeler, S. W., Mihalic, S. F., Rone, L., Thomas, C., & Timmons-Mitchell, J. (1998). *Blueprints for violence prevention, book six: Multisystemic therapy*. Boulder, CO: Center for the Study and Prevention of Violence.

Robin, A. L., & Foster, S. L. (1989). *Negotiating parent-adolescent conflict: A behavioral-family systems approach*. New York: Guilford Press.

Glossary

A

across-time correlations — the extent to which a person's test scores remain in a similar rank compared to others across time (e.g., a highly stable test might have Suzy score high on three separate testings, Sam moderate, and Jean low)

amygdala — a brain structure that plays a role in emotional behavior, such as aggression, motivation, and memory functions

antipsychotics — (also referred to as neuroleptics) tranquilizing medications, especially those used in treating mental disorders

antisocial behavior — behavior that violates fundamental social rules and/or the basic rights of others

B

baseline — the period of time prior to the beginning of a therapeutic intervention

C

case manager — a person, typically a social worker, who oversees all aspects of the patient's treatment program

clinically significant — a pattern of behavioral and/or psychological symptoms that has become established enough, severe enough, and impairing enough to interfere with a child's day-to-day functioning in the home, the school, and/or the community

conscious — within the person's awareness

contingency contracting — a plan for the positive and negative consequences that follow specific child behaviors

contingency management program — a system for rewarding good behaviors and providing costs for misbehaviors

comorbid — the simultaneous presence of two or more disorders

correlates — the extent to which two scores are linearly related to each other (e.g., as one score goes up, the other tends to go up or down)

D

developmental history — significant events and milestones during childhood such as age the child first walked or talked

deviant peer groups — groups of youths who behave outside of socially accepted norms

dysfunctional — patterns of behavior that have distressing and problematic outcomes

DSM-IV (TR) — the *Diagnostic and Statistical Manual of Mental Disorders, Fourth Edition, Text Revision,* published by the American Psychiatric Association

F

face valid — the content of test items directly assesses a self-evident psychological construct

family roles — the way that parents and children relate with one another in terms of power, allegiance, and function

H

homeostasis — equilibrium or balance

hypothalamus — a brain structure involved in the control of body temperature, heart rate, blood pressure, etc.

I

inter-interviewer reliability — degree of agreement among the ratings of various interviewers

internal reliability — the extent to which the various items on a test are related to one another

inter-observer reliability — degree of agreement among the ratings of various observers

inter-parental agreement — the degree of agreement on test scores between parents

M

MAOI medications — monamine oxidase inhibitors, which are used to treat depression and other psychiatric disorders

mental disorder — a clinically significant pattern of behavioral or psychological symptoms associated with one or more major negative outcomes (e.g., distress, pain, injury, disability, confinement)

monitoring — hour-to-hour each day, a parent knows whom their son or daughter is with, where he or she is, and what he or she is doing

N

negative reinforcement — the discontinuation of an undesired event (e.g., parents fighting) following a behavior (e.g. child hits sibling) rewards the occurrence of that behavior (i.e. the hit)

neuroleptics — tranquilizing medications, especially those used in treating mental disorders

neurotransmitters — chemical agents that carry information between nerve cells in the body and affect behavior, mood, and thoughts

P

positive reinforcement — the delivery of a desired event (e.g., parent says, "Great job, Joe!" and gives Joe a hug) following a behavior (e.g., child playing nicely with sibling), which results in an increase of that behavior

prosocial — responsible, socially considerate behavior

psychosocial history — history of significant social development such as family and peer interaction and adjustment at school

psychotropic — broadly, a substance that impacts the behavior, emotions, and/or thoughts of an individual

R

rate-per-minute — the average number of specific behaviors of interest occurring in one minute

recidivism — A tendency to lapse into a previous pattern of behavior, especially a pattern of criminal habits associated with repeat arrests

relational aggression — harm perpetrated against others using indirect, non-physical means such as manipulation, threats, and exclusion

respite care — short-term out-of-home placements (e.g., a weekend)

reuptake — reabsorption of a neurotransmitter into the cell that released it

S

stimulants — medications that increase the arousal of the central nervous system

synapse — the space between individual nerve cells in the brain

T

test-retest reliability — the extent to which those tested obtain similar scores relative to each other on each administration of the test

titration — slow increase in medication until significant effects on the problem behaviors are noticed

token economy system — a program of earning points or other currency that can be traded in for specific rewards

W

wandering — spending time in unstructured settings without adult supervision

References

1. Robins, L. N. (1981). Epidemiological approaches to natural history research: Antisocial disorders in children. *Journal of the American Academy of Child Psychiatry, 20*, 566–580.

2. Eddy, J. M., & Swanson-Garbskov (1997). Juvenile justice and delinquency prevention in the United States: The influence of theories and traditions on policies and practices. In T. P. Gullota, G. R. Adams, & R. Montemayor (Eds.), *Delinquent Violent Youth* (pp. 12–52). Thousand Oaks, CA: Sage.

3. Wolff, S. (1961). Symptomatology and outcome of preschool children with behavior disorders attending a child guidance clinic. *Journal of Child Psychology and Psychiatry, 2*, 269–276.

4. Kazdin, A. E. (1994). Interventions for aggressive and antisocial children. In L. D. Eron, J. H. Gentry, & P. Schlegel (Eds.), *Reason to hope: A psychological perspective on violence and youth* (pp. 341–382). Washington, DC: American Psychological Association.

5. Reid, J. B., Patterson, G. R., & Snyder, J. (2002). *Antisocial behavior in children and adolescents: A developmental analysis and model for intervention.* Washington, DC: American Psychological Association.

6. Loeber, R. (1982). The stability of antisocial and delinquent behavior: A review. *Child Development, 53*, 1431–1446.

7. Huesmann, L. R., Eron, L. D., Lefkowitz, M. M., & Walder, L. O. (1984). The stability of aggression over time and generations. *Developmental Psychology, 20*, 1120–1134.

8. American Psychiatric Association (1994). *Diagnostic and Statistical Manual of Mental Disorders, Fourth Edition.* Washington, DC, American Psychiatric Association.

9. Offord, D. R., Boyle, M. C., & Racine, Y. A. (1991). The epidemiology of antisocial behavior in childhood and adolescence. In D. J. Peplar, & K. H. Rubin (Eds.), *The development and treatment of childhood aggression* (pp. 31–54). Hillsdale, NJ: Lawrence Erlbaum Associates.

10. Rutter, M., Cox, A., Tupling, C., Berger, M., & Yule, W. (1975). Attainment and adjustment in two geographical areas. I. The prevalence of psychiatric disorder. *British Journal of Psychiatry, 126*, 493–509.

11. McGee, R., Feehan, M., Williams, S., & Anderson, J. (1992). DSM-III disorders from age 11 to age 15 years. *Journal of the American Academy of Child and Adolescent Psychiatry, 31*, 50–59.

12. Cohen, P. (1993). An epidemiological study of disorders in late childhood and adolescence: I. Age- and gender-specific prevalence. *Journal of Child Psychology and Psychiatry and Allied Disciplines, 34*, 851–867.

13. McGee, R., Feehan, M., Williams, S., & Partridge, R. (1990). DSM-III disorders in a large sample of adolescents. *Journal of the American Academy of Child and Adolescent Psychiatry, 29*, 611–619.

14. Rutter, M. (1981). The city and the child. *American Journal of Orthopsychiatry, 51*, 610–625.

15. Patterson, G. R., Reid, J. B., & Dishion, T. J. (1992). *Antisocial boys.* Eugene, OR: Castalia Publishing.

16. Loeber, R., & Dishion, T. J. (1983). Early predictors of male delinquency: A review. *Psychological Bulletin, 94*, 68–99.

17. Lipsey, M. W., & Derzon, J. H. (1999). Predictors of violent or serious delinquency in adolescence and early adulthood: A synthesis of longitudinal research. In R. Loeber & D.P. Farrington (Eds), *Serious and Violent Juvenile Offenders.* (pp.86–105). Thousand Oaks, CA: Sage

18. Olweus, D. (1979). Stability of aggressive reaction patterns in males: A review. *Psychological Bulletin, 86*, 852–875.

19. Farrington, D. P. (1987). Early precusors of frequent offending. In J. Q. Wilson & G. C. Loury (Eds.), *From children to citizens, vol. 3: Families, schools, and delinquency prevention.* (pp. 27–50). New York: Springer-Verlag.

20. Robins, L. N. (1966). *Deviant children grown up: A sociological and psychiatric study of sociopathic personality.* Baltimore: Williams and Wilkins.

21. Rutter, M., & Giller, H. (1983). *Juvenile delinquency: Trends and perspectives.* New York: Penguin Books.

22. Loeber, R. (1990). Development and risk factors of juvenile antisocial behavior and delinquency. *Clinical Psychology Review, 10*, 1–41.

23. Kazdin, A. E. (1987). *Conduct disorder in childhood and adolescence.* Newbury Park, CA: Sage.

24. Lipsey, M. W.; & Derzon, J. H. (1998). Predictors of violent or serious delinquency in adolescence and early adulthood: A synthesis of longitudinal research. In R. Loeber & D. P. Farrington (Eds.), *Serious & violent juvenile offenders: Risk factors and successful interventions.* (pp. 86–105). Thousand Oaks, CA: Sage Publications, Inc.

25. Offord, D. R., Sullivan, K., Allen, N., & Abrams, N. (1979). Delinquency and hyperactivity. *Journal of Nervous and Mental Disorders, 167,* 734–741.

26. Waschbusch, D. A. (2002). A meta-analytic examination of comorbid hyperactive-impulsive-attention problems and conduct problems. *Psychological Bulletin, 128*(1), 118–150.

27. LeBlanc, M., & Frechette, M. (1989). *Male offending from latency to adulthood.* New York: Springer-Verlag.

28. Patterson, G. R., & Capaldi, D. C. (1994). *Frequency of offending and violent behavior.* Unpublished manuscript. Eugene, OR: Oregon Social Learning Center.

29. Dodge, K. A., Dishion, T. J., & Lansford, J. E. (Eds.) (in press). *Deviant by design: Interventions and policies that aggregate deviant youth, and strategies to optimize outcomes.* New York: Guilford Press.

30. Loeber, R. (1988). Natural histories of conduct problems, delinquency, and associated substance use: Evidence for developmental progressions. In B. B. Lahey & A. E. Kasdin (Eds.), *Advances in clinical child psychopathology, 11,* (pp. 73–124). New York: Plenum.

31. Patterson, G. R., DeBaryshe, B. D., & Ramsey, E. A. (1989). A developmental perspective on antisocial behavior. *American Psychologist, 44,* 329–335.

32. Robins, L. N. (1991). Conduct disorder. *Journal of Child Psychology and Psychiatry, 20,* 566–680.

33. Robins, L. N. (1970). The adult development of the antisocial child. *Seminars in Psychiatry, 6,* 420–434.

34. Robins, L. N., & Ratcliff, K. S. (1978–1979). Risk factors in the continuation of childhood antisocial behaviors into adulthood. *International Journal of Mental Health, 7,* 96–116.

35. Farrington, D. P. (1983). Offending from 10 to 25 years of age. In K. T. Van Dusen, & S. A. Mednick (Eds.), *Prospective studies of crime and delinquency.* (pp. 17–37). Boston: Kluwer-Nijhoff.

36. Serbin, L. A., Moskowitz, D. S., Schwartzman, A. E., & Ledingham, J. E. (1991). Aggressive, withdrawn, and aggressive/withdrawn children in adolescence: Into the next generation. In D. J. Peplar, & K. H. Rubin (Eds.), *The development and treatment of childhood aggression.* (pp. 55–70). Hillsdale, NJ: Erlbaum.

37. Hubbard, D. J., & Pratt, T. C. (2002). A meta-analysis of the predictors of delinquency among girls. *Journal of Offender Rehabilitation, 34*(3), 1–13.

38. Robins, L. N. (1978). Sturdy childhood predictors of adult antisocial behavior: Replications from longitudinal studies. *Psychological Medicine, 8,* 611–622.

39. Eron, L. D., Huesmann, L. R., & Zelli, A. (1991). The role of parental variables in the learning of aggression. In D. J. Peplar, & K. H. Rubin (Eds.), *The development and treatment of childhood aggression.* (pp. 169–188). Hillsdale, NJ: Lawrence Erlbaum Associates.

40. Farrington, D. P. (1991). Childhood aggression and adult violence: Early precursors and later life outcomes. In D. J. Peplar, & K. H. Rubin (Eds.), *The development and treatment of childhood aggression.* (pp. 5–29). Hillsdale, NJ: Lawrence Erlbaum Associates.

41. Capaldi, D. M., & Clark, S. (1998). Prospective family predictors of aggression toward female partners for young at-risk males. *Developmental Psychology, 34,* 1175–1188.

42. Costello, E. J., Edelbrock, C. S., Costello, A. J., Dulcan, M. K., Burns, B. J., & Brent, D. (1988). Psychopathology in pediatric primary care: The new hidden morbidity. *Pediatrics, 82,* 415–424.

43. Sleater, E. K., & Ullmann, R. L. (1981). Can the physician diagnose hyperactivity in the office? *Pediatrics, 67,* 13–17.

44. Stoolmiller, M. S. (1994). Antisocial behavior, delinquent peer association, and unsupervised wandering for boys: Growth and change from childhood to early adolescence. *Multivariate Behavioral Research, 29,* 263–288.

45. Wilson, H. (1980). Parental supervision: A neglected aspect of delinquency. *British Journal of Criminology, 20,* 203–254.

46. Crick, N. R., & Grotpeter, J. K. (1995). Relational aggression, gender, and social-psychological adjustment. *Child Development, 66,* 710–722.

47. Fesbach, S. (1970). Sex differences in children's modes of aggressive responses toward outsiders. *Merrill-Palmer Quarterly, 15,* 249–258.

48. Putallaz, M., & Bierman, K. L. (Eds.) (2004). *Aggression, antisocial behavior, and violence among girls.* New York: Guilford Press.

49. Patterson, G. R., Capaldi, D., & Bank, L. (1991). An early starter model for predicting delinquency. In D. J. Peplar & K. H. Rubin (Eds.), *The development and treatment of childhood aggression.* (pp. 139–168). Hillsdale, NJ: Lawrence Erlbaum Associates.

50. Patterson, G. R., Yoerger, K., & Stoolmiller, M. S. (in press). A developmental model for late-onset delinquency. In D. Stoff, J. Maser, & J. Breiling (Eds.), *Handbook of antisocial behavior.* New York: John Wiley & Sons.

51. Patterson, G. R., Duncan, T. E., Reid, J. B., & Bank, L. (1994). *Systematic maternal errors in predicting son's future arrests.* Unpublished manuscript, Oregon Social Learning Center, Eugene.

52. Reid, J. B., Kavanagh, K., & Baldwin, D. V. (1987). Abusive parents' perceptions of child problem behaviors: An example of parental bias. *Journal of Abnormal Child Psychology, 15,* 457–466.

53. Lorber, T. (1981). *Parental tracking of childhood behavior as a function of family stress.* Unpublished doctoral dissertation, University of Oregon, Eugene.

54. Holleran, P. A., Littman, D. C., Freund, R., Schmaling, K., & Heeren, J. (1982). A signal detection approach to social perception: Identification of negative and positive behaviors by parents of normal and distressed children. *Journal of Abnormal Child Psychology, 10,* 547–557.

55. Barkley, R. A. (1990). *Attention deficit hyperactivity disorder: A handbook for diagnosis and treatment.* New York: Guilford Press.

56. Patterson, G. R., Reid, J. B., Jones, R. R., & Conger, R. E. (1975). A social learning approach to family intervention, vol. 1: *Families with aggressive children.* Eugene, OR: Castalia Publishing.

57. Achenbach, T. M. (1991). *Manual for the Child Behavior Checklist/4–18 and 1991 profile.* Burlington, VT: University of Vermont Department of Psychiatry.

58. Pelham, W. E., Gnagy, E. M., Greenslade, K. E., & Milich, R. (1992). Teacher ratings of DSM-III-R symptoms for the disruptive behavior disorders. *Journal of the American Academy of Child and Adolescent Psychiatry, 31,* 210–218.

59. Sandberg, D. E., Meyer-Bahlburg, H. F. L., & Yager, T. J. (1991). The Child Behavior Checklist nonclinical standardization samples: Should they be utilized as norms? *Journal of the American Academy of Child and Adolescent Psychiatry, 30,* 124–134.

60. Achenbach, T. M., Bird, H. R., Canino, G., & Phares, V. (1990). Epidemiological comparisons of Puerto Rico and U. S. mainland children: Parent, teacher, and self-reports. *Journal of the American Academy of Child and Adolescent Psychiatry, 29,* 84–93.

61. Achenbach, T. M. (1991). *Manual for the Teacher's Report Form and 1991 profile.* Burlington, VT: University of Vermont Department of Psychiatry.

62. Achenbach, T. M. (1991). *Manual for the Youth Self-Report and 1991 profile.* Burlington, VT: University of Vermont Department of Psychiatry.

63. Pelham, W. E., Evans, S. W., Gnagy, E. M., & Greenslade, K. E. (1992). Teacher ratings of DSM-III-R symptoms for the disruptive behavior disorders: Prevalence, factor analyses, and conditional probabilities in a special education sample. *School Psychology Review, 21,* 285–299.

64. Kovacs, M. (1980). Ratings scales to assess depression in school aged children. *Acta Paedopsychiatrica, 46,* 305–315.

65. Woodcock, R. W. (1977). Woodcock-Johnson Psycho-Educational Battery: *Technical report.* Allen, TX: DLM Teaching Resources.

66. Schaffer, D., Fisher, P., Dulcan, M., Davies, M., Piacentini, J., Schwab-Stone, M., Lahey, B., Bourdon, K., Jensen, P., Bird, H., Canino, G., & Regier, D. (1995). The NIMH Diagnostic Interview Schedule for Children (DISC 2.3): Description, acceptability, prevalences, and performance in the MECA study. *Unpublished manuscript,* New York State Psychiatric Institute, New York.

67. Costello, A. J., Edelbrock, C., Dulcan, M. K., Kalas, R., & Klaric, S. H. (1984). Development and testing of the NIMH Diagnostic Interview Schedule for Children in a clinic population. *Final report (Contract No. RFP-DB-81-0027)*. Rockville, MD: Center for Epidemiologic Studies, National Institutes of Mental Health.

68. Weschler, D. (1991). *The Wechsler Intelligence Scale for Children —Third edition*. New York: The Psychological Corporation.

69. Fisher, P., Shaffer, D., Wicks, J., & Piacentini, J. (1989). A users' manual for the DISC-2 (Diagnostic Interview Schedule for Children, Version 2). *Unpublished manual*, New York State Psychiatric Institute, New York, NY.

70. Piacentini, J., Shaffer, D., Fisher, P., Schwab-Stone, M., Davies, M., & Gioia, P. (1993). The Diagnostic Interview Schedule for Children — Revised (DISC-R): III. Concurrent criterion validity. *Journal of the American Academy of Child and Adolescent Psychiatry, 32,* 658–665.

71. Edelbrock, C., & Costello, A. J. (1988). Structured psychiatric interviews for children. In M. Rutter, A. H. Tuma, & I. S. Lann (Eds.), *Assessment and diagnosis in child psychopathology.* (pp. 87–112). New York: Guilford Press.

72. Edelbrock, C., Costello, A. J., Dulcan, M. K., Conover, N .C., & Kalas, R. (1986). Parent-child agreement on child psychiatric symptoms assessed via structured interview. *Journal of Child Psychology and Psychiatry, 27,* 181–190.

73. Costello, E. J., Edelbrock, C., & Costello, A. J. (1985). The validity of the NIMH Diagnostic Interview Schedule for Children: A comparison between pediatric and psychiatric referrals. *Journal of Abnormal Child Psychology, 13,* 579–595.

74. Exner, J. E. (1993). *The Rorschach: A comprehensive system: Volume I: Basic foundations.* Somerset, NJ: John Wiley & Sons.

75. Hathaway, S. R., Butcher, J. N., & McKinley, J. C. (1989). *Minnesota Multiphasic Personality Inventory - 2.* Minneapolis: University of Minnesota Press.

76. Kraemer, H. C., & Thiemann, S. (1989). A strategy to use soft data effectively in randomized controlled clinical trails. *Journal of Consulting and Clinical Psychology, 57*(1), 148–154.

77. Eddy, J. M., Stoolmiller, M. S., Reid, J. B., Dishion, T. J., & Bank, L. (1995, November). *A method for the development of reliable measures of change.* Paper presented at the 29th annual convention of the Association for the Advancement of Behavior Therapy. Washington, DC.

78. Chamberlain, P. (1994). *Family connections: A treatment foster care model for adolescents with delinquency.* Eugene, OR: Castalia Publishing.

79. Chamberlain, P., & Reid, J. B. (1987). Parent observation and report of child symptoms. *Behavioral Assessment, 2,* 97–109.

80. Sanders, M. R., & Dadds, M. R. (1993). *Behavioral family intervention.* Boston: Allyn & Bacon.

81. Hanley, G. P., Iwata, B. A., & McCord, B. E. (2003). Functional analysis of problem behavior: A review. *Journal of Applied Behavior Analysis, 36*(2), 147–185.

82. O'Neil, R. E., Horner, R. H., Albin, R. W., Storey, K., & Sprague, J. R. (1990). *Functional analysis of problem behavior: A practical assessment guide.* Sycamore, IL: Sycamore.

83. Patterson, G. R. (1982). *Coercive family process.* Eugene, OR: Castalia Publishing.

84. McMahon, R. J., & Forehand, R. (1988). Conduct Disorders. In E. J. Mash & L. G. Terdal (Eds.), *Behavioral assessment of childhood disorders.* (pp. 105–156). New York: Guilford Press.

85. Robin, A. L., & Foster, S. L. (1989). *Negotiating parent-adolescent conflict: A behavioral-family systems approach.* New York: Guilford Press.

86. McConaughy, S. H., & Achenbach, T. M. (1988). *Practical guide for the Child Behavior Checklist and related materials.* Burlington, VT: University of Vermont, Department of Psychiatry.

87. Sattler, J. M. (1990). *Assessment of children,* (3rd Ed.). San Diego: Jerome Sattler.

88. Patterson, G. R., & Bank, L. (1986). Bootstrapping your way in the nomological thicket. *Behavioral Assessment, 8,* 49–73.

89. McConaughy, S. H., Achenbach, T. M., & Gent, C. L. (1988). Multiaxial empirically based assessment: Parent, teacher, observational, cognitive, and personality correlates of Child Behavior Profiles for 6-11 year-old boys. *Journal of Abnormal Child Psychology, 16,* 485–509.

90. Weinrott, M. R., Reid, J. B., Bauske, R. W., & Brummet, B. (1981). Supplementing naturalistic observations with observer impressions. *Behavioral Assessment, 3,* 151–159.

91. Horne, A. M., & Sayger, T. V. (1990). *Treating conduct and oppositional defiant disorders in children.* New York: Pergammon Press.

92. Dunford, F. W., & Elliot, D. S. (1982). *Identifying career offenders with self-report data* (Grant No. MH27552). Washington, DC: National Institute of Mental Health.

93. Anderson, J. C., Williams, S. M., McGee, R., & Silva, P. A. (1987). DSM-III disorders in preadolescent children: Prevalence in a large sample from the general population. *Archives of General Psychiatry, 44,* 69–76.

94. Feldman, R. A., Caplinger, T. E., & Wodarski, J. S. (1983). *The St. Louis conundrum: The effective treatment of antisocial youths.* Englewood Cliffs, NJ: Prentice Hall.

95. Williams, J. R., & Gold, M. (1972). From delinquent behavior to official delinquency. *Social Problems, 20,* 209–229.

96. O'Neil, R. E., Horner, R. H., Albin, R. W., Storey, K., & Sprague, J. R. (1990). *Functional analysis of problem behavior: A practical assessment guide.* Sycamore, IL: Sycamore.

97. McConaughy, S., H. (1993, February). *Comorbidity of DSM disorders and empirically derived syndromes in general population and clinically referred samples.* Paper presented at the fifth annual meeting of the Society for Research in Child and Adolescent Psychopathology, Santa Fe, NM.

98. Coccaro, E., Schmidt, C. A., Samuels, J. F., & Nestadt, G. (2004). Lifetime and 1-month prevalence estimates of Intermittent Explosive Disorder in a community sample. *Journal of Clinical Psychiatry, 65*(6), 820–824.

99. Olvera, R. L. (2002). Intermittent Explosive Disorder: Epidemiology, diagnosis, and management. *CNS Drugs, 16*(8), 517–526.

100. Loney, J., & Milich, R. (1982). Hyperactivity, inattention, and aggression in clinical practice. In D. Routh & M. Wolraich (Eds.), *Advances in developmental and behavioral pediatrics.* (Vol. 3, pp. 113–147). Greenwich, CT: JAI Press.

101. Angold, A., Costello, E. J., & Erkanli, A. (1999). Comorbidity. *Journal of Child Psychology and Psychiatry, 40*(1), 57–87.

102. Costello, E. J., Mustillo, S., Erkanli, A., Keeler, G., & Angold, A. (2003). Prevalence and development of psychiatric disorders in childhood and adolescence. *Archives of General Psychiatry, 60,* 837–844.

103. Hinshaw, S. P. (1987). On the distinction between attentional deficits/hyperactivity and conduct problems/aggression in child psychopathology. *Psychological Bulletin, 101,* 443–463.

104. Geller, B., Sun, K., Zimmerman, B., Luby, J., Frazier, J., & Williams, M. (1995). Complex and rapid-cycling in bipolar children and adolescents: A preliminary study. *Journal of the Affective Disorders, 34,* 259–268.

105. Kovacs, M., & Pollock, M. (1995). Bipolar disorder and cormorbid conduct disorder in childhood and adolescence. *Journal of the American Academy of Child and Adolescent Psychiatry, 34,* 715–723.

106. Geller, B., & Luby, J. (1997). Child and adolescent bipolar disorder: A review of the past 10 years. *Journal of the American Academy of Child and Adolescent Psychiatry, 36,* 1168–1176.

107. Lewinsohn, P. M., Hops, H., Roberts, R. E., Seeley, J. R., &Andrews, J. A. (1993). Adolescent psychopathology. I. Prevalence and incidence of depression and other DSM-III-R disorders in high school students. *Journal of Abnormal Psychology, 102,* 133–144.

108. Robins, L. N., & McEvoy, L. (1990). Conduct problems as predictors of substance abuse. In L. N. Robins & M. Rutter (Eds.), *Straight and devious pathways from childhood to adulthood.* (pp. 182–204). Cambridge: Cambridge University Press.

109. Myers, M. G., Stewart, D. G., & Brown, S. A. (1998). Progression from conduct disorder to antisocial personality disorder following treatment for adolescent substance use. *American Journal of Psychiatry, 155*(4), 479–485.

110. Tomlinson, K. L., Brown, S. A., & Abrantes, A. (2004). Psychiatric comorbidity and substance use treatment outcomes of adolescents. *Psychology of Addictive Behaviors, 18*(2), 160–169.

111. Kazdin, A. E. (1988). *Child psychotherapy: Developing and identifying effective treatments.* New York: Pergammon Press.

112. Schaefer, C. E., & Millman, H. L. (Eds.) (1977). *Therapies for children.* San Francisco: Jossey Bass.

113. Kazdin, A. E. (1997). Practitioner reviews: Psychosocial ties for conduct disorder in children, *Journal of Child Psychology & Psychiatry and Allied Disciplines 38*(2), 161–178.

114. Brestan, E. V. & Eyberg, S. M. (1998). Effective psychosocial ties of conduct disorder in children and adolescents: 29 years, 82 studies, 5272 kids. *Journal of Clinical Child Psychology, 27*(2), 180–189.

115. Kazdin, A. E. (1998). Psychosocial treatments for conduct disorder in children. In P. M. Nathan & J. M. Gorman (Eds.), *A guide to treatments that work.* (pp. 65–89). London: Oxford University Press.

116. Kazdin, A. E., & Weisz, J. R. (Ed.) *Evidence-based psychotherapies for children and adolescents.* New York: Guilford Press.

117. Kazdin, A. E. (2004). Evidence-based treatments: Challenges and priorities for practice and research. *Child and Adolescent Psychiatric Clinics of North America, 13,* 923–940.

118. Littell, J. H. (2005). Lessons from a systematic review of effects of multisystemic therapy. *Children and Youth Services Review, 27*(4), 445–463.

119. Campbell, M., Gonzalez, N. M., & Silva, R. R. (1992). The pharmacologic treatment of conduct disorders and rage outbursts. *Psychiatric Clinics of North America, 15,* 69–85.

120. Dodge, K. (1980). Social cognition and children's aggressive behavior. *Child Development, 51,* 162–170.

121. McMahon, R. J., & Wells, K. C. (1989). Conduct disorders. In E. J. Mash & R. A. Barkley (Eds.), *Treatment of childhood disorders.* (pp. 73–134). New York: Guilford Press.

122. Greenberg, M. T., & Speltz, M. L. (1988). Attachment and the ontogeny of conduct problems. In J. Belsky & T. Nezworski (Eds.), *Clinical implications of attachment.* (pp. 177–218). Hillsdale, NJ: Lawrence Erlbaum Associates.

123. Tolman, A. (1995). *Major depressive disorder: The latest assessment and treatment strategies.* Kansas City, MO: Compact Clinicals.

124. Bank, L., Marlowe, J. H., Reid, J. B., Patterson, G. R., & Weinrott, M. R. (1991). A comparative evaluation of parent training interventions for families of chronic delinquents. *Journal of Abnormal Child Psychology, 19,* 15–33.

125. Brestan, E. V., & Eyberg, S.M. (1998). Effective psychosocial treatments of conduct-disordered children and adolescents: 29 years, 82 studies, and 5,272 kids. *Journal of Clinical Child Psychology, 27*(2), 180–189.

126. Bloomquist, M. L., & Schnell, S. V. (2002). *Helping children with aggression and conduct problems: Best practices for intervention.* New York: Guilford Press.

127. Kazdin, A. E., & Weisz, J. R. (Eds.) (2003). *Evidence-based psychotherapies for children and adolescents.* New York: Guilford Press.

128. Nathan, P. M., & Gorman, J. M. (Eds.). (2002). *A guide to treatments that work* (2nd ed.). London: Oxford University Press.

129. Pelham, W. E., Wheeler, T., & Chronis, A. (1998). Empirically supported psychosocial treatments for ADHD. *Journal of Clinical Child Psychology, 27,* 190–205.

130. Webster-Stratton, C., & Hammond, M. (1997). Treating children with early-onset conduct problems: A comparison of child and parent training interventions. *Journal of Consulting & Clinical Psychology, 65(1),* 93–109.

131. Webster-Stratton, C. (1998). Parent training with low-income families: Promoting parental engagement through a collaborative approach. In J. R. Lutzker (Ed.), *Handbook of child abuse research and treatment, Issues in clinical child psychology.* (pp. 183–210). New York: Plenum Press.

132. Webster-Stratton, C. (1998). Preventing conduct problems in Head Start children: Strengthening parenting competencies. *Journal of Consulting & Clinical Psychology, 66*(5), 715–730.

133. Webster-Stratton, C., & Hancock, L. (1998). Training for parents of young children with conduct problems: Content, methods, and therapeutic processes. In J. M. Briesmeister & C. E. Schaefer (Eds.), *Handbook of parent training: Parents as co-therapists for children's behavior problems.* (2nd ed., pp. 98–152). New York: John Wiley & Sons, Inc.

134. Patterson, G. R., Chamberlain, P., & Reid, J. B. (1982). A comparative evaluation of a parent training program. *Behavior Therapy, 13,* 638–650.

135. Miller, G. E., & Prinz, R. J. (1990). The enhancement of social learning family interventions for childhood conduct disorder. *Psychological Bulletin, 108,* 291–307.

136. Griest, D. L., & Wells, K. C. (1983). Behavioral family therapy with conduct disorders in children. *Behavior Therapy, 14,* 37–53.

137. Webster-Stratton, C. , Hollingsworth, T., & Kolpacoff, M. (1989). The long-term effectiveness of treatment and clinical significance of three cost-effective training programs for families with conduct problem children. *Journal of Consulting and Clinical Psychology, 57,* 550–553.

138. Baum, C. G., & Forehand, R. (1981). Long-term follow-up assessment of parent training by use of multiple-outcome measures. *Behavior Therapy, 12,* 643–652.

139. Patterson, G. R., & Fleischman, M. J. (1979). Maintenance of treatment effects: Some considerations concerning family systems and follow-up data. *Behavior Therapy, 10,* 168–185.

140. Walker, H. M., Colvin, G., & Ramsey, E. (1995). *Antisocial behavior in school: Strategies and best practices.* Pacific Grove, CA: Brooks/Cole.

141. Hops, H., & Walker, H. M. (1988). *CLASS: Contingencies for Learning Academic and Social Skills.* Seattle, WA: Educational Achievement Systems.

142. Walker, H., Hops, H., & Greenwood, C. (1993). *RECESS: A program for reducing negative-aggressive behavior.* Seattle, WA: Educational Achievement Systems.

143. DuPaul, G. J., & Eckert, T. L. (1997). The effects of school-based interventions for attention deficit hyperactivity disorder: A meta-analysis. *School Psychology Review, 26,* 134–143.

144. Pelham, W. E. (2002). Psychosocial interventions for ADHD. In Jensen, P. S., & Cooper, J. R. (Eds.) *Attention Deficit Hyperactivity Disorder: State of the science, best practices.* (pp. 12–1 to 12–36). Kingston, NJ: Civic Research Institute.

145. Hops, H., Walker, H. M., Fleischman, D., Nagoshi, J., Omura, R., Skinrud, K., & Taylor, J. (1978). CLASS: A standardized in-class program for acting-out children. II. Field test evaluations. *Journal of Educational Psychology, 70,* 636–644.

146. Chamberlain, P., & Reid, J. B. (1998). Comparison of two community alternatives to incarceration for chronic juvenile offenders. *Journal of Consulting and Clinical Psychology, 66*(4), 624–633.

147. Eddy, J. M., Whaley, R. B., & Chamberlain, P. (2004). The prevention of violent behavior by chronic and serious male juvenile offenders: A 2-year follow-up of a randomized clinical trial. *Journal of Emotional and Behavioral Disorders, 12*(1), 2–8.

148. Eddy, J. M., & Chamberlain, P. (2000). Family management and deviant peer association as mediators of the impact of treatment condition on youth antisocial behavior. *Journal of Consulting and Clinical Psychology, 68*(5), 857–863.

149. Springelmeyer, P. G., Smith, D. K., and Chamberlain, P. (2002). *Adapting the Oregon Multidimensional Treatment Foster Care program for delinquent adolescent females.* (Manuscript in preparation.)

150. Leve, L. D., Chamberlain, P., & Reid, J. B. (in press). Intervention outcomes for girls referred from juvenile justice: Effects on delinquency. *Journal of Consulting and Clinical Psychology.*

151. Fisher, P. A., Burraston, B., & Pears, K. (2005). The Early Intervention Foster Care Program: Permanent placement outcomes from a randomized trial. *Child Maltreatment, 10,* 61–71.

152. Meyers, A. W., & Craighead, W. E. (Eds.) (1984). *Cognitive behavior therapy with children.* New York: Plenum.

153. Dodge, K. A. (1991). The structure and function of proactive and reactive aggression. In D. J. Peplar, & K. H. Rubin (Eds.), *The development and treatment of childhood aggression.* (pp. 201–218). Hillsdale, NJ: Lawrence Erlbaum Associates.

154. Camp, B. W., & Bash, M. A. S. (1985). *Think aloud: Increasing social and cognitive skills — A problem solving program for children.* Champaign, IL: Research Press.

155. Spivak, G., Platt, J. J., & Shure, M. B. (1976). *The problem-solving approach to adjustment.* San Francisco: Jossey-Bass.

156. Peplar, D. J., King, G., & Byrd, W. (1991). A social-cognitively based social skills training program for aggressive children. In D. J. Peplar & K. H. Rubin (Eds.), *The development and treatment of childhood aggression.* (pp. 361–386). Hillsdale, NJ: Lawrence Erlbaum Associates.

157. Guevermont, D. (1990). Social skills and peer relationship training. In R. A. Barkley (Ed.), *Attention Deficit Hyperactivity Disorder: A handbook for diagnosis and treatment.* (pp. 540–572). New York: Guilford Press.

158. Kendall, P. C., Ronan, K. R., & Epps, J. (1991). Aggression in children/adolescents: Cognitive-behavioral treatment perspectives. In D. J. Peplar & K. H. Rubin (Eds.), *The development and treatment of childhood aggression.* (pp. 341–360). Hillsdale, NJ: Lawrence Erlbaum Associates.

159. Feldman, R. A., & Caplinger, T. E. (1983). The St. Louis experiment: Treatment of antisocial youths in prosocial peer groups. In J. R. Kluegel (Ed.), *Evaluating juvenile justice.* (pp. 121–148). Beverly Hills, CA: Sage.

160. Catterall, J. S. (1987). An intensive group counseling dropout prevention intervention: Some cautions on isolating at-risk adolescents within high schools. *American Education Research Journal, 24,* 521–540.

161. Dishion, T. J., & Andrews, D. W. (1995). Preventing escalation in problem behaviors with high-risk young adolescents: Immediate and 1-year outcome. *Journal of Consulting and Clinical Psychology, 63,* 538–548.

162. Lochman, J. E., Burch, P. R., Curry, J. F., & Lampon, L. B. (1984). Treatment and generalization effects of cognitive-behavioral and goal-setting interventions with aggressive boys. *Journal of Consulting and Clinical Psychology, 52,* 915–916.

163. Oden, S., & Asher, S. R. (1977). Coaching children in social skills training for friendship making. *Child Development, 48,* 495–506.

164. Ladd, G. W. (1981). Effectiveness of a social learning method for enhancing children's social interaction and peer acceptance. *Child Development, 52,* 171–178.

165. Kendall, P. C., Kane, M., Howard, B., & Siqueland, L. (1989). Cognitive-behavioral therapy for anxious children: Treatment manual. *Available from the author,* Department of Psychology, Temple University, Philadelphia, PA 19122.

166. Meichenbaum, D. H., & Goodman, J. (1971). Training impulsive children to talk to themselves as a way of developing self-control. *Journal of Abnormal Child Psychology, 77,* 115–126.

167. Taylor, T. K., Eddy, J. M., & Biglan, A. (1999). Interpersonal skills training to reduce aggressive and delinquent behavior. Limited evidence and the need for an evidence-based system of care. *Clinical Child and Family Psychology Review, 2,* 169–182.

168. Kazdin, Esveldt-Dawson, French, & Unis, 1987). Effects of parent management and problem-solving skills training combined in the treatment of child antisocial behavior. *Journal of the American Academy of Child and Adolescent Psychiatry, 26,* 416–424.

169. Kendall, P. C., Reber, M., McCleer, S., Epps, J., & Ronan, K. R. (1990). Cognitive-behavioral treatment of conduct disordered children. *Cognitive Therapy and Research, 14,* 279–297.

170. Kazdin, A. E., Esveldt-Dawson, K., French, N. H., & Unis, A. S. (1987). Problem-solving skills training and relationship therapy in the treatment of antisocial child behavior. *Journal of Consulting and Clinical Psychology, 55,* 76–85.

171. Derzon, J. H., & Lipsey, M. W. (2000). *Family features and problem, aggressive, criminal, or violent behavior: A meta-analytic inquiry.* Manuscript submitted for publication.

172. Walsh, W. M. (1980). *A primer in family therapy.* Springfield, IL: Charles C. Thomas.

173. Alexander, J. F. (1973). Defensive and supportive communications in normal and deviant families. *Journal of Consulting and Clinical Psychology, 40,* 223–231.

174. Kazdin, A. E. (1985). *Treatment of antisocial behavior in children and adolescents.* Homewood, IL: Dorsey Press.

175. Jacob, T. (1975). Family interaction in disturbed and normal families: A methodological and substantive review. *Psychological Bulletin, 82,* 33–65.

176. Jacob, T. (Ed.) (1987). *Family interaction and psychopathology: Theories, methods, & findings.* New York: Plenum Press.

177. Bateson, G., Jackson, D. D., Haley, J., & Weakland, J. (1956). Toward a theory of schizophrenia. *Behavioral Science, 1,* 251–264.

178. Alexander, J. F., & Parsons, B. V. (1973). Short-term behavioral intervention with delinquent families: Impact on family process and recidivism. *Journal of Abnormal Psychology, 81,* 219–225.

179. Klein, N. C., Alexander, J. F., & Parsons, B. V. (1977). Impact of family systems intervention on recidivism and sibling delinquency: A model of primary prevention and program evaluation. *Journal of Consulting and Clinical Psychology, 45,* 469–474.

180. Alexander, J. F., Waldron, H. B., Newberry, A. M., & Liddle, N. (1988). Family approaches to treating delinquents. In E. W. Nunnally, C. S. Chilman, & F. M. Cox (Eds.), *Mental illness, delinquency, addictions, and neglect.* Newbury Park, CA: Sage.

181. Gordon, D. A., Arbuthnot, J., Gustafson, K. E., & McGreen, P. (1988). Home-based behavioral systems family therapy with disadvantaged juvenile delinquents. *American Journal of Family Therapy, 163,* 243–255.

182. Henggeler, S. W. (1990). *Family therapy and beyond: A multisystemic approach to treating the behavior problems of children and adolescents.* Pacific Grove, CA: Brooks/Cole.

183. Randall, J., & Henggeler, S. W. (1999). Multisystemic therapy: Changing the social ecologies of youths presenting serious clinical problems and their families. In S. Walker Russ, & T. H. Ollendick (Eds.), *Handbook of psychotherapies with children and families, Issues in clinical child psychology.* (pp. 405–418). New York: Kluwer Academic/Plenum.

184. Henggeler, S. W., Cunningham, P. B., Pickrel, S. G., Schoenwald, S. K., & Brondino, M. J. (1999). Multisystemic therapy: An effective violence prevention approach for serious juvenile offenders. *Journal of Adolescence, 19,* 47–61.

185. Cunningham, P. B., & Henggeler, S. W. (1999). Engaging multiproblem families in treatment: Lessons learned throughout the development of multisystemic therapy. *Family Process, 38* (2), 265–286.

186. Bourdin, C. M., Mann, B. J., Cone, L., Henggeler, S. W., Fucci, B. R., Blaske, D. M., & Williams, R. A. (1992). *Multisystemic treatment of adolescents referred for serious and repeated antisocial behavior.* Unpublished manuscript, Medical University of South Carolina, Charleston.

187. Henggeler, S. W., Melton, G. B., & Smith, L. A. (1992). Family preservation using multisystemic therapy: An effective alternative to incarcerating serious juvenile offenders. *Journal of Consulting and Clinical Psychology, 60,* 953–961.

188. Feldman, R. A. (1992). The St. Louis experiment: Effective treatment of antisocial youths in prosocial peer groups. In J. McCord & R. E. Tremblay (Eds.), *Preventing antisocial behavior.* (pp. 232–252). New York: Guilford Press.

189. Pelham, W. E., & Hoza, B. (1993, February). Comprehensive treatment for ADHD: A proposal for intensive summer treatment programs and outpatient follow-up. *Paper presented at the fifth annual meeting of The Society for Research in Child and Adolescent Psychopathology.* Santa Fe, NM.

190. Arnold, L. E., Abikoff, H. B., Cantwell, D. P., Conners, C. K., Elliott, G. R., Greenhill, L. L., Hechtman, L., Hinshaw, S. P., Hoza, B., Jensen, P. S., Kraemer, H. C., March, J. S., Newcorn, J. H., Pelham, W. E., Richters, J. E., Schiller, E., Severe, J. B., Swanson, J. M., Vereen, D., Wells, K. C. (1997). NIMH collaborative multimodal treatment study of children with ADHD (MTA): Design, methodology, and protocol evolution. *Journal of Attention Disorders, 2*(3), 141–158.

191. Richters J. E., Arnold, L. E., Jensen, P. S., Abikoff, H., et al. (1995). NIMH collaborative multisite multimodal treatment study of children with ADHD: I. Background and rationale. *Journal of the American Academy of Child & Adolescent Psychiatry, 34*(8), 987-1000.

192. Jensen, P. S. et al. (2001). ADHD comorbidity findings from MTA Study: Comparing comorbid subgroups. *Journal of the American Academy of Child and Adolescent Psychiatry, 40*(2), 147–158.

193. Conners, K. C. et al. (2001). Multimodal treatment of ADHD in the MTA: An alternative outcome analysis. *Journal of the American Academy of Child and Adolescent Psychiatry, 40*(2), 159–167.

194. Swanson, J. M. et al. (2001). Clinical relevance of the primary findings of the MTA: Success rates based on severity of ADHD and ODD symptoms at the end of treatment. *Journal of the American Academy of Child and Adolescent Psychiatry, 40*(2), 168–179.

195. Swanson, J. M. et al. (2001) Response to commentary on the Multidomal Treatment Study of ADHD (MTA): Mining the meaning of the MTA. *Journal of Abnormal Child Psychology, 30*(4), 327–332.

196. Wells, K. C. et al. (2001). Psychosocial treatment strategies in the MTA Study: Rationale, methods, and critical issues in design and implementation. *Journal of Abnormal Child Psychology, 30*(4), 483–505.

197. Hinshaw, S. P. et al. (2000). Family processes and treatment outcomes in the MTA: Negative/ineffective parenting practices in relation to multimodal treatment. *Journal of Abnormal Child Psychology, 28 (6)*, 555–568.

198. Jensen P. S. (1999). Fact versus fancy concerning the multimodal treatment study for attention-deficit hyperactivity disorder. *Canadian Journal of Psychiatry, 44(10)*, 975–980.

199. Multimodal Treatment Study of Children with ADHD Cooperative Group (1999). A 14-month random-ized clinical trial of treatment strategies for attention-deficit/hyperactivity disorder. *Archives of General Psychiatry, 56(12)*, 1073–1086.

200. Pelham, W. E., Jr. (1999). The NIMH multimodal treatment study for attention-deficit hyperactivity disorder: Just say yes to drugs alone? *Canadian Journal of Psychiatry, 44(10)*, 981–990.

201. Boyle, M.H. and Jadad, A.R. (1999). Lessons from large trials: The MTA study as a model for evaluation of the treatment of childhood psychiatric disorder. *Canadian Journal of Psychiatry, 44*(10), 991–998.

202. Main, M., Kaplan, N., & Cassidy, J. (1985). Security in infancy, childhood, and adulthood: A move to the level of representation. IN I. Bretherton & E. Waters (Eds.), Growing points of attachment theory and research. *Monographs of the Society for Research in Child Development, 50* (1–2, Serial No. 209).

203. Bowlby, J. (1973). Attachment and loss: Vol. 2. *Separation.* New York: Basic Books.

204. Sroufe, L. A., & Flesson, J. (1986). Attachment and the construction of relationships. In W. Hartup & Z. Rubin (Eds.), *Relationships and development.* (pp. 51–71). Hillsdale, NJ: Lawrence Erlbaum Associates.

205. Speltz, M. L. (1990). The treatment of preschool conduct problems: An integration of behavioral and attachment concepts. In M. T. Greenberg, D. Cicchetti, & M. Cummings (Eds.), *Attachment in the preschool years: Theory, research, and intervention.* (pp. 399–426). Chicago: University of Chicago Press.

206. Marvin, R., Cooper, G., Hoffman, K. & Powell, B. (2002). The Circle of Security Project: Attachment-based intervention with caregiver-pre-school child dyads. *Attachment & Human Development, 4*(1), 107–124.

207. Cloninger, C. R., & Gottesman, I. I. (1987). Genetic and environmental factors in antisocial behavior disor-ders. In S. A. Mednick, T. E. Moffit, & S. A. Stack (Eds.), *The causes of crime: New biological approaches.* (pp. 92–109). New York: Cambridge University Press.

208. Albert, D. J., Walsh, M. L., Jonik, R. H. (1994). Aggression in humans: What is its biological foundation? *Neuroscience and Biobehavioral Reviews, 17,* 405–425.

209. Fishbein, D. H. (1992). The psychobiology of female aggression. *Criminal Justice and Behavior, 10*(2), 99–126.

210. Raine, A. (2002). Biosocial studies of antisocial and violent behavior in children and adults: A review. *Journal of Abnormal Child Psychology, 30 (4),* 311–326.

211. Gilligan, J., and Bandy, L., (2004). The psychopharmacologic treatment of violent youth. *Ann NY Acad Sci 103*: 356–381.

212. Lorber, M. F. (2004). Psychophysiology of aggression, psychopathy, and conduct problems: A meta-analysis. *Psychological Bulletin, 130*(4), 531–552.

213. Hutchings, B., & Mednick, S. A. (1974). Registered criminality in the adoptive and biological parents of registered male criminal adoptees. In R. R. Frieve, D. Rosenthal, & H. Brill (Eds.), *Genetic research in psychiatry.* Baltimore: Johns Hopkins University Press.

214. Mednick, S. A., Gabrielli, W. F., & Hutchings, B. (1984). Genetic influences in criminal convictions: Evidence from an adoption cohort. *Science, 224,* 891–894.

215. Cadoret, R. J., Cain, C. A., Crowe, R. R. (1983). Evidence for gene-environment interaction in the develop-ment of adolescent antisocial behavior. *Behavior Genetics, 13,* 301–310.

216. Bohman, M., Cloninger, C. R., Sigvardsoon, S., & von Knorring, A. (1982). Predisposition to petty criminality in Swedish adoptees: I. Genetic and environmental heterogeneity. *Archives of General Psychiatry, 39,* 1233–1241.

217. Dalgard, O. S., & Kringlen, E. (1976). A Norwegian twin study of criminality. *British Journal of Criminology, 16,* 213–232.

218. Bohman, M. (1978). Some genetic aspects of alcoholism and criminality. *Archives of General Psychiatry, 35,* 269–276.

219. Loeber, R., Stouthamer-Loeber, M., & Green, S. M. (1991). Age of onset of problem behavior in boys and later disruptive and delinquent behavior. *Criminal Behavior and Mental Health, 1,* 229–246.

220. Goodman, R., & Stevenson, J. (1989). A twin study of hyperactivity: II. The etiological role of genes, family relationships, and perinatal adversity. *Journal of Child Psychology and Psychiatry, 30,* 691–709.

221. Fishbein, D. (2000). The importance of neurobiological research to the prevention of psychopathology. *Prevention Science, 1*(2), 89–106.

222. Plomin, R., & Hershberger, S. (1991). Genotype-environment interaction. In T. D. Wachs & R. Plomin (Eds.), *Conceptualization and measurement of organism-environment interaction.* (pp. 29–43). Washington, DC: American Psychological Association.

223. Searight, H.R., Rottnek, F., Abby, S.L., (2001). Conduct disorder: Diagnosis and treatment in primary care. *American Family Physician,* www.aafp.org/afp/20010415/1579.html.

224. Bassarath, L., (2003). Medication strategies in childhood aggression: A review. *Can J Psychiatry 48*: 367–373

225. Conner, D.F., Glat, S.J., Lopez, I.D.l Jackson, D., Melloni, R.H., Jr. (2002). Psychopharmacology and aggression. I: A meta-analysis of stimulant effects on overt/covert aggression-related behaviors in ADHD. *Journal of the American Academy of Child and Adolescent Psychiatry, 41*(3), 253–61.

226. Snyder, R., Turgay, A., A,am, M., Binder, C., Fisman, S., Carroll, A. (2002). Effects of risperidone on conduct and disruptive behavior disorders in children with subaverage IQs. *American Academy Child Adolescents Psychiatry, 41*(9), 1026–36

227. Aman, M.G., Desmedt, G., Derivan, Alk Lyons, B., Findling, R.L. (2002). Double-blind placebo-controlled study of risperidone for the treatment of disruptive behaviors in children with subaverage intelligence. *American Journal of Psychiatry, 159*(9), 1337–46.

228. Pelham, W. E. (1993). Pharmacotherapy for children with attention-deficit hyperactivity disorder. *School Psychology Review, 22*(2), 199–227.

229. Pelham, W. E. (1993). Recent developments in pharmacological treatment for child and adolescent mental health disorders: Annotated bibliography. *School Psychology Review, 22*(2), 252–253.

230. Safer, D. J., & Krager, J. M. (1988). A survey of medication treatment for hyperactive/inattentive students. *Journal of the American Medical Association, 260,* 2256–2258.

231. Wilens, T. E., & Biederman, J. (1992). The stimulants. *Psychiatric Clinics of North America, 15,* 191–222.

232. DuPaul, G. J., & Barkley, R. A. (1990). Medication therapy. In R. A. Barkley (Ed.), *Attention deficit hyperactivity disorder: A handbook for diagnosis and treatment.* (pp. 573–612). New York: Guilford Press.

233. Greenhill, L. L. (2002). Stimulant medication treatment of children with attention deficit hyperactivity disorder. In Jensen, P. S., & Cooper, J. R. (Eds.) *Attention deficit hyperactivity disorder: State of the science, best practices.* (pp. 9–1 to 9–27). Kingston, NJ: Civic Research Institute.

234. Solanto, M. V. (1998). Neuropsychopharmacological mechanisms of stimulant drug action in attention-deficit hyperactivity disorder: A review and integration. *Behavioural Brain Research, 94*(1), 127–152.

235. Elia, J., Stoff, D. M., & Coccaro, E. F. (1992). Biological correlates of impulsive behavior disorders: Attention deficit hyperactivity disorder, conduct disorder, and borderline personality disorder. In E. Peschel, R. Peschel, C. W. Howe, & J. W. Howe (Eds.), *Neurobiological disorders in children and adolescents.* (pp. 51–57). San Francisco, CA: Jossey-Bass.

236 Steiner, H., Petersen, M.L., Saxena, K., Ford, S., Matthews, Z. (2003). Divalproex sodium for the treatment of conduct disorder: A randomized controlled clinical trial. *Journal of Clinical Psychiatry, 64*(10), 1183–91.

237. Hinshaw, S., Heller, T., & McHale, J. (1992). Covert antisocial behavior in boys with attention-deficit hyperactivity disorder: External validation and effects of methylphenidate. *Journal of Consulting and Clinical Psychology, 60,* 274–281.

238. Klein, R., Abikoff, H., Klass, E., Ganales, D., Seese, L., & Pollack, S. (1997). Clinical efficacy of methylphenidate in conduct disorder with and without attention deficit hyperactivity disorder. *Archives of General Psychiatry, 54,* 1073–1080.

239. Hazell, P.L., Stuart, J.E. (2003) A randomized controlled trial of clonidine added to psychostimulant medication for hyperactive and aggressive children. *Journal of the American Academy of Child and Adolescent Psychiatry, 42*(8), 886–94.

240. Greenhill, L. L., (1992). Pharmacologic treatment of attention deficit hyperactivity disorder. *Psychiatric Clinics of North America, 15,* 1–27.

241. Whitaker, A., & Rao, U. (1992). Neuroleptics in pediatric psychiatry. *Psychiatric Clinics of North America, 15,* 243–276.

242. Sprague, R. L., & Sleator, E. K. (1977). Methylphenidate in hyperkinetic children: Differences in dose effects on learning and social behavior. *Science, 198,* 1274–1276.

243. Pelham, W. E., & Hoza, J. (1987). Behavioral assessment of psychostimulant effects on ADD children in a summer day treatment program. In R. Prinz (Ed.), *Advances in behavioral assessment of children and families.* (Vol. 3, pp. 3–33). Greenwich, CT: JAI Press.

244. Barkley, R. A. (1977). A review of stimulant drug research with hyperactive children. *Journal of Child Psychology and Psychiatry, 18,* 137–165.

245. Gittelman, K. (1987). Pharmacotherapy of childhood hyperactivity: An update. In Meltzer, H. Y. (Ed.), Psychopharmacology: *The third generation of progress.* (pp. 1215–1224). New York: Raven.

246. Rains, A., & Scahill, L. (2004). New long-acting stimulants in children with ADHD. *JCAPN, 17*(4), 177–179.

247. Campbell, M., Small, A.M., Green, W. H., et al. (1984). Behavioral efficacy of haloperidol and lithium carbonate: A comparison in hospitalized aggressive children with conduct disorder. *Archives of General Psychiatry, 41,* 650–656.

248. Donovan, S.J., Stewart, J.W., Nunes, et al. (2000). Divalproex treatment for youth with explosive temper and mood lability: A double-blind, placebo-controlled crossover design. *Am J Psychiatry 157(6)*: 1038.

249. Armenteros, J.L. & Lewis, J.E. (2002). Citalopram treatment for impulsive aggression in children and adolescents: An open pilot study. *Journal of the American Academy of Child and Adolescent Psychiatry, 41*(5), 522–529.

250. Jacobvitz, D., Sroufe, L. A., Stewart, M. et al. (1990). Treatment of attentional and hyperactivity problems in children with sympathomimetic drugs: A comprehensive review. *Journal of the American Academy of Child and Adolescent Psychiatry, 29(5),* 677–688.

Index

T

Telephone interviews 14, 18, 19, 20, 32
   See also Parent daily report (PDR)
Time out 35, 37–38, 38, 42, 43, 56, 57
Titration 70
Treatment *See* Medication;
   Psychological treatments
      Plan 13, 14, 23, 24, 55

V

Violent behavior *See* Aggression

W

Weschler Intelligence Scale for Children-
   Third Edition (WISC-III) 19

Z

Ziprasidone 65, 70

We Want Your Opinion!

Comments about **Conduct Disorders**:

_____

_____

_____

_____

_____

Other titles you would like Compact Clinicals to offer:

_____

_____

_____

_____

To be placed on our mailing list, please provide the following:

Name: _____

Address: _____

_____

_____

E-mail: _____

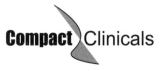

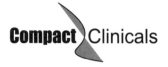

Order in 3 easy steps:

▶ 1   Provide complete billing and shipping information

Name _____   Company_____

Profession_____   Dept./Mail Stop_____

Street Address/P.O. Box_____

City/State/Zip_____

Telephone_____   ☐ Ship to Residence   ☐ Ship to Business

▶ 2   Choose Titles

For Clinicians:

	Qty.	Unit Price	Total
Attention Deficit Hyperactivity Disorder *The latest assessment and treatment strategies*		$16.95	
Bipolar Disorder *The latest assessment and treatment strategies*		$16.95	
Borderline Personality Disorder *The latest assessment and treatment strategies*		$16.95	
Conduct Disorders *The latest assessment and treatment strategies*		$16.95	
Depression in Adults *The latest assessment and treatment strategies*		$16.95	
Obsessive Compulsive Disorder *The latest assessment and treatment strategies*		$16.95	
Post-Traumatic and Acute Stress Disorders *The latest assessment and treatment strategies*		$16.95	

For Physicians:

Bipolar Disorder: Treatment and Management		$18.95	

Continuing Education credits
available for mental health professionals.
Call 1-800-408-8830 for details.

Subtotal	
Tax (Add 7.975% in MO)	
Shipping ($3.75 first book/ $1.00 per additional book)	
TOTAL	

▶ 3   Choose Payment Method

Please charge my: ☐ Visa   ☐ MasterCard   ☐ Discover   ☐ American Express   ☐ Check Enclosed

Account # __ __ __ __ — __ __ __ __ — __ __ __ __ — __ __ __ __   Exp. Date __ __ / __ __

Name on Card _____   Cardholder Signature _____

Postal Orders: Compact Clinicals, 7205 NW Waukomis Dr., Suite A, Kansas City, MO 64151

Telephone Orders: Toll Free 1-800-408-8830   **Fax Orders:** 1(816)587-7198

We Want Your Opinion!

Comments about **Conduct Disorders**:

_____

_____

_____

_____

_____

Other titles you would like Compact Clinicals to offer:

_____

_____

_____

_____

To be placed on our mailing list, please provide the following:

Name: _____

Address: _____

_____

_____

E-mail: _____

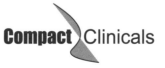

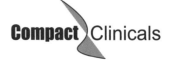

Order in 3 easy steps:

▶ 1   Provide complete billing and shipping information

Name _____   Company _____

Profession _____   Dept./Mail Stop _____

Street Address/P.O. Box _____

City/State/Zip _____

Telephone _____   ☐ Ship to Residence   ☐ Ship to Business

▶ 2   Choose Titles

For Clinicians:

	Qty.	Unit Price	Total
Attention Deficit Hyperactivity Disorder *The latest assessment and treatment strategies*		$16.95	
Bipolar Disorder *The latest assessment and treatment strategies*		$16.95	
Borderline Personality Disorder *The latest assessment and treatment strategies*		$16.95	
Conduct Disorders *The latest assessment and treatment strategies*		$16.95	
Depression in Adults *The latest assessment and treatment strategies*		$16.95	
Obsessive Compulsive Disorder *The latest assessment and treatment strategies*		$16.95	
Post-Traumatic and Acute Stress Disorders *The latest assessment and treatment strategies*		$16.95	

For Physicians:

Bipolar Disorder: Treatment and Management		$18.95	

	Subtotal
Continuing Education credits *available for mental health professionals.* *Call 1-800-408-8830 for details.*	**Tax** (Add 7.975% in MO)
	Shipping ($3.75 first book/ $1.00 per additional book)
	TOTAL

▶ 3   Choose Payment Method

Please charge my: ☐ Visa   ☐ MasterCard   ☐ Discover   ☐ American Express   ☐ Check Enclosed

Account # __ __ __ __ — __ __ __ __ — __ __ __ __ — __ __ __ __   Exp. Date __ __ / __ __

Name on Card _____   Cardholder Signature _____

Postal Orders: Compact Clinicals, 7205 NW Waukomis Dr., Suite A, Kansas City, MO 64151

Telephone Orders: Toll Free 1-800-408-8830   **Fax Orders:** 1(816) 587-7198

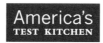

Also by the Editors at America's Test Kitchen

The Complete Cooking for Two Cookbook

The America's Test Kitchen Cooking School Cookbook

The Cook's Illustrated Baking Book

The Cook's Illustrated Cookbook

The Science of Good Cooking

The America's Test Kitchen Menu Cookbook

The America's Test Kitchen Quick Family Cookbook

The America's Test Kitchen Healthy Family Cookbook

The America's Test Kitchen Family Baking Book

The America's Test Kitchen Family Cookbook

THE AMERICA'S TEST KITCHEN LIBRARY SERIES AND THE TEST KITCHEN HANDBOOK SERIES:

Slow Cooker Revolution Volume 2

The Six-Ingredient Solution

Pressure Cooker Perfection

Comfort Food Makeovers

The America's Test Kitchen D.I.Y. Cookbook

Pasta Revolution

Simple Weeknight Favorites

Slow Cooker Revolution

The Best Simple Recipes

THE COOK'S COUNTRY SERIES:

From Our Grandmothers' Kitchens

Cook's Country Blue Ribbon Desserts

Cook's Country Best Potluck Recipes

Cook's Country Best Lost Suppers

Cook's Country Best Grilling Recipes

The Cook's Country Cookbook

America's Best Lost Recipes

THE TV COMPANION SERIES:

The Complete Cook's Country TV Show Cookbook

The Complete America's Test Kitchen TV Show Cookbook 2001–2014

America's Test Kitchen: The TV Companion Cookbook (2002–2009 and 2011–2014 Editions)

AMERICA'S TEST KITCHEN ANNUALS:

The Best of America's Test Kitchen (2007–2014 Editions)

Cooking for Two (2010–2013 Editions)

Light & Healthy (2010–2012 Editions)

THE BEST RECIPE SERIES:

The New Best Recipe

More Best Recipes

The Best One-Dish Suppers

Soups, Stews & Chilis

The Best Skillet Recipes

The Best Slow & Easy Recipes

The Best Chicken Recipes

The Best International Recipe

The Best Make-Ahead Recipe

The Best 30-Minute Recipe

The Best Light Recipe

The Cook's Illustrated Guide to Grilling and Barbecue

Best American Side Dishes

Cover & Bake

Steaks, Chops, Roasts & Ribs

Baking Illustrated

Italian Classics

American Classics

FOR A FULL LISTING OF ALL OUR BOOKS OR TO ORDER TITLES:

CooksIllustrated.com

AmericasTestKitchen.com

or call 800-611-0759

Praise for Other America's Test Kitchen Titles

"Ideal as a reference for the bookshelf and as a book to curl up and get lost in, this volume will be turned to time and again for definitive instruction on just about any food-related matter."
PUBLISHERS WEEKLY ON *THE SCIENCE OF GOOD COOKING*

"The perfect kitchen home companion. The practical side of things is very much on display. . . . cook-friendly and kitchen-oriented, illuminating the process of preparing food instead of mystifying it."
THE WALL STREET JOURNAL ON *THE COOK'S ILLUSTRATED COOKBOOK*

"A wonderfully comprehensive guide for budding chefs. . . . Throughout are the helpful tips and exacting illustrations that make ATK a peerless source for culinary wisdom."
PUBLISHERS WEEKLY ON *THE COOK'S ILLUSTRATED COOKBOOK*

"This book upgrades slow cooking for discriminating, 21st-century palates—that is indeed revolutionary."
THE DALLAS MORNING NEWS ON *SLOW COOKER REVOLUTION*

"There are pasta books . . . and then there's this pasta book. Flip your carbohydrate dreams upside down and strain them through this sieve of revolutionary, creative, and also traditional recipes."
SAN FRANCISCO BOOK REVIEW ON *PASTA REVOLUTION*

"If this were the only cookbook you owned, you would cook well, be everyone's favorite host, have a well-run kitchen, and eat happily every day."
THECITYCOOK.COM ON *THE AMERICA'S TEST KITCHEN MENU COOKBOOK*

"The strength of the Best Recipe series lies in the sheer thoughtfulness and details of the recipes."
PUBLISHERS WEEKLY ON THE BEST RECIPE SERIES

"Expert bakers and novices scared of baking's requisite exactitude can all learn something from this hefty, all-purpose home baking volume."
PUBLISHERS WEEKLY ON *THE AMERICA'S TEST KITCHEN FAMILY BAKING BOOK*

"If you're hankering for old-fashioned pleasures, look no further."
PEOPLE MAGAZINE ON *AMERICA'S BEST LOST RECIPES*

"This tome definitely raises the bar for all-in-one, basic, must-have cookbooks. . . . Kimball and his company have scored another hit."
PORTLAND OREGONIAN ON *THE AMERICA'S TEST KITCHEN FAMILY COOKBOOK*

"A foolproof, go-to resource for everyday cooking."
PUBLISHERS WEEKLY ON *THE AMERICA'S TEST KITCHEN FAMILY COOKBOOK*

"These dishes taste as luxurious as their full-fat siblings. Even desserts are terrific."
PUBLISHERS WEEKLY ON *THE BEST LIGHT RECIPE*

"The best instructional book on baking this reviewer has seen."
THE LIBRARY JOURNAL (STARRED REVIEW) ON *BAKING ILLUSTRATED*

"Further proof that practice makes perfect, if not transcendent. . . . If an intermediate cook follows the directions exactly, the results will be better than takeout or mom's."
THE NEW YORK TIMES ON *THE NEW BEST RECIPE*

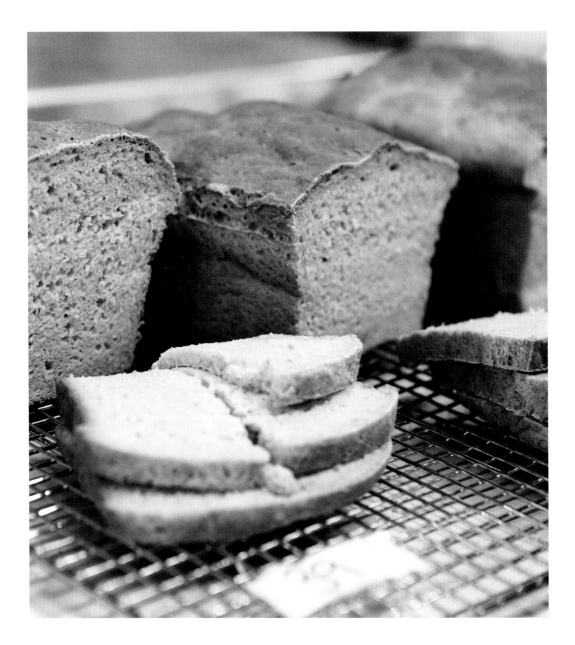

THE HOW CAN IT BE GLUTEN FREE COOKBOOK

REVOLUTIONARY TECHNIQUES.

GROUNDBREAKING RECIPES.

BY THE EDITORS AT
America's Test Kitchen

AMERICA'S TEST KITCHEN
17 Station Street, Brookline, MA 02445

Library of Congress
Cataloging-in-Publication Data
The how can it be gluten free cookbook : revolutionary techniques, groundbreaking recipes / by the editors at America's Test Kitchen. -- 1st ed.
     pages cm
 Includes index.
 ISBN 978-1-936493-61-6
1. Gluten-free diet--Recipes. 2. Gluten-free foods. I. America's Test Kitchen (Firm)
 RM237.86.U48 2014
 641.3--dc23
                                  2013038636

Manufactured in the United States of America

10 9 8 7 6 5 4 3 2 1

Paperback: $26.95 US
Distributed by America's Test Kitchen
17 Station Street, Brookline, MA 02445

EDITORIAL DIRECTOR: Jack Bishop
EDITORIAL DIRECTOR, BOOKS: Elizabeth Carduff
EXECUTIVE FOOD EDITOR: Julia Collin Davison
SENIOR EDITORS: Louise Emerick and Suzannah McFerran
EDITORIAL ASSISTANT: Melissa Herrick
TEST COOKS: Danielle DeSiato-Hallman, Sara Mayer, and Stephanie Pixley
ASSISTANT TEST COOK: Meaghen Walsh
ASSOCIATE EDITOR: Andrew Janjigian
DESIGN DIRECTOR: Amy Klee
ART DIRECTOR: Greg Galvan
DESIGNERS: Taylor Argenzio and Allison Pfiffner
PHOTOGRAPHY: Carl Tremblay
STAFF PHOTOGRAPHER: Daniel J. van Ackere
ADDITIONAL PHOTOGRAPHY: Steve Klise
PHOTO EDITOR: Steve Klise
FOOD STYLING: Daniel Cellucci and Marie Piraino
PHOTOSHOOT KITCHEN TEAM:
    ASSOCIATE EDITOR: Chris O'Connor
    TEST COOK: Daniel Cellucci
    ASSISTANT TEST COOK: Cecelia Jenkins
ILLUSTRATIONS: Jay Layman
PRODUCTION DIRECTOR: Guy Rochford
SENIOR PRODUCTION MANAGER: Jessica Quirk
PROJECT MANAGEMENT DIRECTOR: Alice Carpenter
PRODUCTION AND TRAFFIC COORDINATORS: Brittany Allen and Britt Dresser
WORKFLOW AND DIGITAL ASSET MANAGER: Andrew Mannone
SENIOR COLOR AND IMAGING SPECIALIST: Lauren Pettapiece
PRODUCTION AND IMAGING SPECIALISTS: Heather Dube and Lauren Robbins
COPYEDITOR: Jeff Schier
PROOFREADER: Ann-Marie Imbornoni
INDEXER: Elizabeth Parson

PICTURED ON FRONT COVER: Oatmeal-Honey Sandwich Bread
PICTURED ON BACK COVER: Cranberry-Orange Pecan Muffins and Blueberry Muffins, Chicken Pot Pie, Chocolate Layer Cake

CONTENTS

Welcome to the Test Kitchen

This book has been tested, written, and edited by the folks at America's Test Kitchen, a very real 2,500-square-foot kitchen located just outside of Boston. It is the home of *Cook's Illustrated* magazine and *Cook's Country* magazine and is the Monday-through-Friday destination for more than three dozen test cooks, editors, food scientists, tasters, and cookware specialists. Our mission is to test recipes over and over again until we understand how and why they work and until we arrive at the "best" version.

We start the process of testing a recipe with a complete lack of conviction, which means that we accept no claim, no theory, no technique, and no recipe at face value. We simply assemble as many variations as possible, test a half-dozen of the most promising, and taste the results blind. We then construct our own hybrid recipe and continue to test it, varying ingredients, techniques, and cooking times until we reach a consensus. The result, we hope, is the best version of a particular recipe, but we realize that only you can be the final judge of our success (or failure). As we like to say in the test kitchen, "We make the mistakes, so you don't have to."

All of this would not be possible without a belief that good cooking, much like good music, is indeed based on a foundation of objective technique. Some people like spicy foods and others don't, but there is a right way to sauté, there is a best way to cook a pot roast, and there are measurable scientific principles involved in producing perfectly beaten, stable egg whites. This is our ultimate goal: to investigate the fundamental principles of cooking so that you become a better cook. It is as simple as that.

If you're curious to see what goes on behind the scenes at America's Test Kitchen check out our daily blog, AmericasTestKitchenFeed.com, which features kitchen snapshots, exclusive recipes, video tips, and much more. You can watch us work (in our actual test kitchen) by tuning in to *America's Test Kitchen* (AmericasTestKitchen.com) or *Cook's Country from America's Test Kitchen* (CooksCountryTV.com) on public television. Tune in to *America's Test Kitchen Radio* (AmericasTestKitchen.com) on public radio to listen to insights, tips, and techniques that illuminate

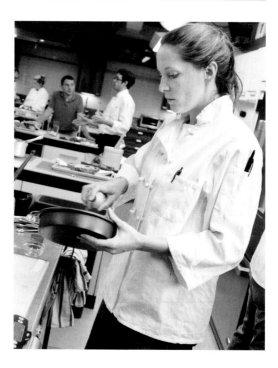

the truth about real home cooking. Want to hone your cooking skills or finally learn how to bake—from an America's Test Kitchen test cook? Enroll in a cooking class at our online cooking school at OnlineCookingSchool.com. And find information about subscribing to *Cook's Illustrated* magazine at CooksIllustrated.com or *Cook's Country* magazine at CooksCountry.com. Both magazines are published every other month. However you choose to visit us, we welcome you into our kitchen, where you can stand by our side as we test our way to the best recipes in America.

facebook.com/AmericasTestKitchen
twitter.com/TestKitchen
youtube.com/AmericasTestKitchen
instagram.com/TestKitchen
pinterest.com/TestKitchen
americastestkitchen.tumblr.com
google.com/+AmericasTestKitchen

Preface

Let me start with the sad truth. The vast majority of gluten-free recipes either do not work or the results are so second-rate that you would be hard-pressed to eat them. Muffins are gritty and crumbly. Cookies spread all over the baking sheet. Cakes are dense, gummy, and overly sweet. Pizza crusts are cracker-like. And, in general, baked goods are greasy.

Gluten-free cooking represents the pinnacle of recipe development since replacing wheat flour is tricky business. Gluten is formed when two wheat flour proteins—glutenin and gliadin—form cross-links when they are hydrated. This creates gluten, a protein that stretches to hold gas and therefore provides lift during baking. It also produces good chew.

Unfortunately, simply substituting a gluten-free flour blend for regular flour doesn't work. We needed to completely rethink each and every recipe, employing a host of tricks and techniques to get the results we wanted. We started with our own unique blend of flours and starches. (You can use gluten-free flour blends made by King Arthur or Bob's Red Mill if you like, although in some instances the results will be a bit different.)

Our first discovery was that some batters, such as those for quick breads, are best mixed vigorously instead of gently, breaking all the usual rules. We also found that many batters and doughs are better when rested for 30 minutes; this eliminated grittiness in the final baked goods. It also provided more time for the starches in the gluten-free flour blend to absorb liquid, which helps texture.

Vinegar helped to produce a flaky, tender pie pastry. Melted white chocolate added to a yellow layer cake allowed us to cut back on butter but still turn out a rich, but not greasy, cake. We also discovered that using less butter but adding cream cheese to a pound cake recipe made for a lighter, better cake since cream cheese does not easily separate into water and fat during baking.

One of the Holy Grails of gluten-free baking is the everyday sandwich bread. (As you probably know, the frozen supermarket offerings are a far cry from the real thing.) Our solution included powdered psyllium husk for structure, milk powder for browning, and oat flour to boost protein levels. We also added a lot of water to the dough to produce extra steam for better rising. Potato flakes, not gluten-free bread, were the perfect binder for better meatballs. We also developed great recipes for lasagna (only one brand of gluten-free noodles worked), eggplant Parmesan, and pizza dough, perhaps the most difficult challenge ever faced by our test kitchen.

My most vivid childhood memories were gathered in the kitchen of the Yellow Farmhouse, the home of Marie Briggs who was the de facto cook and baker in our small town in Vermont. In those days, Vermont had its own distinctive patchouli: wood smoke from the dark green Kalamazoo wood cookstove, wet dog, yeast, molasses cookies, green wood, anadama bread, and deep-fried nutmeg doughnuts. There is no need to leave those memories behind, even in a world where so many can no longer eat those foods. With this cookbook in hand, Saturday morning pancakes, a fat slice of chocolate cake, a blueberry muffin, and even high-quality sandwich bread are back on the menu.

That reminds me of our bird dog, Kili, who liked to chase cars. The problem was that she had no idea what to do with the car if she ever caught it. The world of gluten-free baking and cooking has been much the same—everyone has been chasing an unattainable goal.

So, hear the good news! Pies, breads, muffins, biscuits, cakes, etc., are back on the table where they belong. Yes, you can have your cake and eat it too. Enjoy!

CHRISTOPHER KIMBALL
Founder and Editor,
Cook's Illustrated and *Cook's Country*
Host, *America's Test Kitchen* and
Cook's Country from America's Test Kitchen

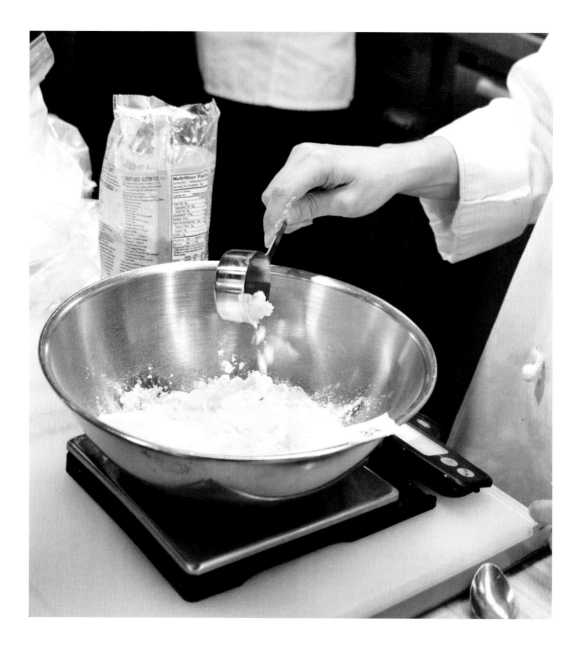

THE BASICS OF GLUTEN-FREE COOKING

Introduction

Our test kitchen works for you, our readers, as well as our television viewers, Web users, and radio listeners. We ask for—and we get—a lot of feedback every single day. We send out hundreds of recipes to readers before publication in order to measure their success. We also get plenty of comments about our publications; these include many unsolicited requests, and in the past few years many of you have asked for gluten-free recipes. This book is our test kitchen's attempt to help home cooks when wheat-based ingredients are no longer in the pantry.

There are many reasons why someone might be interested in a gluten-free diet. Our test kitchen isn't in the business of prescribing diets or offering up medical advice. We do, however, know how to test our way into foolproof recipes.

You already have hundreds, if not thousands, of gluten-free recipes in your home library. Most vegetable dishes are gluten-free, as are many seafood, poultry, and meat preparations. We didn't feel the need to include "gluten-free" recipes for roast beef or steamed broccoli. Our mission for this book was to solve more pressing problems faced by the home cook who is no longer eating dishes made with wheat-based ingredients. We identified four goals when we started this project.

DEVELOP gluten-free recipes for favorite foods that typically rely on wheat in some form. In addition to the obvious cakes, cookies, breads, and pizzas, we wanted to tackle recipes like fried chicken (usually made with a flour coating) and eggplant Parmesan (with a bread-crumb coating).

CREATE a versatile alternative to all-purpose flour—an America's Test Kitchen Gluten-Free Flour Blend. We wanted a blend that could be used not only in the recipes in this book, but as a starting point for reworking your favorite recipes—the ones already in your recipe box.

RATE key gluten-free supermarket ingredients that would make cooking—and eating—easier, including the wide variety of gluten-free pastas and sandwich breads now on the market. We also explored substitutions for pantry staples, like soy sauce, that are typically made with wheat.

TEACH readers about the wide range of gluten-free grains (everything from oat berries to millet) now sold in supermarkets. Many cooks are unfamiliar with these grains, and our test kitchen explains how to buy, store, and cook them, offering up approachable, appealing recipes for the most versatile grains.

As the test kitchen was working on this book, we sent the most important (and most difficult) recipes out to volunteer recipe testers—home cooks like you. In all, we received more than 2,000 written reports from this army of gluten-free testers. Thank you. Your feedback helped identify techniques that needed to be described in more detail as well as recipes that needed to be reworked.

If you have comments or questions about this book, we'd love to hear from you. E-mail us at **glutenfree@ americastestkitchen.com**.

The Science of Gluten

Before you attempt to cook without gluten, it's helpful to understand what gluten does in various recipes. Let's start with the most common source of gluten—wheat flour—which is the main ingredient in everything from pasta and pizza to cakes and cookies.

WHEAT FLOUR 101

Flour is milled from wheat berries, which contain starches, proteins, and fats. There are two main proteins in wheat flour—glutenin and gliadin. Glutenin is a very large, loosely coiled protein, while gliadin is a much smaller and tightly coiled sphere. Glutenin provides most of the strength and elasticity in dough, allowing it to bounce back after it has been stretched. Gliadin, on the other hand, provides the stretch.

DEFINING GLUTEN

In dry flour, these proteins are basically lifeless strands wrapped around granules of starch. But they begin to change shape when they come in contact with water, a process called hydration. Once moistened, the individual protein molecules (the glutenin and gliadin) begin to link up with one another to form long, elastic chains called gluten. These strands of gluten combine to form a membrane-like network. The network engulfs swollen starch granules and gas bubbles (created by yeast, chemical leaveners like baking powder, or foams like whipped egg whites), stretching as the batter or dough rises and then bakes, giving the finished cake or loaf its structure and chew.

GLUTEN DEVELOPMENT

There are several factors that can affect gluten development. The first is the flour itself. Bread flour is milled from high-protein wheat, which means it's capable of developing more gluten, or structure, which is perfect for chewy artisan loaves. In contrast, cake flour is made from soft wheat with a low protein content. As a result, cake flour produces less gluten, making it perfect for tender cakes. All-purpose flour has a relatively high protein content of 10 to 12 percent, depending on the brand. Bread flours have even more protein, generally 12 to 14 percent. Cake flour has just 6 to 8 percent protein.

Second, the amount of water can affect gluten development. Basically, the more water in a dough or batter, the stronger and more elastic the gluten strands. Why does this matter? If the gluten strands are strong and elastic, they can support the starch granules and air bubbles that hydrate and swell as the dough rises and bakes, producing an airier bread with good chew.

The third variable is the mixing time. A muffin batter that is gently stirred will develop less gluten than a bread dough beaten in a stand mixer for 10 minutes. More stirring equals more gluten, which equals more structure and chew.

What Is Gluten?

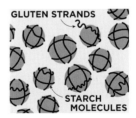

Wheat flour contains two types of protein strands, glutenin and gliadin, wrapped around starch granules.

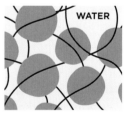

When flour is combined with water, the protein strands unwind and link together to form a membrane-like network, which is called gluten.

Strategies for Replacing Wheat Flour

The cook who wants to remove the flour from favorite recipes needs to consider the role the flour is playing in that recipe in order to devise a successful substitute. Remember that flour contains both protein and starch, and the kind of substitute you will need when trying to convert a recipe to be gluten-free will vary because some recipes rely on one but not the other element. Let's look at the three most common roles played by wheat flour.

FLOUR THICKENS

In sauces, gravies, soups, and stews, wheat flour plays the role of thickener. When the starch granules in the flour are heated in these dishes, they absorb water, swell, and eventually burst, releasing a starch molecule called amylose that diffuses throughout the solution, trapping additional water and forming a gelatinous network. This is how a few tablespoons of flour turn chicken stock into gravy.

Some thickeners, like cornstarch, are pure starches and contain more amylose than other thickeners, like flour, that contain components other than starch molecules. (Remember, flour also contains proteins and fats, and the starch content is about 75 percent.) Purity affects not only thickening power but performance.

Cornstarch is actually more fickle than flour. For instance, overwhisking pastry cream can break the bonds of the starch gel and thin out the custard. In contrast, the proteins and lipids in flour dilute its capacity to form starch gels, so that more flour is needed for thickening. But these non-starch compounds also act as binders, ensuring that the liquid not only thickens but also stays that way.

For these reasons, simply replacing flour with a pure starch doesn't always work. Large quantities of pure starch can impart a gritty texture to dishes. We had this problem when developing our recipe for pot pie—the amount of cornstarch needed to thicken the filling to the proper consistency gave the sauce a gritty mouthfeel. Luckily, there are other gluten-free starches besides cornstarch, including arrowroot (derived from a tropical tuber of the same name), potato starch, and tapioca starch (derived from cassava, another tropical tuber). In the end, we didn't find a single replacement for flour as a thickener, but given all the options we had no trouble finding an excellent work-around.

FLOUR COATS

In addition to its use as a thickener, flour can also be used as a coating in dishes like fried chicken or pan-fried pork chops. The starches in the flour are responsible for most of the browning and crisping, while the proteins in the flour help the coating cling to the surface of the food. The proteins also create chew or texture in the fried or baked coating.

When looking for a replacement for wheat flour, it's easy enough to deal with the starch component. Cornstarch is traditionally used as a coating in many recipes, everything from tempura to onion rings. Replacing the wheat flour with cornstarch was a start in many recipes. However, since cornstarch contains almost no protein, we had to rely on other ingredients to help the coating adhere and/or to create a chewy texture in the coating.

In our pan-fried pork chop recipe, we used the sticky proteins in the meat itself to help bind the coating to the chops. Simply cutting a very shallow crosshatch pattern into the meat released these sticky proteins and ensured that the crisp cornstarch and cornflake crust stayed put. In our fried chicken recipe, we added cornmeal (a good source of protein) as well as an egg to the coating. Some baking powder and baking soda also helped the coating to puff in the hot oil and create a crisp crust with the requisite chew.

Finally, in recipes like eggplant Parmesan and chicken fingers that rely on a bread-crumb coating, we were able to use gluten-free sandwich bread (dried in the oven first to make the crumbs less sticky) in combination with cornstarch (which improved overall coverage and increased browning and crispness). In the end, we didn't find a single replacement for flour as a coating ingredient, but here, too, given all the options we had no trouble finding an excellent work-around.

FLOUR BUILDS STRUCTURE

Finally, the main use for flour in the home kitchen is as a structural agent in baked goods. It's here that the gluten performs an essential function, as the ability of the proteins in wheat flour to expand and trap gas bubbles is key in many baked goods. In contrast to our efforts to come up with substitutions for wheat flour's other uses as a thickener or a coating, finding a replacement to replicate these structural functions using gluten-free ingredients was especially challenging because most options contain less protein.

In a baked good such as a muffin, the starch granules in the flour absorb moisture and swell as the batter is being prepared. The strands of gluten bond together and surround the starch granules. Gluten is particularly elastic and strong, especially when heated. This highly organized and strong network of gluten gives the muffin its structure and shape. Compared with wheat flour, gluten-free flours generally contain less protein, so they don't do as good of a job of organizing and holding the swollen starch granules. These proteins are also less elastic than gluten. In order to replace wheat flour with a lower-protein flour, such as rice flour, you must boost the effectiveness of that protein.

Xanthan gum acts like glue, helping cement the protein network in gluten-free flour. Another option is something that can help the flour to hydrate more readily, something that will promote the swelling of the starch granules and the bonding of the protein strands. An emulsifier such as nonfat milk powder can be used for this task. Emulsifiers can also make gluten-free flour more compatible with fat—something that wheat flour does better than other flours. Why is this important? Many baked goods (think cookies, cakes, even muffins) contain a lot of fat for flavor and moistness. If the flour doesn't absorb fat well, the baked good can be greasy (from the unabsorbed fat) and dry (because the starches are not properly coated with fat).

There's one more issue to consider when replacing wheat flour in baked goods. Wheat flour

TIPS FOR SUCCESSFULLY MAINTAINING A GLUTEN-FREE DIET

If you're new to a gluten-free diet, you will want to pick up some good resources to help teach you how to read a product label and find hidden sources of gluten. Here are the key challenges, in brief.

Check Ingredients: Many foods are made with an ingredient that contains gluten. This list includes the obvious (traditional sandwich bread and Italian pasta) and the less obvious (such as soy sauce—which is typically made with soybeans and wheat—and some brands of baking powder). You will need to learn which ingredients are typically made with wheat-based ingredients, and then to read labels carefully.

Review Processing: Other foods can be processed in facilities that also handle wheat and as a result may contain trace amounts of gluten—even though the food contains no wheat. This can be an issue with foods like cornmeal or oats. If you have celiac disease or other reason to avoid foods with even trace amounts of gluten, you need to read labels carefully to make sure naturally gluten-free foods, like oats, have not been processed in the same machines used to grind wheat.

Separate and Safe: Likewise, as a cook, you need to think about cross-contamination if you're trying to eliminate all gluten, even trace amounts, from your diet. If you're preparing dishes with wheat as well as gluten-free recipes in the same kitchen, you need to be vigilant about washing measuring tools, bowls, cutting boards, and your hands.

contains a starch content of roughly 75 percent. Most gluten-free flours contain an even higher starch content, which means they can impart a gritty texture to baked goods. In effect, there's too much starch and not enough protein. As we developed baked goods for this book, much of our testing was aimed at solving both grittiness and weak structure.

Key Test Kitchen Discoveries

During the year we spent in the kitchen testing gluten-free recipes, we learned that cooking without wheat really is different. In many cases, we had to reinvent recipes and employ new techniques. Here are some of the key discoveries, which may be helpful if you are trying to adapt recipes already in your repertoire to work without wheat flour.

COOKING TIPS

Thickening stays the same: In recipes where a tablespoon or two of flour is used as a thickener, you can generally use a gluten-free flour blend in a one-to-one replacement. This includes most stews and pan sauces. As with wheat flour, let the gluten-free flour cook for a minute before whisking in the liquid. This will cook out some of the raw, starchy flavor in the flour.

If you use cornstarch: You can also thicken liquids with cornstarch rather than flour. However, you must first turn cornstarch into a slurry by mixing it with cold water, and then use this slurry at the end of the cooking process. In general, you will need less cornstarch than flour.

For dusting proteins: Many breaded foods (everything from fried chicken and pork chops to eggplant Parmesan) are made with a bound breading—that is, they are dusted with flour, dipped in eggs or dairy, and then coated with crumbs. For the "dusting" part of the equation, cornstarch is a good replacement for the flour.

Make your own breading: We weren't terribly impressed with the brands of gluten-free bread crumbs that we tested. We had better luck taking our top-rated gluten-free sandwich bread and then grinding it into crumbs. Note that fresh bread crumbs should be dried in the oven before being used as a coating (see page 139 for more information).

Consider cornflakes: Cornflakes (as long as they are produced in a gluten-free facility) are another option that can be used in place of bread crumbs to top casseroles and such, though they are a bit sweeter than bread crumbs.

Replace soy sauce with tamari: Any recipe made with soy sauce (which generally contains wheat) can be made with tamari sauce (which generally does not contain wheat). A one-to-one replacement will work in most recipes.

BAKING TIPS

Cut the butter and oil: Gluten-free flours don't absorb liquid fat as readily as wheat flour does. In high-fat recipes, such as cookies or cakes, simply replacing the wheat flour with an equal amount of gluten-free flour doesn't work. The baked goods are often much too greasy, which not only makes them unappetizing but can affect how cookies spread in the oven or determine whether pie dough holds its shape when baked. When reworking conventional recipes with gluten-free flour, we often trimmed a few tablespoons of butter or oil.

Look elsewhere for richness: While using less butter or oil solved the greasiness problem in many recipes, this also made them less rich. In some cases, we compensated by adding another rich ingredient, such as cream cheese, sour cream, white chocolate, or even almond flour.

Increase the leavener to lighten the load: Less protein means batters and doughs can't hold on to air bubbles as well, and the end result can be heavy and dense. Gluten-free recipes often benefit from a bit more baking powder, baking soda, or yeast as compared with traditional recipes. Yeast bread often benefits from the addition of baking powder or baking soda.

Add a binder for structure and elasticity: A binder (xanthan gum, guar gum, or psyllium) helps in most baked goods. A little goes a long way, especially xanthan. See page 16 for more details on our testing of these three binders and when to use each one.

Boost browning: Gluten-free flour doesn't brown as well as wheat flour. To improve browning as well as add richness, we included milk powder in our blend. A few recipes, such as sandwich bread, benefited from the addition of even a bit more milk powder. We sometimes added baking soda to help with browning, and often we sprinkled sugar on top of things (such as muffins) to encourage browning.

Add additional liquid: The high starch content of gluten-free flour can impart a gritty texture to baked goods. Many gluten-free batters and doughs need more liquid to hydrate properly.

Give it a rest: Many batters and doughs benefit from a 30-minute rest before baking. The starches have time to hydrate before they go into the oven, and the final texture is much improved. Longer resting times are not recommended, especially as this can affect the performance of leaveners. Also, recipes that require a lengthy baking time don't need to rest because the flour will have time to hydrate in the oven.

Extend the baking time: If you have added more liquid to help hydrate the flour blend, you will need to extend the baking time to help dry out baked goods, especially breads.

Don't make too much: Gluten-free baked goods don't last as long as regular baked goods, so don't make big batches of cookies or muffins and expect them to stay fresh for days. We provide storage guidelines for various types of baked goods throughout the book.

Troubleshooting When Baking

After hundreds of kitchen tests, we have a sense of what problems are likely to occur when you attempt to make a conventional baked good gluten-free. The Baking Tips on this page and the previous page offer general advice that applies to many baked goods, while this chart lists problems specific to smaller subsets of recipes. We've included the solution that most often fixed these more specific problems. Note that every baking recipe is a unique formula, so these solutions won't work in all cases. Think of this information as a starting point when problem solving in your kitchen.

TYPE OF RECIPE	COMMON PROBLEM	POSSIBLE SOLUTIONS
Pancakes	Dense, heavy texture	Fold in whipped egg whites
	Gummy center	Lower burner or griddle temperature (so pancakes have more time to cook through)
Muffins/Quick Breads	Crumbly texture	Add extra egg and use binder, like xanthan gum
	Dense texture	Use more leavener
	Gritty texture	Let batter rest for 30 minutes before baking
Drop Cookies	Excessive spread	Add binder and let dough rest
	Gritty texture	Let dough rest for 30 minutes before baking
	Overly hard texture	Use more brown sugar, less white sugar
	Airy, hollow texture	Use less butter and melt butter instead of creaming it
Cakes	Greasy mouthfeel	Swap in oil for some or all of butter
	Dense crumb	Use less fat or more stable fat like chocolate or cream cheese
	Gummy center	Extend baking time to set starches in flour
Pie/Tart Dough	Crumbly texture	Add binder, such as xanthan gum
	Overly tough and not flaky enough	Add small amount of vinegar
Yeast Breads	Squat loaves	Use more liquid, add higher-protein flour, and wrap loaf pan with foil collar
	Dense crumb with insufficient chew	Add psyllium
	Gummy, wet crumb	Extend baking time

The Appeal of a Gluten-Free Flour Blend

Unfortunately, no single gluten-free flour or starch behaves like wheat flour. To pull off the same (or at least similar) results, you need to use a combination of gluten-free flours and starches. Both flours and starches are ground from various parts (including seeds and tubers) of various plants. We use the term flour for those products that contain protein as well as starch. We use the term starch for those products that contain just starch.

Most home cooks don't want to stock a dozen flours and starches and use a customized blend for each recipe. A single blend—with several flours and starches—that can be used in place of wheat flour in most recipes clearly has tremendous appeal. We decided to develop as many recipes as possible using one gluten-free flour blend.

COMMERCIAL OR HOMEMADE?

Many supermarkets now sell "all-purpose" or "multipurpose" gluten-free flour. We decided to test the most widely available brands knowing that we would also want to explore buying several flours and making a homemade blend. That said, there are two challenges with either approach.

HOW TO TEST APPLES AND ORANGES

It's hard to evaluate individual flour blends because they often contain very different ingredients so you're not comparing apples to apples. In addition, even brands or homemade blends with the same ingredients use them in different ratios.

FINDING THE RIGHT RECIPES

The second challenge is figuring out how to evaluate various gluten-free flour blends. You can't taste them as is—you need to use them in a recipe. But many blends are meant to be used with recipes specifically formulated for that blend. But if we tested these flours in different recipes we'd be evaluating the recipes as much as (if not more than) the flours. Frankly, there was no good way to resolve this dilemma. For this first round of testing, we decide to test all the various blends in our published recipes developed with all-purpose flour. We chose three established test kitchen recipes—drop biscuits, sugar cookies, and yellow sheet cake—and substituted the blends for the all-purpose flour in each recipe. We knew that the results wouldn't be perfect since we were working with recipes developed around wheat flour. But all flour blends would be at an equal disadvantage and there would be no variables, other than the brand of gluten-free flour.

TESTING STORE-BOUGHT FLOUR BLENDS

We started by choosing five store-bought blends that varied in their ingredients and were somewhat widely available. We settled on blends from King Arthur, a well-established, respected company in the flour and baking products world; Bob's Red Mill, a brand available at most supermarkets and a company with a strong focus on gluten-free baking and cooking products; Cup4Cup, a blend developed by Lena Kwak and Thomas Keller (who is also a leading chef and owner of the French Laundry and Per Se) that is sold exclusively through Williams-Sonoma; Pamela's, a California-based company focused on gluten-free baking mixes with a national distribution; and Dakota Prairie, a brand sold online, primarily at the wholesale level to well-known gluten-free product manufacturers.

THE RESULTS

In the end, no single blend was a clear favorite. One brand made the best cookies, a different brand made the best biscuits, and yet another brand made the preferred cake. (For detailed notes on each flour blend, see the chart on the opposite page.) And while all five blends produced cookies, biscuits, and cakes that looked the part (or at least came close), there were a lot of textural and flavor problems. The vast majority of the samples were noticeably gritty, dry, and crumbly, or they were dense and gummy. The cookies, biscuits, and cakes almost universally had an unappealing starch flavor that lingered. Tasters noticed off-flavors in several samples (metallic and fishy notes were common complaints), and, across the board, decent browning was a rare occurrence.

Evaluating Commercial Flour Blends

We tested five widely available gluten-free flour blends in three applications—biscuits, sugar cookies, and yellow cake. Flours are listed in alphabetical order.

BRAND	INGREDIENTS	TASTERS' COMMENTS
BOB'S RED MILL GF All-Purpose Baking Flour PRICE: $4.29/1.5-lb bag ($2.86/lb)	Garbanzo Bean Flour, Potato Starch, Tapioca Flour, Sorghum Flour, Fava Bean Flour	Our tasters did not like the distinctive and "off-putting" taste of bean flour in their baked goods. There were numerous complaints that items tasted "like fish," and most panelists picked up strong "earthy" notes. However, structurally and texturally, this blend performed especially well. Biscuits, cookies, and cakes were slightly more dense than desired but pretty good.
CUP4CUP Gluten-Free Flour PRICE: $19.95/3-lb bag ($6.65/lb)	Cornstarch, White Rice Flour, Brown Rice Flour, Nonfat Milk Powder, Tapioca Flour, Potato Starch, Xanthan Gum	The high level of cornstarch (the number one ingredient in this blend) left a starchy coating on the tongue and produced a "tight" texture in baked goods. Many tasters complained about a "starch bomb in your mouth." The sugar cookies fared better than the biscuits and cake, in part because the sugar seemed to mask the presence of the cornstarch.
DAKOTA PRAIRIE Gluten-Free All-Purpose White Flour PRICE: $13.99/5-lb bag ($2.80/lb)	White Rice Flour, Potato Starch, Cornstarch, Tapioca Flour, Xanthan Gum	This was the only blend we tested that did not have a whole-grain flour in it—and tasters could tell. Many described the baked goods it produced as bland and "barely OK" in terms of flavor (this was particularly noticeable in the biscuits, likely because there are so few ingredients). It had a lot of textural issues as well, producing rubbery muffins, crumbly biscuits, and a dense cake.
KING ARTHUR Gluten-Free Multi-Purpose Flour PRICE: $7.95/1.5-lb box ($5.30/lb)	White Rice Flour, Tapioca Flour, Potato Starch, Brown Rice Flour. Calcium Carbonate, Niacinamide (a B vitamin), Reduced Iron Thiamin Hydrochloride (vitamin B1), Riboflavin (vitamin B2)	Across the board this blend performed well, in terms of both delivering good structure and having a neutral, not-too-starchy flavor. It finished in the top three for all tests. A few tasters found it too sweet in cakes and cookies, but overall it won out for tasting like "the real thing." Many noted a grainy, gritty texture, but not enough to push it to the bottom of any tastings.
PAMELA'S Artisan Flour Blend PRICE: $7.98/1.5-lb bag ($5.31/lb)	Brown Rice Flour, Tapioca Flour, White Rice Flour, Potato Starch, Sorghum Flour, Arrowroot Flour, Sweet Rice Flour, Xanthan Gum	This blend fared pretty well, delivering a "wheaty" biscuit that took first place. The cake won points for being moist, but it had a starchy, gritty texture. The "ugly" muffin didn't rise much compared with the others in the lineup.

Developing Our Own Flour Blend

Given our mixed success with store-bought blends, we felt it was worth pursuing the option of making our own blend. To make the transition from store-bought to homemade blend, we started by selecting a variety of published recipes for homemade blends, then ran them through the same biscuit, cookie, and cake tests. We saw a lot of the same issues that we had observed in our store-bought blend tests. The vast majority of baked goods were similarly gritty and crumbly, and others were dense and gummy. The unappealing starch flavor once again was an issue. Earthy flavors that seemed out of place for an all-purpose flour substitute were noticeable in multiple samples. And decent browning was rare. It was time to build our own blend from the ground up.

WHAT WE HAD LEARNED

At this point, we recognized that the blends (whether store-bought or homemade) were based on one of three ingredients—rice, sorghum, or bean. We didn't love the bean-based blends; while they worked well structurally, we didn't like the off-flavors. And while we liked how sorghum flour worked structurally in recipes, its earthy flavor made these blends taste more like whole-wheat flour and less like a classic all-purpose white flour. Rice flour was clearly the best choice for building our own versatile flour blend that could be used in place of all-purpose wheat flour.

In addition to rice flour, we knew that any homemade blend would need another source of starches because the starches in rice flour don't behave the same way that starches in wheat flour do. Individual plant starches absorb water, swell, and gel at different temperatures and to different degrees, creating more or less structure, more or less readily. Using rice flour, along with pure starches like tapioca starch or potato starch, is a way of combining different properties for different applications. Previous testing had convinced us that cornstarch made baked goods very starchy, so it was out of the mix.

TESTING FLOURS AND STARCHES

White rice flour made a logical starting point for our base because of its neutral flavor, but blends that relied on it as the sole flour component tasted overly starchy and produced a tight crumb. Adding brown rice flour reduced the starchiness in baked goods and added some nice flavor notes. However, as with whole-wheat and white flour, brown rice flour is coarser than white rice flour, and too much brown rice flour made baked goods gritty and coarse. In the end, we

found that three parts white rice flour to one part brown rice flour was best.

After more testing, we decided to use both tapioca and potato starches in our blend. They worked well in combination and are widely available. Tapioca starch provided chew, elasticity, and structure, while potato starch helped contribute tenderness and binding power. We found that too much starch overall led to a rubbery, chewy texture, so ultimately we settled on roughly three parts flour to one part starch as the best ratio. In determining the ratio of the two starches, we discovered that too much tapioca starch made cookies and muffins dense, rubbery, and bready, while samples with too much potato starch and not enough tapioca were too crumbly. We ended up using about twice as much potato starch as tapioca starch to balance out the various pros and cons.

WHAT ABOUT XANTHAN GUM?

Many flour blends include xanthan gum to help with structure and stability. Those without it note to add a specific amount to recipes when swapping in their gluten-free blend. We decided early in the development process to omit gums from our blend—even a mere ⅛ teaspoon could make a marked difference in a recipe. It seemed best to customize the amount of gum to the needs of each particular recipe rather than lock them all into a set amount by putting xanthan gum in our blend. For more information on using xanthan and other binders, see page 16.

MORE PROTEIN, PLEASE

Our working recipe was based on white rice flour; brown rice flour helped balance the starchiness and add wheaty flavor; tapioca starch lent elasticity and

THE AMERICA'S TEST KITCHEN GLUTEN-FREE FLOUR BLEND
MAKES 42 OUNCES (ABOUT 9⅓ CUPS)

Be sure to use potato starch, not potato flour. Tapioca starch is also sold as tapioca flour; they are interchangeable. See notes at right about shopping for rice flours and substituting soy milk powder.

- 24 ounces (4½ cups plus ⅓ cup) white rice flour
- 7½ ounces (1⅔ cups) brown rice flour
- 7 ounces (1⅓ cups) potato starch
- 3 ounces (¾ cup) tapioca starch
- ¾ ounce (3 tablespoons) nonfat milk powder

Whisk all ingredients together in large bowl until well combined. Transfer to airtight container and refrigerate for up to 3 months.

BUYING RICE FLOURS

We used rice flours made by Bob's Red Mill during our testing process. We found some rice flours (including those made by Arrowhead Mills, another widely available brand) to be a bit coarser, which can negatively impact the texture of baked goods. We strongly recommend that you buy Bob's Red Mill white and brown rice flours. See page 19 for more detail on our testing of rice flours.

USING MILK POWDER

If dairy is part of your diet, we strongly recommend adding the nonfat milk powder. (We use nonfat, rather than whole-milk, powder because it is more readily available.) If you prefer, use an equal amount of soy milk powder. You can omit the milk powder altogether, however baked goods won't brown quite as well and they will taste a bit less rich, especially in recipes without a lot of fat.

structure; and potato starch was in the mix for tenderness and some binding power. But we were still having some structural problems in baked goods. We suspected our flour blend needed a protein boost. (All-purpose flour has a protein content of 10 to 12 percent and rice flours contain about half that.)

TESTING "SECRET" INGREDIENTS

We considered three ingredients that had potential to boost the protein level: calcium carbonate, powdered egg whites, and nonfat milk powder.

We'd seen calcium carbonate listed as an ingredient in one commercial flour blend, and calcium in various forms is also added to many gluten-free breads. In the everyday world, calcium carbonate is sold at drugstores as a calcium supplement and an antacid (it's the active ingredient in Tums). According to our science editor, calcium carbonate could unlock the proteins in rice flour and thus contribute a more tender crumb to baked goods. We located some calcium carbonate tablets, crushed them, and added them to our blend. In several applications, tasters did

in fact notice a tenderizing effect, but ultimately we decided the hassle factor outweighed the benefit.

Egg whites are mostly water with a decent protein content, but the powdered version is nearly all protein. As we hoped, powdered egg whites added a big boost in terms of structure, but no one in the test kitchen liked the meringuelike flavor they imparted.

The nonfat milk powder was the only "secret" ingredient to make the cut. It helped with structure and tenderness, added richness and buttery flavor, and contributed to browning. (Milk powder contains both sugars and proteins, the two building blocks necessary for the Maillard reaction, which creates browning and additional flavors.) The milk powder also seemed to temper the starchiness in baked goods.

After two months of testing we finally had a blend, which consisted of roughly 57 percent white rice flour, 18 percent brown rice flour, 17 percent potato starch, 7 percent tapioca starch, and 2 percent nonfat milk powder. It sounds so simple (and it is), but don't tell that to the team that tasted hundreds of baked goods to arrive at this formula.

Deciding Whether to Make or Buy a Flour Blend

We think you should make our blend. It produces excellent results—and in many recipes those results are superior to anything possible with a store-bought blend. In a few cases (rolled holiday cookies, for example), the results with store-bought blends were so inferior that we can't recommend using them. In addition to producing superior results, our homemade blend is cheaper than commercial blends, which cost an average of $4.50 per pound. Our blend costs about $2 per pound for the first batch, and subsequent batches will be even cheaper because there will be leftovers of some ingredients.

SAME RECIPE, DIFFERENT FLOURS

Almost all of the recipes in this book can be made with our blend (page 13) or blends made by King Arthur or Bob's Red Mill. However, the fact that all three flour options will provide good results doesn't mean they produce identical results. Below are yellow cupcakes (see recipe on page 286) made with each of the three flour blends. You can see appearance differences, and our tasters noted textural and flavor differences, too.

ATK BLEND
Cupcake rises extremely well, with slight doming. Crumb is fine and very tender.

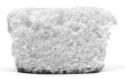

KING ARTHUR
Cupcake is denser and doesn't rise as well as other samples. Slight starchy taste.

BOB'S RED MILL
Cupcake rises well but crumb is more coarse and crumbly. Distinct bean flavor.

BUT IF YOU'RE GOING TO BUY A BLEND

The King Arthur blend is the closest (in terms of ingredients) to our blend and is our top choice for those cooks who want to buy a blend. Unfortunately, the distribution of this blend isn't universal. About one-third of the volunteer testers who vetted recipes for this book reported they couldn't find this flour in their local markets.

While we don't like the bean flavors in the Bob's Red Mill blend (this is a bigger issue in plain recipes but less so in recipes with a lot of sugar or other strong flavors), we like the structural properties of this blend, and our testers report that this product is very easy to find. For these reasons, we decided to test all recipes in this book with our homemade blend as well as with King Arthur and Bob's Red Mill.

PAY ATTENTION TO G-F TESTING LAB

If you are using a store-bought blend, pay careful attention to this feature that accompanies recipes in this book. We use this feature to explain any noticeable structural or flavor issues resulting from the use of either of these two commercial flours in a specific recipe. Also, we will warn you about a few recipes that can't successfully be made with a commercial blend.

ONE LAST WARNING

Given the increasing number of commercial flour blends on the market, we simply couldn't test every recipe in this book with all of the various options. Therefore, we can't guarantee your results unless you use our blend (our preference) or the blends made by King Arthur and Bob's Red Mill.

Measuring Gluten-Free Flour

All brands of wheat flour contain the same ingredients, so they measure out the same. However, different brands of gluten-free flour contain different ingredients and, as a result, these flours will pack differently. How fine or coarse the individual ingredients in a blend are ground also impacts how these gluten-free flours will pack into measuring cups. For this reason, weight-to-volume equivalencies vary from brand to brand, as illustrated in the information below. (Refer to page 314 for a complete weight-to-volume conversion chart for all three of these flours.)

FLOUR BLEND	CONVERSION
ATK Gluten-Free Flour Blend	1 cup = 4.5 ounces
	2 cups = 9 ounces
	3 cups = 13.5 ounces
Bob's Red Mill GF All-Purpose Baking Flour	1 cup = 5.0 ounces
	2 cups = 10.0 ounces
	3 cups = 15.0 ounces
King Arthur Gluten-Free Multi-Purpose Flour	1 cup = 5.5 ounces
	2 cups = 11 ounces
	3 cups = 16.5 ounces

As you can see, one cup of Bob's Red Mill contains 11 percent more flour than one cup of the ATK flour blend. And one cup of King Arthur contains a whopping 22 percent flour than one cup of our flour blend. That kind of variance is enough to cause serious problems in a recipe. So what should you do?

You can easily avoid this problem if you simply weigh your flour, and we strongly recommend that you do this when cooking from this book. Ten ounces of gluten-free flour blend is the same, no matter the brand. All recipes in this book are written with ounce measurements for the flour. Invest in a good scale, please! Even if you're using our flour blend, a scale will ensure accuracy when you measure.

However, we know that many cooks prefer to use cup measures. If you're measuring flour by volume, please follow the technique outlined in the photos below.

And if you're using Bob's Red Mill or King Arthur, you will need to refer to the G-F Testing Lab notes in each recipe for the proper volume conversion.

How to Measure Gluten-Free Flour

If you're not weighing gluten-free flour, use the following technique to measure out flour by volume. Note that the dip-and-sweep method that we typically use in the test kitchen doesn't work well with the small bag or box sizes of gluten-free flours.

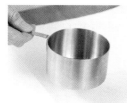

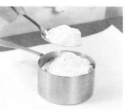

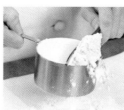

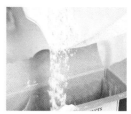

1. Place sheet of paper towel on counter and set measuring cup in center.

2. Spoon flour into cup, occasionally shaking cup to settle flour, until flour is mounded over rim. Do not tap cup or pack flour.

3. Using flat edge (like back of butter knife), scrape away excess flour to level.

4. Use paper towel to help funnel excess flour back into bag/container.

The Use of Binders

Because there is less protein in gluten-free flours than in wheat flours, gluten-free flours are not capable of forming the strong network required to stretch and surround starch granules. In our testing, we found that gluten-free flours required some help from a binder, generally in the form of xanthan gum, guar gum, or powdered psyllium husk. (See page 21 for detailed descriptions of each.) These ingredients strengthen protein networks in baked goods and make them more elastic. In effect, they act as the glue that gives gluten-free baked goods the proper shape. Below is a summary of the test kitchen's experiences using each binder in a wide range of recipes.

XANTHAN GUM AND GUAR GUM

We tested both xanthan gum and guar gum in muffins, cakes, cookies, brownies, and fresh pasta as well as in pie dough and tart dough, and we preferred xanthan gum in every application. In many cases the differences were slight, but the guar gum produced baked goods that were a bit more pasty and/or starchy. Also, baked goods made with xanthan had a longer shelf life than those made with guar. That said, guar gum produced good results in almost every case other than tart dough and fresh pasta.

PSYLLIUM IN YEASTED RECIPES

Powdered psyllium husk is especially effective at creating a more open and airy crumb. In extensive kitchen tests, we found it was the only choice in yeast breads and pizza. It produced breads with a bit of chew and a better rise. And its earthy flavor (which might seem out of place in a sugar cookie) worked beautifully in bread recipes. So why does psyllium work better than either gum in yeast breads? It binds more effectively with water, and there's a lot of water in bread dough. As a result, psyllium does a better job of strengthening the protein network so it is capable of holding in lots of gas and steam during baking.

PSYLLIUM IN NON-YEASTED RECIPES

We tried psyllium in nearly a dozen other recipes. In most cases it worked fine but not quite as well as xanthan, in part because so much more of it is required. In recipes with less moisture than bread dough (like muffins, cookies, fresh pasta, pie dough, or tart dough), the psyllium produced a drier texture and a coarser crumb, and its hearty flavor seemed a little out of place in some cases (especially shortbread and fresh

pasta). That said, it was a good substitute for xanthan if you want a more "natural" option.

OUR APPROACH

Other than our yeast breads, which rely on psyllium, the majority of the baked goods in this book call for a small amount of xanthan gum. We don't recommend replacing the psyllium in our bread recipes with xanthan or guar gum. Breads made with either gum will be dense and heavy.

We know that some people have a hard time digesting xanthan, so we did a lot of testing to devise guidelines for those bakers who want to use something else in our recipes that call for it. We found you can replace xanthan with an equal amount of guar or twice as much psyllium in most recipes in this book. The one exception is drop cookies, where xanthan does a better job of controlling spread. (Since drop cookies are baked "free-form," the dough can spread too much unless you add sufficient binder.) In chocolate chip, oatmeal, and other drop cookies, we suggest replacing xanthan with three times as much guar or five times as much psyllium.

Substitution Formulas

	SUBSTITUTIONS
Baked Goods (except Drop Cookies)	1 teaspoon xanthan gum =
	1 teaspoon guar gum =
	2 teaspoons psyllium powder
Drop Cookies	1 teaspoon xanthan gum =
	3 teaspoons guar gum =
	5 teaspoons psyllium powder

Making Ingredient Substitutions

Many people on a gluten-free diet have additional health issues or nutritional concerns. We aren't able to address all of these individual challenges in this book. Our approach is to focus on replacing the gluten while relying on the other ingredients we typically use in traditional recipes.

As a result, many of the baked goods in this book contain butter, and we generally rely on granulated sugar and brown sugar. Many cakes call for milk. And we use nuts and nut flours liberally in recipes where they make sense, and sometimes even where they wouldn't seem logical but proved to be the surprise solution, like almond flour in our sugar cookies. That said, the test kitchen can offer some advice on making substitutions to meet particular dietary needs beyond the scope of this book.

Although it may sound obvious, a small change is more likely to succeed than a radical change. Also, remember that substitutions affect both flavor and texture. While you might think that canola oil spread tastes fine on toast, it will behave quite differently than butter in a cookie recipe, affecting how the cookies spread and brown.

MILK

Unsweetened soy milk is usually a good substitute for cow's milk. Since soy milk generally contains about half the fat of whole milk, finished dishes will be a bit less rich. You will hardly notice the difference in a cake recipe with a lot of butter, but a pudding that relies on milk may taste a bit hollow or wan. (The same thing can happen when you replace whole cow's milk with low-fat cow's milk.) In savory applications, we find the flavor of the soy milk to be overpowering and not terribly appealing. Finally, soy milk can curdle if it gets too hot, so don't boil pureed soups once soy milk has been added.

BUTTERMILK

You can spike soy milk (rather than our recommended cow's milk) with lemon juice to replace buttermilk in many recipes. See page 43 for details.

SOUR CREAM/YOGURT

In general, you can use sour cream and whole-milk yogurt interchangeably in recipes, with some modest differences in richness in the final dish. Since whole-milk yogurt already contains far less fat than sour cream, don't attempt to use low-fat or nonfat yogurt in place of sour cream. Unless otherwise specified, all recipes in this book were developed using American-style yogurt. Because of its low moisture content, Greek yogurt can make baked goods a bit dry if you use it as a one-to-one substitute for American-style yogurt. To use Greek yogurt in our recipes, try this

formula: To replace 1 cup of regular yogurt, use ⅔ cup Greek yogurt combined with ⅓ cup water.

BUTTER

Oil-based spreads don't taste or behave like butter. Vegetable oil is a better option in many recipes, although flavor will be affected.

EGGS

Since eggs add richness and structure, you can't easily omit them from gluten-free recipes. The structure that eggs provide is especially important because gluten-free flour is low in protein, and eggs are an excellent source of protein. For this reason, many recipes in this book call for more eggs than you might find in a conventional recipe.

SWEETENERS

Sugar affects both the flavor and the texture of baked goods. We find that most substitutes impart an undesirable off-flavor. (Agave and honey are exceptions.) Perhaps even more important, alternative sweeteners, including honey and agave, will affect the moisture level and texture in baked goods. Cookies that are nice and chewy when made with brown sugar might be dry and stale when made with Splenda or another substitute like stevia (commonly sold as Truvia). Sweetener changes can also affect browning and spread. In general, alternate sweeteners will be most successful in liquid-based recipes such as puddings.

The Gluten-Free Pantry

Flours and starches are two of the most important ingredients in the gluten-free pantry. Below are the flours and starches that have found a place in the test kitchen's pantry. We've also included other helpful ingredients, such as leaveners and binders, that are essential when preparing gluten-free baked goods.

Many of the ingredients listed in this section are sold in all supermarkets. Other items (like rice flour) are sold in natural food stores and well-stocked supermarkets, or you can buy them online directly from manufacturers. Bob's Red Mill makes many of the flours and starches listed below and is the brand we stock in the test kitchen. Amazon also sells most of the products listed below.

FLOURS

Because protein is an important component in any flour, we have included this information below. (The percentage will vary according to how the flour is processed.) Wheat flour has 6 to 13 percent protein.

Almond Flour: Almond flour has a mild flavor that is subtly sweet and nutty. It is high in protein and has a coarse texture. Almond flour is usually made with blanched almonds, while almond meal can be made with blanched almonds or almonds with their skins on. That said, some manufacturers, including Bob's Red Mill, use both terms on their packaging, so read labels carefully. We prefer flour (or meal) made from blanched almonds since the lighter color tends to be more versatile. Almond flour is a good choice for rustic cakes, and we have found that it is particularly helpful to cookie recipes, where a small amount contributes richness, heft, and fat without adding a noticeable flavor. You can make your own almond flour by grinding blanched almonds in the food processor.

Protein: 21%
Best Use: Cookies and rustic cakes
Where to Store It: Refrigerator or freezer

Buckwheat Flour: Buckwheat, despite its name, is not related to wheat but is in fact an herb. Made by grinding the plant's triangular seeds, buckwheat flour (and all buckwheat products) has a noticeably earthy flavor and dark color. Its most familiar uses are in the traditional Russian yeast-raised pancakes known as blini and as the base of soba noodles. It is also a good option for making crêpes. Because of its strong flavor, it is best used in combination with another flour. (See also Buckwheat Groats and Kasha on page 28.)

Protein: 13%
Best Use: Pancakes
Where to Store It: Refrigerator or freezer

Chickpea (Garbanzo Bean) Flour: Made by grinding whole dried chickpeas, this flour has a distinct bean flavor and darker color and is more often seen in dishes outside the United States, particularly in the Middle East, France, and Italy.

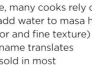

Protein: 20%
Best Use: Unleavened crêpes known as socca
Where to Store It: Refrigerator or freezer

Masa Harina: This fine flour is made from dried masa, the corn-flour dough used throughout Latin America. Masa is made from hominy (dried corn kernels) that are cooked in water with slaked lime until tender. The wet corn kernels are then ground to a flour, and mixed with more water and fat (usually lard or shortening) to form a dough. Since fresh masa has a short life, many cooks rely on the masa harina. You simply add water to masa harina (which has a mild corn flavor and fine texture) to make masa. Maseca (the name translates as "dried masa") is sold in most supermarkets.

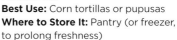

Protein: 11%
Best Use: Corn tortillas or pupusas
Where to Store It: Pantry (or freezer, to prolong freshness)

Oat Flour: Made by grinding oats to a powder, this flour has a subtle, slightly sweet, whole-grain flavor. It adds a welcome wheatiness to sandwich bread, and because it is high in protein it helps build structure in breads. You can grind old-fashioned rolled oats in a food processor or spice grinder for about 1 minute to make your own oat flour.

Protein: 17%
Best Use: Breads
Where to Store It: Refrigerator or freezer

TESTING RICE FLOURS

All-purpose wheat flour has the same smooth consistency no matter the brand, but this is not the case for white and brown rice flours. Depending on the brand, the grind can range from very fine to sort of fine to a tad gritty. These differences can significantly affect the performance of our flour blend and the success of the recipes in which it is used. To better understand this variable, we conducted a series of tests with our Red Velvet Cupcakes and Chocolate Chip Cookies using four different brands of white rice flour and six different brands of brown rice flour. Here's what we learned.

- Because our flour blend contains three times more white rice flour than brown rice flour, the brand of white rice flour has a bigger impact on the success of any baked good.

- Some brands don't absorb liquid and fat as well as others. As a result, many cookies spread too much or had an unpleasant greasy feel. Cookies made with Arrowhead Mills seemed to almost fry while baking in the fat that was not absorbed.

- Because they are baked in a contained vessel, the cupcakes were more forgiving. That said, cupcakes made with Arrowhead Mills didn't rise as well and were both gritty (from the coarser grind) and mushy (because the flour wasn't absorbing liquid as well).

- Flours that are more coarsely ground impart a starchy, gritty texture you can taste. This was most apparent with Arrowhead Mills white and brown rice flours as well as Hodgson Mills brown rice flour (this company doesn't make white rice flour).

- Some brands of brown rice flour have an odd earthy flavor. Now Foods was the biggest offender.

- We found Bob's Red Mill (the most widely available brand of white and brown rice flour) to be the best, although several other flours were acceptable, including EnerG (white and brown), Living Now (white), and King Arthur (brown). If using another brand of rice flour, the texture should be close to that of cornstarch, with no more than a hint of grit.

BOB'S RED MILL RICE FLOURS
These cookies spread nicely and had just the right balance of crispy edges and chewy centers.

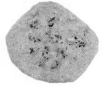

ARROWHEAD MILLS RICE FLOURS
These cookies spread too much and seemed to fry in unabsorbed fat, resulting in a candy-like texture.

Rice Flour, Brown: Since it still contains the bran, brown rice flour has more fiber, fat, and protein than white rice flour. It has a sandy texture like white rice flour, but a nuttier, earthier flavor (just like brown rice in comparison to white rice). Because of its fat content, brown rice flour has a short shelf life and should not be stored in the pantry. Look for brown rice flour that is as finely ground as possible.
Protein: 7%
Best Use: Our flour blend and fresh pasta
Where to Store It: Refrigerator or freezer

Rice Flour, White: Made from rice after the bran and germ have been removed, white rice flour has a neutral flavor, light color, and somewhat sandy texture. It is affordable, fairly easy to find, and has a long shelf life. Look for white rice flour that is as finely ground as possible, with little or no grit. For best results when making recipes in this book, we recommend using Bob's Red Mill white and brown rice flours.
Protein: 5%
Best Use: Our flour blend
Where to Store It: Pantry

STARCHES

Like the flours, each starch behaves differently—they are not interchangeable. Most of these starches are already familiar to you, and you'll find that you use them in a variety of roles for both cooking and baking applications.

Cornstarch: This refined product, made from the starchy endosperm of corn, has a neutral flavor and has long been used as a thickener for sauces and gravies. Some gluten-free recipes use it in large quantities in baked goods, but we found this approach sometimes imparted a starchy texture. In addition, cornstarch isn't the most nutritious ingredient, so using it by the cupful isn't terribly appealing.
Best Use: Thickener for sauces; dusted onto meat, poultry, and fish to absorb moisture and to encourage breading to cling; component in the frying/breading coating itself to encourage browning and crispness
Where to Store It: Pantry

Potato Starch: Made by dehydrating a slurry of water and peeled potatoes, potato starch provides structure, along with tenderness and binding power. However, it requires a higher baking temperature (and thus more time and moisture) than tapioca starch (see below) to reach its maximum viscosity. This makes it most useful in longer-cooking baked goods that have more moisture, like muffins or quick breads (tapioca starch is more effective in cookies). Do not confuse it with potato flour, which is made from cooked unpeeled potatoes and has a definite potato flavor.
Best Use: Our flour blend
Where to Store It: Pantry

Tapioca Starch: Made from the starchy tuberous root of the cassava plant, this white powder provides chew, elasticity, and structure to baked goods. Tapioca starch is sometimes labeled tapioca flour even though it contains no protein and is a pure starch. Either product can be used in our recipes.
Best Use: Our flour blend and moist breads such as cornbread and Brazilian cheese bread
Where to Store It: Pantry

OTHER HELPFUL INGREDIENTS

In the absence of gluten's structural power, you'll find that leaveners become absolutely critical in creating the necessary amount of lift and browning in your baked goods. Many of the recipes in this book rely on multiple leaveners and, in some cases, in comparatively large quantities. Binders such as xanthan gum, guar gum, and psyllium husk are essential in replacing that now-missing structure typically provided by gluten. See page 16 for more information on our testing of these three binders.

Baking Soda: Containing just bicarbonate of soda, baking soda provides lift to cakes, muffins, and other baked goods both traditional and gluten-free. When baking soda, which is alkaline, encounters an acidic ingredient (such as sour cream, buttermilk, or brown sugar), carbon and oxygen combine to form carbon dioxide. The tiny bubbles of carbon dioxide then lift up the dough. In addition to lift, baking soda helps cookies spread and improves browning in everything from cornbread to fried chicken.
Best Use: Baked goods including muffins, pancakes, cookies, and cakes as well as breaded or fried coatings
Where to Store It: Pantry

Baking Powder: Baking powder creates carbon dioxide to provide lift to baked goods. Cooks use baking powder rather than baking soda when there is no natural acidity in the batter. The active ingredients in baking powder are baking soda and an acidic element, such as cream of tartar. It also contains cornstarch to absorb moisture and keep the powder dry. These three ingredients are naturally gluten-free, so there should be nothing to worry about in theory. However, wheat starch is sometimes used in place of the cornstarch, so make sure to check the ingredient list on the nutritional label when buying baking powder. Also note that some brands may be produced in a facility that also processes wheat, and if this is the case then this information will also be noted on the label. As with baking soda, baking powder is sometimes added to savory breaded or fried coatings for improved texture and chew.
Best Use: Baked goods including muffins, pancakes, cookies, and cakes as well as breaded or fried coatings
Where to Store It: Pantry

Yeast: Active dry yeast is the most commonly called-for type of yeast. In order to use active dry yeast, the granules must first be proofed, or dissolved in liquid. Instant, or rapid-rise, yeast does not require proofing and can be added directly to the dry ingredients when making bread—hence the name "instant." Our recipes call for instant yeast because it's easier to use.

To substitute active dry for instant yeast, use 25 percent more active dry. For example, if the recipe calls for 1 teaspoon of instant yeast, use 1¼ teaspoons of active dry. And don't forget to proof the active dry yeast—that is, dissolve it in a portion of the water from the recipe, heated to 105 degrees.

Best Use: Breads, rolls, and coffee cakes

Where to Store It: Refrigerator (and pay attention to the expiration date)

Cream of Tartar: This fine white powder is sold in small bottles in the spice aisle, but it's not actually a spice. Cream of tartar is a byproduct of the wine-making process. It is used to help stabilize egg whites when they are whipped. This is especially important in gluten-free recipes, which often depend on whipped egg whites for structure and height. How does cream of tartar work? As an acid, it lowers the pH of the egg whites. This slows down the process by which the proteins link up and form a foam. The longer it takes for the proteins to link up, the stronger the foam will be—and a stable foam is key to tall cakes and sturdy meringues.

Best Use: Dishes with whipped egg whites, including yellow layer cake and pavlova

Where to Store It: Pantry

Nonfat Milk Powder: This shelf-stable dehydrated dairy product is incredibly helpful in gluten-free baking. It acts as an emulsifier, which contributes to structure by helping proteins and starches hydrate more readily so that they can then swell and form networks more effectively. It also helps gluten-free flours become more compatible with fat (gluten-free flours can't absorb fat as much as wheat flour can). It also adds dairy flavor, and the lactose sugar and milk proteins help with browning.

Best Use: Our flour blend and some yeast breads

Where to Store It: Pantry

Xanthan Gum: Made by using the microorganism *Xanthomonas campestris* to ferment simple sugars, xanthan gum is used widely as a thickener and stabilizer in commercial products like prepared salad dressings and toothpaste. It serves many roles in gluten-free baking. Because gluten-free flours have less protein than wheat flours and are not capable of forming the same network required to stretch and surround starch granules, they need reinforcement. Xanthan gum strengthens these networks and also makes them more elastic. Essentially, adding xanthan gum is like adding glue to the proteins in gluten-free flour. It also increases the shelf life of baked goods. Yes, xanthan gum is expensive, but you only need a little bit.

Best Use: Most baked goods to add structure and increase shelf life; see page 16 for more information

Where to Store It: Refrigerator or freezer

Guar Gum: A powder derived from the ground endosperm of guar seeds, guar gum is high in fiber so it is often sold as a laxative. It works like xanthan gum in adding structure and thickener, although it does impart a slightly starchy texture to baked goods. We prefer to use xanthan rather than guar gum, but the two are interchangeable in most recipes.

Best Use: See page 16 for information on using guar gum in place of xanthan gum

Where to Store It: Pantry

Powdered Psyllium Husk: Psyllium seed husk powder is one of the major components of Metamucil and Colon Cleanse. Its high viscosity makes it a very good laxative. Its chemical composition is similar to that of xanthan gum, but it has a higher viscosity, so it is able to bind water even more effectively. We have found that psyllium interacts strongly with the proteins in gluten-free flours, creating a sturdy network capable of holding in lots of gas and steam during baking, and it provides a strong enough structure to support highly leavened bread once the bread cools. It adds wheat flavor that works well in breads where "whole-wheat" flavor is appropriate.

Best Use: Yeast breads; see page 16 for more information

Where to Store It: Pantry

Gluten-Free Sandwich Bread

When you're avoiding gluten, it's tough to give up toast and sandwiches. Enter gluten-free bread: a multi-billion-dollar industry that's rapidly expanding as the trend of avoiding gluten for dietary reasons continues to grow. Hoping to find a loaf that was a serviceable alternative to (not a sacrifice compared with) regular sandwich bread, we tasted eight national brands of gluten-free white sandwich bread both plain and toasted with butter.

THE BAD NEWS

Almost all of the breads were very unappealing straight out of the packaging. Toasting and buttering turned a few inedible samples palatable, but most were still subpar by our sandwich bread standards. The exception: our winning bread, whose "light wheatiness" and "yielding" chew were impressively close to that of regular white bread. So what was this manufacturer doing differently?

HOW TO REPLACE GLUTEN

First we reviewed how gluten works in bread. When the proteins in wheat flour (and other grain flours like barley and rye) are combined with water and kneaded, they link into a network that strengthens dough. This linked structure helps baking bread trap gas as it rises, allowing the loaf to expand and achieve a lighter, springier crumb and satisfying chew. Replacing gluten is tricky because alternative flours don't contain these structure-building proteins.

THE GOOD NEWS

However, when we compared the nutrition labels on all eight loaves (to make even comparisons among samples with different serving sizes, we converted all nutrition values to base them on a 100-gram serving), we noticed that our winner contained far more protein than the competing breads—as much as 72 percent more. Its source? Lots of protein-rich egg whites. Like gluten, egg whites build structure by trapping air in the baking bread. Our gluten-free winner also adds chemical leaveners and, of course, yeast, which contribute to more lift, along with a goodly amount of salt (our favorite regular sandwich loaf contains 43 percent less sodium), which boosts flavor.

LOOK IN FREEZER CASE

We also looked into why gluten-free breads are sold from the freezer case. It turns out that most of these products are high in moisture (as much as 55 percent compared with roughly 36 percent for regular sandwich bread) and starch—qualities that make them stale easily due to a process called retrogradation. The more water and starch in the bread, the more susceptible its starch molecules are to moving around and crystallizing (trapping water inside the crystals), which renders the crumb dry. Freezing halts the staling process since the frozen starch molecules can't move around. (The lone product that wasn't frozen came vacuum-sealed with a sell-by date six months away.) What's more, gluten-free bread turnover in supermarkets is slow, so freezing makes sense.

THE BOTTOM LINE

If you're looking for a gluten-free option, our winner has a clean, yeasty flavor and a moderate amount of chew, making it the best—and only worthwhile—alternative to regular sandwich bread.

WHAT ABOUT COOKING?

We use regular sandwich bread as a binder for meatballs and meatloaf and as a coating for chicken cutlets. When making a panade for meatballs or meatloaf, gluten-free sandwich breads did not turn into the necessary smooth paste and never disappeared into the meat. Simply put, don't use gluten-free sandwich bread this way. We had better results turning gluten-free sandwich bread into fresh crumbs for coating chicken, although browning varied significantly because of the different ingredients used to make each brand. And we needed to toast the crumbs before using them as a coating in order to make them less sticky. For best results when breading foods, we recommend that you stick with our top-rated sandwich bread.

Rating Sandwich Breads

Our tasting panel tasted each sample twice—straight from the package (defrosted per directions provided, when necessary) and toasted with butter. The scores from the two tastings were averaged to determine overall rankings.

RECOMMENDED

UDI'S Gluten Free White Sandwich Bread
PRICE: $5.00 for 12-oz loaf
PROTEIN: 8.2 g in 100 g
SODIUM: 612 mg in 100 g
TASTERS' COMMENTS: Thanks to its high protein and salt levels, this bread "looked good," "smelled nice," and boasted an "airy texture." Toasted, it was "crunchy yet yielding"—"close to 'real' bread."

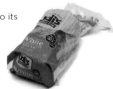

RECOMMENDED WITH RESERVATIONS

CANYON BAKEHOUSE Mountain White Gluten Free Bread
PRICE: $5.00 for 18-oz loaf
PROTEIN: 5.9 g in 100 g
SODIUM: 324 mg in 100 g
TASTERS' COMMENTS: This bread tasted "a little boring but not actually bad." Its texture, however, was noticeably inferior. Even after toasting, it was "mushy," "gummy," "stretchy," and "rubbery"—like "toast-flavored chewing gum"—with a "slightly gritty finish."

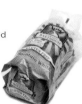

NOT RECOMMENDED

KINNIKINNICK White Bread, Gluten Free
PRICE: $4.99 for 16-oz loaf
PROTEIN: 3.5 g in 100 g
SODIUM: 351 mg in 100 g
TASTERS' COMMENTS: "As bland as white Minute Rice." "Very fragile, papery, gums up in the mouth." Toasting gave it a "very crisp crust," but its texture was still problematic: "The butter wasn't absorbed by the toast—it floated on the surface!" while the crumb "sticks to your teeth."

SCHÄR Classic White Bread Gluten-Free Wheat-Free
PRICE: $6.29 for 14.1-oz loaf
PROTEIN: 6.7 g in 100 g
SODIUM: 400 mg in 100 g
TASTERS' COMMENTS: "This is not bread," one taster declared. "This is . . . sad." Its "very yeasty smell" was deceiving, as the slices were "dry" and "sandy," and toasting only made them "gummy" and "dense," with the flavor of "sourdough Play-Doh."

NOT RECOMMENDED (continued)

GENIUS BY GLUTINO Gluten Free White Sandwich Bread
PRICE: $5.99 for 14.1-oz loaf
PROTEIN: 6.9 g in 100 g
SODIUM: 483 mg in 100 g
TASTERS' COMMENTS: Beyond its "brittle foam" crumb that "disintegrated in your mouth," tasters bemoaned this bread's blandness: "I can't comment on flavor because there is none." Except when it was toasted: Then tasters thought it tasted like "fake popcorn."

RUDI'S Gluten Free Organic Original
PRICE: $6.29 for 18-oz loaf
PROTEIN: 2.7 g in 100 g
SODIUM: 405 mg in 100 g
TASTERS' COMMENTS: Tasters picked up on the honey and molasses in this bread but found it "cloying"—like a "burnt marshmallow." Its texture was a turnoff, too: "very dry but with a finer crumb, like sweet, soft sand" that "breaks into a million pieces the minute it hits your mouth."

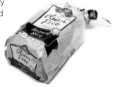

FOOD FOR LIFE Gluten Free White Rice Bread
PRICE: $6.79 for 24-oz loaf
PROTEIN: 2.3 g in 100 g
SODIUM: 535 mg in 100 g
TASTERS' COMMENTS: A measly amount of protein left this bread with "no structure at all," not to mention "hard, with a grainy, seedy texture" that was "not the least bit edible." Its flavor was "super-stale," with a "horrible aftertaste."

ENERG Gluten Free Tapioca Loaf, Regular Sliced
PRICE: $5.79 for 16-oz loaf
PROTEIN: 3.6 g in 100 g
SODIUM: 446 mg in 100 g
TASTERS' COMMENTS: This bread didn't just taste like "cardboard." It was "flat" and "dense," like a "coaster." Several tasters had to force themselves to eat more than one bite and regretted the "insanely dense," "scratchy" texture. In sum: "Why bother?"

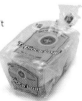

Gluten-Free Pasta

Just because you're no longer eating wheat doesn't mean that pasta is off the menu. There are two routes you can take—Asian noodles that traditionally don't contain wheat, or gluten-free approximations of classic Italian pasta.

SOBA NOODLES

Shopping: Soba noodles possess a rich, nutty flavor and delicate texture. They get their flavor from buckwheat flour. Be aware that many brands also contain wheat, which not only keeps the price down but gives the noodles more structure. Make sure to read the label and look for those that contain buckwheat flour only.

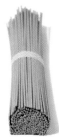

Cooking: Soba noodles should be cooked like Italian-style pasta. Since they are often used in Asian-inspired recipes that include salty ingredients like tamari, there is often no need to salt the water.

To cook soba noodles: Bring 4 quarts water to boil in large pot. Add noodles and cook, stirring often, until tender. Reserve ½ cup cooking water (for thinning sauce, if necessary) and drain noodles.

RICE NOODLES

Shopping: This delicate pasta, made from rice flour and water, is used in a variety of dishes in Southeast Asia and southern China. Flat rice noodles come in several widths; we use a medium-width (¼-inch-wide) noodle in Pad Thai with Shrimp (page 126), but like a larger (⅜-inch-wide) noodle in other recipes. Round rice noodles also come in a variety of sizes, but we prefer the thinner rice vermicelli, which are used in Singapore Noodles with Shrimp (page 124).

Cooking: Don't follow the package directions, which often call for boiling. Such treatment will turn these delicate noodles into a gummy, mushy, unappealing mess. You'll get the most reliable results by steeping these noodles in hot water.

To rehydrate rice noodles: Place noodles in very large bowl, cover with very hot tap water, and stir to separate. Let noodles soak until they are softened, pliable, and limp but not fully tender, 20 minutes for vermicelli or narrow flat noodles or 35 to 40 minutes for wide flat noodles. Drain noodles and use as directed.

LASAGNA NOODLES

Shopping: Gluten-free lasagna noodles are available in both no-boil and boil-before-use forms. We found that no-boil gluten-free noodles varied considerably; some brands were thick and cooked up gummy, while others were thin and fragile. We had better luck using noodles that we boiled. There are just a few brands on the market. We had the most success with Tinkyada; they were tender once cooked and held up well, while other brands were incredibly fragile.

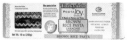

Cooking: Boil them for a bit less time than the package instructions indicate so they don't fall apart.

To prepare lasagna noodles: Bring 4 quarts water to boil in large pot. Add noodles and 1 tablespoon salt and cook, stirring frequently, until just tender. Drain noodles, return them to pot, and toss with 1 teaspoon olive oil. Spread oiled noodles out in single layer on baking sheet to prevent sticking.

DRIED ITALIAN-STYLE PASTA

Shopping: We ran an extensive taste test of gluten-free spaghetti (see following pages). In subsequent work in the test kitchen, we had excellent results with other shapes manufactured by Jovial, winner of our spaghetti tasting.

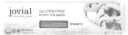

Cooking: As with wheat pasta, we found that cooking times listed on packages of gluten-free pasta are often inaccurate. You must taste pasta often as it cooks. Also note that gluten-free pasta goes from al dente to mush even faster than wheat-based pasta, so err on the side of undercooking the noodles. Our recipes often call for reserving some of the starchy cooking water to help loosen sauces. Place a measuring cup in the colander so you remember not to pour all the cooking water down the drain.

To cook dried pasta: Bring 4 quarts water to boil in large pot. Add pasta and 1 tablespoon salt and cook, stirring often, until tender. Reserve cooking liquid as directed and drain.

Italian-Style Dried Pasta

In traditional Italian-style dried pasta, gluten is critically important. This protein matrix provides the structure that keeps noodles intact and pleasantly springy. For people who are avoiding gluten in their diets, finding good wheat-free pasta with the right texture and flavor is a challenge, one which has been met in a variety of ways by pasta manufacturers. We sampled eight brands of gluten-free spaghetti made from substitute grains—mainly rice, quinoa, and corn—that lack the specific proteins necessary to form gluten. Each pasta was boiled and tasted with olive oil, then with tomato sauce in a second round.

ONE STANDOUT

The results were unambiguous: Most brands absolutely failed to meet our standards. Tomato sauce provided some distraction that improved scores, but not by much. Most of these pastas disappointed with textures that managed, despite careful cooking, to be both "mushy" and "gritty." And many tasters complained about flavors that ranged from "bland" to "fishy." But there was a lone standout that tasters described as "clean" and "springy."

CORN, NO THANKS

We examined the labels, looking for clues to our preferences. Our first discovery was that two brands that billed themselves as "quinoa" pasta were frankly misleading: one contained more rice flour than quinoa; the other was principally made of corn. We definitely didn't enjoy any of the pastas containing corn; all three fell in the bottom half of our rankings.

HIGH FIBER, HIGH PROTEIN

Our favorite pasta is made with brown rice, and it contains a relatively high combined total of fiber and protein (the combined total matters more than the amount of either fiber or protein alone). It turns out that protein and fiber keep the noodles intact during cooking, forming a barrier around the starch molecules, which prevents them from escaping and leaving the cooked pasta sticky and soft. If the protein network fails, the starch leaches into the cooking water, turning it cloudy—something we observed when cooking the lower-rated brands. In addition, we also learned that corn proteins are more water-soluble than those in rice, leaving even less protein to surround and control the starch. No surprise, then, that we gave thumbs-down to the texture of corn-based pasta.

DRYING MATTERS

Just as important, our winning brand uses a low-temperature drying method, which helps preserve flavor and ensures that the proteins coagulate and provide structure for the starch. Our favorite pasta is dried in a 70-degree room for 12 to 14 hours. In contrast, lower-rated brands are dried quickly, in as little as 3½ hours in rooms heated as high as 160 degrees. Our favorite wheat-based pasta likewise uses a similar drying method, which takes more time (and money), but it does seem to make a difference in the final product, whether made with wheat or brown rice.

THE BOTTOM LINE

High-protein, high-fiber brown rice makes a stronger pasta, and the flavor is surprisingly close to that of whole-wheat pasta. Jovial Gluten Free Brown Rice Spaghetti tasted "pretty close to the real deal." Other brands, however, were disappointing.

Rating Italian-Style Dried Pastas

Pastas were boiled in abundant salted water until al dente and then promptly drained. Our tasting panel tasted each sample twice—once tossed with olive oil and once with a basic tomato sauce. The scores from the two tastings were averaged to determine overall rankings.

RECOMMENDED

JOVIAL Gluten Free Brown Rice Spaghetti
PRICE: $3.99 for 12 oz ($0.33 per oz)
INGREDIENTS: Organic brown rice flour, water
TASTERS' COMMENTS: Thanks to a relatively high combined total of fiber and protein and a low, slow drying process, these "delicate and thin" brown rice strands were "springy" and "clean," with none of the gumminess or off-flavors that plagued other brands.

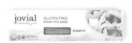

RECOMMENDED WITH RESERVATIONS

ANDEAN DREAM Gluten Free Quinoa Spaghetti
PRICE: $4.39 for 8 oz ($0.55 per oz)
INGREDIENTS: Organic rice flour, organic quinoa flour
TASTERS' COMMENTS: Several tasters noted that this "slightly translucent," "plastic"-looking rice and quinoa pasta was "rubbery," like "Twizzlers," and a few noted that its generally "neutral," "bland" flavor took on a "fishy," "ashy" aftertaste when eaten plain. At least tomato sauce camouflaged some of those off-flavors.

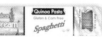

NOT RECOMMENDED

BIONATURAE Gluten Free Organic Spaghetti
PRICE: $3.99 for 12 oz ($0.33 per oz)
INGREDIENTS: Organic rice flour, organic rice starch, organic potato starch, organic soy flour
TASTERS' COMMENTS: The "soft," "super-mushy" texture of this pasta was likely due to high-temperature drying, which can cause the dough's protein structure to break down. It was also "utterly bland"—a flaw that was helped only moderately by adding sauce.

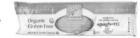

ANCIENT HARVEST Gluten Free Quinoa Spaghetti
PRICE: $3.29 for 8 oz ($0.41 per oz)
INGREDIENTS: Organic corn flour, organic quinoa flour
TASTERS' COMMENTS: This so-called quinoa spaghetti actually contains more corn than quinoa—so much so that its color is "neon yellow," and one taster likened it to eating a "boiled corn muffin." Tasters also universally panned its texture—the "gritty," "gummy" strands "dissolve and break apart," they complained.

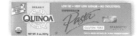

NOT RECOMMENDED (continued)

TINKYADA Brown Rice Pasta Spaghetti Style Gluten Free
PRICE: $3.59 for 1 lb ($0.22 per oz)
INGREDIENTS: Brown rice, rice bran, and water
TASTERS' COMMENTS: These brown rice strands elicited far fewer complaints for their "neutral"—if a bit "metallic"—flavor than they did for their texture. Most tasters couldn't get past the "very thick chew" of these "rubbery ropes," even when they were covered with tomato sauce.

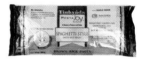

RUSTICHELLA Gluten Free Spaghetti Pasta—100% Corn
PRICE: $8.80 for 8.8 oz ($1.00 per oz)
INGREDIENTS: Organic corn flour, water
TASTERS' COMMENTS: There was no debating what these strands were made of. They tasted like "raw corn flour," one taster complained, while another compared their flavor to "sawdust" and found them "gritty" and even "gluey," perhaps as a result of the high-temperature drying process. Plus, their "abnormally yellow" color was "alarming."

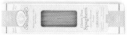

DELALLO Gluten-Free Pasta Corn/Rice Spaghetti
PRICE: $4.99 for 12 oz ($0.42 per oz)
INGREDIENTS: Corn flour, rice flour
TASTERS' COMMENTS: Due to the lack of fiber and protein and the brief, hot drying process, this corn- and rice-based spaghetti cooked up "sticky" and "mushy"; some tasters even complained that it "fell apart and clumped together" into "one big starch ball." Worse, the flavor was "flat" and "corn-ish."

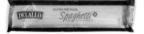

DEBOLES Gluten Free Rice Spaghetti-Style Pasta
PRICE: $3.99 for 8 oz ($0.50 per oz)
INGREDIENTS: Rice flour, rice bran extract
TASTERS' COMMENTS: "Gummy," "mushy," and "gluey" were the watchwords for this rice-based pasta that contained almost no fiber. Tasters also complained about a "weird, bitter wet paper flavor" that gave way to an "awful aftertaste." In sum: "This is not pasta."

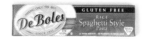

Gluten-Free Grains

The world of grains is a big one—which is a great thing for those who can't eat gluten. True, there are a number of familiar grains, like wheat berries, barley, and farro, that are off-limits, but the list of grains that are gluten-free is notably long. Rice is an obvious starting point; in that category alone there are a number of options. And there is plenty beyond rice, with enough variety in flavor and texture that repetition and boredom certainly won't be an issue. Below are the grains we use in this book; make sure to look at the recipes in chapter 2. For basic cooking directions, see page 30. The following grains can all be found in natural food stores and well-stocked supermarkets.

BROWN RICE

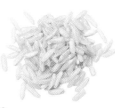

All rice (except wild) starts out as brown rice. Each grain of rice is made up of an endosperm, germ, bran, and a protective outer hull or husk. Brown rice is rice that has been simply husked and cleaned. Considered a whole grain, brown rice has more fiber and vitamins than white rice, along with a firmer texture and a nuttier, earthier flavor. Keep in mind that the bran and germ contain oils that shorten the rice's shelf life. Brown rice takes longer to cook than white rice because it requires more time to allow water to penetrate the bran.

Brown rice comes in a variety of grain sizes: short, medium, and long. Long-grain brown rice, the best choice for pilafs, cooks up fluffy with separate grains. (See page 71 for shopping recommendations.) Medium-grain brown rice is a bit more sticky, perfect for risotto, paella, and similar dishes. Short-grain brown rice is the most sticky, ideal for sushi and other Asian dishes where getting the grains to clump together is desired.

WHITE RICE

Like brown rice, white rice has been husked and cleaned, but then it is processed a step further by removing the germ and bran. This makes the rice cook up faster and softer, and it's more shelf-stable, but the process also removes much of the fiber, protein, and other nutrients, as well as flavor.

Like brown rice, white rice can be long-, medium-, or short-grained. Long-grain is a broad category and includes generic long-grain rice as well as aromatic varieties such as basmati and jasmine (see below for more about these three varieties). The grains are slender and elongated and measure four to five times longer than they are wide. Long-grain white rice cooks up light and fluffy, with firm, distinct grains, making it good for pilafs and salads.

Medium-grain white rice includes a wide variety of specialty rices used to make risotto (Arborio; see following page) and paella (Valencia), as well as many Japanese and Chinese brands. The grains are fat and measure two to three times longer than they are wide. Medium-grain white rice cooks up a bit sticky, and when simmered the grains clump together, making this rice a common choice in Chinese restaurants.

With the exception of sushi, we don't eat much shortgrain white rice in this country. The grains are almost round, and the texture is quite sticky and soft when cooked.

Avoid converted rice, which is parboiled during processing. This tan-colored rice cooks up too separate in our opinion, and the flavor seems a bit off.

BASMATI RICE

Prized for its nutty flavor and sweet aroma, basmati rice is eaten in pilafs and biryanis and with curries. Indian basmati is aged for a minimum of a year, though often much longer, before being packaged. Aging dehydrates the rice, which translates into grains that, once cooked, expand greatly. We don't recommend American-grown basmati.

JASMINE RICE

From Southeast Asia, jasmine rice has an aroma similar to basmati rice, but the texture is stickier and moister and the grain size is much smaller. Because it clumps together when cooked, jasmine rice works well in stir-fries. It's also nice in soups.

ARBORIO RICE

Arborio, the variety of medium-grain rice that we use in the test kitchen to make risotto, was once grown exclusively in Italy. Now widely available, these stubby, milky grains have a high starch content, which is what enables them to make such creamy risotto. See page 76 for shopping recommendations.

OTHER RICES FOR RISOTTO

Carnaroli and vialone nano are two other varieties of Italian rice often used to make risotto. We have found that carnaroli produces a softer, creamier risotto than Arborio and is a fine substitute (if you can find it); however, while we've read that vialone nano is the popular choice around Venice, where a decidedly lose, soupy texture is the desired consistency for risotto, we find it too soft and pasty, and it lacks the firm center of the other two varieties.

WILD RICE

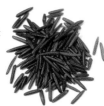

Wild rice is technically not in the same family as other rices; it's actually an aquatic grass. North America's only native grain, it grows naturally in lakes and is cultivated in man-made paddies in Minnesota, California, and Canada. Its smooth grains have a remarkably nutty, savory depth and a distinct chew that make it an ideal choice for a hearty side dish or addition to soup. See page 73 for shopping recommendations.

BUCKWHEAT GROATS AND KASHA

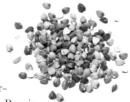

Buckwheat, despite its name, is not related to wheat but is in fact an herb that is related to sorrel and rhubarb. Native to Russia, buckwheat appears in cuisines all over the globe, particularly in Eastern Europe and Japan (think soba noodles).

Buckwheat has an assertive flavor and can be found in several forms. Hulled, crushed buckwheat seeds are known as buckwheat groats, and because of their high carbohydrate content they are generally treated like a grain. Grayish green in color, groats have a mildly earthy flavor. They are often eaten as a staple like rice and are baked into puddings and porridges.

Kasha is buckwheat groats that have been roasted. This process gives kasha a darker color and a noticeably earthier and roasty flavor that some people love, and others don't. Kasha is often served pilaf-style and as a hot cereal and is traditionally used in blintzes, combined with pasta to make a traditional Eastern European Jewish dish called kasha varnishkas, and included as part of a filling for pastries known as knishes.

Buckwheat's triangular seeds can also be ground to make flour; see page 18 for more details.

CORNMEAL

For many consumers, buying cornmeal used to mean picking up a container of Quaker, or perhaps (especially if you lived in the South) a stone-ground local variety. But at most supermarkets today, you've got a lot more options to sort through: fine-, medium-, and coarse-ground; instant and quick-cooking; whole-grain, stone-ground, and regular. What do they all mean, which should you buy, and does it even matter?

Yes, it definitely does matter. Whether you are making Southern-style cornbread, pancakes, polenta, or a rustic Italian-style cake, different recipes require different grinds and types of cornmeal. What you use can make a big difference. Make sure to read—and buy—carefully. See page 149 for shopping recommendations.

MILLET

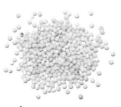

Believed to be the first domesticated cereal grain, this tiny cereal grass seed has a long history and is still a staple in a large part of the world, particularly in Asia and Africa. The seeds can be ground into flour or used whole. Millet has a mellow corn flavor that works well in both savory and sweet applications, including flatbreads, puddings, and pan-fried cakes. It can be cooked pilaf-style or turned into a creamy breakfast porridge or polenta-like dish by slightly overcooking the seeds, which causes the seeds to burst and release starch. To add texture to baked goods, try incorporating a small amount of millet into the batter.

OATS

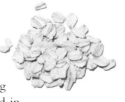

From breakfast table to cookie jar, this nutritious cereal grass is a versatile part of the gluten-free diet. But be careful when buying oats; they're often processed in facilities that also process wheat, which creates cross-contamination issues. It's therefore critical to make sure you are buying oats that are processed in a gluten-free facility. Oats come in several forms: groats (see below), old-fashioned rolled oats, steel cut, and instant. See page 62 for more details on shopping for oats.

STORING GRAINS

To prevent open boxes and bags of grains from spoiling in the pantry, store them in airtight containers and, if you have space, in the freezer. This is especially important for whole grains that turn rancid with oxidation.

OAT BERRIES (OAT GROATS)

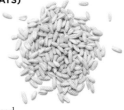

Labeled either oat berries or oat groats, this gluten-free whole grain is simply whole oats that have been hulled and cleaned. They are the least processed oat product (other forms are processed further, such as being rolled flat, cut, or ground). Because they haven't been processed, they retain a high nutritional value. They have an appealing chewy texture and a mildly nutty flavor. Oats are usually thought of as a breakfast cereal, but oat berries make a great savory side dish cooked pilaf-style.

QUINOA

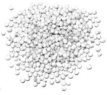

Quinoa originated in the Andes Mountains of South America, and while it is generally treated as a grain, it is actually the seed of the goosefoot plant. Sometimes referred to as a "super grain," quinoa is high in protein, and its protein is complete, which means it possesses all of the amino acids in the balanced amounts that our bodies require. Beyond its nutritional prowess, we love quinoa for its addictive crunchy texture, nutty taste, and ease of preparation. Cooked as a pilaf or for a salad, it can be ready in about 20 minutes. Unless labeled "prewashed," quinoa should always be rinsed before cooking to remove its protective layer (called saponin), which is unpleasantly bitter. Also see page 83 for details about the various colors of quinoas.

Cooking Grains

As you can see, creating variety in your diet with gluten-free grains won't be an issue; however, properly cooking those grains could be if you simply follow the package instructions. While you can get by with decent results doing this, we've spent plenty of time in the test kitchen working with these grains and fine-tuning our techniques to ensure you get the best results every time.

There are two basic ways to cook grains: either with a measured amount of water or in abundant water. The latter method (called the pasta method) is best for larger grains that take a long time to cook. Simply boil them in a big pot of salted water and drain when tender. With so much water in the pot, there's no risk of the pot running dry. And all that water ensures even, thorough cooking. For smaller grains, like rice and millet, we cook them with a measured amount of water in a covered pot over low heat, using either the absorption or the pilaf method (however, we have a unique oven method for cooking brown rice; see our recipe on page 70). Once all the water has been absorbed, the grains are done. In general, we prefer the pilaf method because it adds a nutty, toasted flavor. However, the absorption method can work well in dishes where the grains will be seasoned aggressively once they are cooked.

Most grains should be rinsed before cooking to remove surface starch, detritus, or bitter coatings. (We prefer to buy quinoa labeled "prewashed," but if you're unsure, rinse it anyway to be sure to remove its saponin coating.) In some cases, we go on to dry the grains after rinsing since soggy grains can throw off the water-to-grain ratio. Also, soggy grains are hard to toast, which we do when cooking grains pilaf-style to deepen their flavor.

For the absorption or pilaf method, make sure to use a sturdy, heavy-bottomed saucepan with a tight-fitting lid. Following are the general directions; refer to the chart on the opposite page for specific water amounts.

PASTA METHOD

This method is well suited to larger grains (like oat berries) because it guarantees even cooking. In some cases, toasting the grains before adding the water lends a flavor boost. Grains cooked this way are ready to use in salads and soups. To quickly cool boiled grains for a salad, rinse them with cold running water.

Bring 2 quarts water to boil in Dutch oven. Stir in 1 cup rinsed grains and 1 teaspoon salt. Return to boil, reduce heat to low, and simmer until grains are tender. Drain in strainer in sink. Let sit in strainer for 5 minutes before using (or pat dry with paper towels) to remove excess moisture.

ABSORPTION METHOD

This is the simplest way to prepare small grains like millet and quinoa. It's ideal when using these grains in salads. If you want fluffy rather than sticky grains, place a clean, folded dish towel between the pot and lid during the resting step to absorb excess moisture.

Combine 1 cup rinsed and dried grains, water, and ½ teaspoon salt in medium saucepan. Bring mixture to simmer, then reduce heat to low, cover, and simmer until grains are tender and liquid is absorbed. Off heat, let sit, covered, for 10 minutes. Fluff with fork and serve.

PILAF METHOD

Toasting the grains in fat develops nutty flavor (however, we toast quinoa in a dry pan since toasting in fat makes it taste slightly bitter). You can also sauté spices and aromatics before adding grains; swap in chicken broth for some of the water; and/or stir in fresh herbs before serving. If you want fluffy rather than sticky grains, place a clean, folded dish towel between the pot and lid during the resting step to absorb excess moisture.

Heat 1 tablespoon unsalted butter or oil in medium saucepan over medium-high heat until melted or shimmering, according to recipe. Add 1 cup rinsed and dried grains and toast until lightly golden and fragrant, about 3 minutes. Add ½ teaspoon salt and water. Bring mixture to simmer, then reduce heat to low, cover, and simmer until grains are tender and liquid is absorbed. Off heat, let sit, covered, for 10 minutes. Fluff with fork and serve.

Formulas for Cooking Grains

Use this chart to determine the amount of water and the cooking time needed to prepare 1 cup of grains. If you're using the absorption or pilaf methods, the grains should first be rinsed and dried well; if you're using the pasta method, simply rinse the grains. You can cook 2 or 3 cups of raw grains using the pasta method by increasing the water to 4 quarts; the cooking time will be the same. You can cook 2 cups of grains using the absorption or pilaf method by doubling the amount of water and salt; the cooking time might require a few extra minutes.

GRAIN	METHOD(S)	WATER	SALT	TIME	YIELD
Buckwheat Groats	Pasta	2 quarts	1 teaspoon	10–12 minutes	2¾ cups
Kasha (Roasted Buckwheat Groats)	Absorption or Pilaf	2 cups	½ teaspoon	10–15 minutes	3 cups
Millet	Absorption or Pilaf	2 cups	½ teaspoon	15–20 minutes	2¼ cups
Oat Berries (Oat Groats)	Absorption or Pilaf	1⅓ cups	¼ teaspoon	30–40 minutes	2¾ cups
	Pasta	2 quarts	½ teaspoon	45–50 minutes	2¾ cups
Quinoa (any color)	Absorption or Pilaf	1 cup plus 3 tablespoons	½ teaspoon	18–20 minutes	2¾ cups
Long-Grain White Rice, Jasmine, Basmati	Absorption or Pilaf	1½ cups	½ teaspoon	16–18 minutes	3 cups
	Pasta	2 quarts	1 teaspoon	12–17 minutes	3 cups
Long-Grain Brown Rice	Pasta	2 quarts	1 teaspoon	25–30 minutes	2½ cups
Wild Rice	Pasta	2 quarts	1 teaspoon	35–45 minutes	2½ cups

RINSING AND DRYING GRAINS

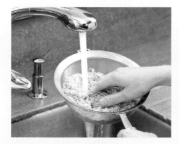

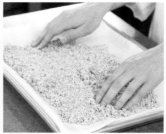

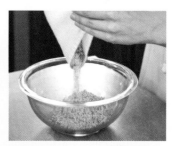

1. Rinse grains in fine-mesh strainer under cool water until water runs clear, occasionally stirring grains around lightly with your hand. Set strainer over bowl to drain until needed.

2. If drying grains, line rimmed baking sheet with clean dish towel and spread rinsed grains over towel. Let grains dry for 15 minutes.

3. To easily and neatly remove grains from towel, pick up towel by corners and gently shake grains into bowl.

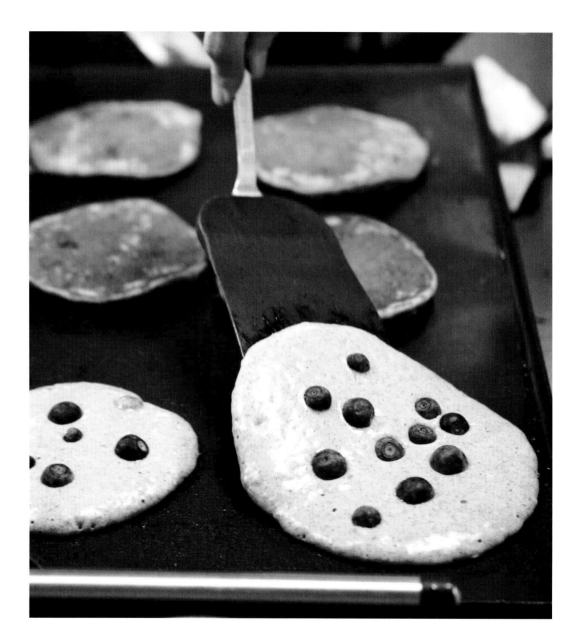

A GOOD START

Buttermilk Pancakes

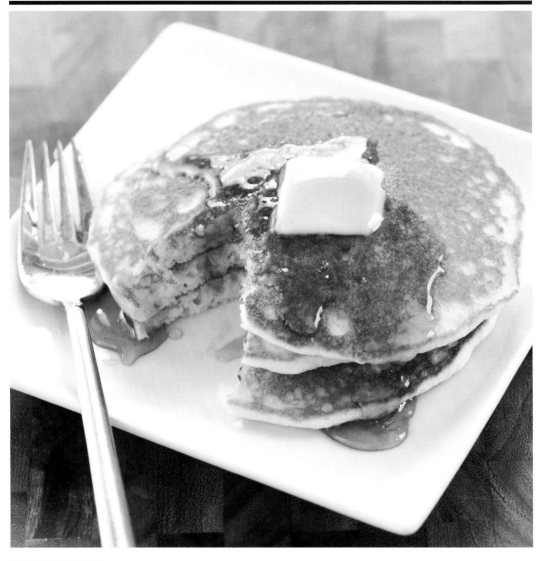

G-F TESTING LAB

FLOUR SUBSTITUTION	King Arthur Gluten-Free Multi-Purpose Flour 10½ ounces = **1⅔ cups plus ¼ cup**	Bob's Red Mill GF All-Purpose Baking Flour 10½ ounces = **2 cups plus 2 tablespoons**

Note that pancakes made with Bob's Red Mill will be flatter and have a distinct bean flavor.

Just because you need to avoid gluten doesn't mean you can't enjoy a leisurely Saturday morning pancake breakfast. But you can't just take a basic traditional recipe and plug in gluten-free flour—the results will be dense and gummy. We found that using both baking powder and baking soda, something we do with traditional pancake recipes as well, was key to keeping our gluten-free pancakes light and tender and ensuring they rose properly. But that wasn't quite enough. Instead of adding whole eggs to the batter, we separated the eggs, whipped the whites to stiff peaks, and gently folded them in. Yes, this step takes a few extra minutes, but it delivers gluten-free pancakes that are light, fluffy, and tender. Buttermilk gives these pancakes a nice tang and helps ensure a light, fluffy texture; see page 43 for buttermilk substitutes. To make blueberry pancakes, sprinkle 1 tablespoon berries over surface of each pancake immediately after adding the batter to the skillet, and cook as directed. You can add raspberries or blackberries the same way, as long as you chop any large berries.

Buttermilk Pancakes
MAKES SIXTEEN 3-INCH PANCAKES; SERVES 6

10½   **ounces (2⅓ cups) ATK Gluten-Free Flour Blend (page 13)**
  1   **teaspoon salt**
  1   **teaspoon baking powder (see page 20)**
  ½   **teaspoon baking soda**
1¾   **cups buttermilk**
  2   **large eggs, separated**
  4   **tablespoons unsalted butter, melted and cooled**
  2   **tablespoons sugar**
1–2   **teaspoons vegetable oil**

1. Adjust oven rack to middle position and heat oven to 200 degrees. Spray wire rack set inside rimmed baking sheet with vegetable oil spray; place in oven. Whisk flour blend, salt, baking powder, and baking soda together in large bowl. In separate bowl, whisk buttermilk, egg yolks, and melted butter until combined.

2. Using stand mixer fitted with whisk, whip egg whites on medium-low speed until foamy, about 1 minute. Increase speed to medium-high and whip whites to soft, billowy mounds, about 1 minute. Gradually add sugar and whip until glossy, stiff peaks form, 2 to 3 minutes.

3. Whisk buttermilk mixture into flour mixture until batter has thickened and no lumps remain, about 1 minute. Gently fold in whipped egg whites until just combined and few streaks remain.

4. Heat 1 teaspoon oil in 12-inch nonstick skillet over medium heat until shimmering, 3 to 5 minutes. Using paper towels, carefully wipe out oil, leaving thin film of oil on bottom and sides of pan. Using ¼ cup batter per pancake, portion batter into skillet and cook until bottoms of pancakes are brown and top surfaces start to bubble, 2 to 3 minutes. Flip pancakes and cook until second side has browned, 1 to 2 minutes longer. Serve immediately or transfer pancakes to wire rack in preheated oven (don't overlap). Repeat with remaining batter, using remaining oil as needed.

TEST KITCHEN TIP
Why Preheating the Skillet Matters

Did you fully preheat your skillet? We call for preheating it (with a teaspoon of oil) for a full 3 to 5 minutes; this step isn't one you can shortcut. A cooking surface that hasn't been allowed to heat up properly will produce pale, dense pancakes. If you aren't sure how hot the cooking surface is, cook a test pancake to get the lay of the land. After a few minutes in the pan, large bubbles should appear in the batter, indicating the pancake is ready to be flipped over. If the pancake isn't browned when flipped, your cooking surface needs to be hotter. Alternatively, if the pancakes are overly browned, you need to turn down the heat. Adjust the heat accordingly, give it a few minutes to preheat properly, and try again. If you own an electric griddle, set it to 325 degrees and lightly grease the cooking surface once it is fully preheated.

Buckwheat Blueberry Pancakes

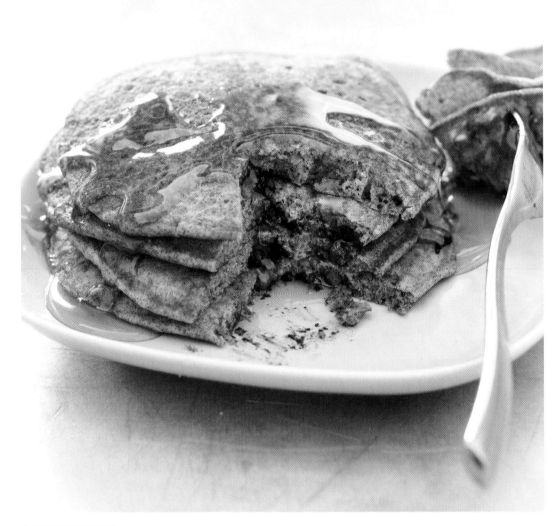

G-F TESTING LAB

FLOUR SUBSTITUTION	King Arthur Gluten-Free Multi-Purpose Flour 7 ounces = 1¼ **cups**	Bob's Red Mill GF All-Purpose Baking Flour 7 ounces = 1¼ **cups plus 2 tablespoons**
	Note that pancakes made with Bob's Red Mill will be flatter and have a distinct bean flavor.	

✔ WHY THIS RECIPE WORKS

Naturally gluten-free buckwheat flour is the main ingredient in Russian blini and can be used to make hearty, slightly savory American-style pancakes. Buckwheat has an assertive flavor, so we knew that substituting just a few ounces for some of the gluten-free flour blend in our Buttermilk Pancakes (page 34) would provide the nutty, slightly earthy flavor we were after without going overboard. Because buckwheat flour is slightly heavier than our gluten-free flour blend (think wheat flour compared to all-purpose), it was no surprise that our first batch of pancakes cooked up flat and gummy. Adding an extra whipped egg white to the batter gave our pancakes the proper rise. The tang of the buttermilk in our original pancake recipe competed with the flavor of the buckwheat, so we swapped it out for whole milk (and dropped the baking soda because it worked in tandem with the buttermilk). Sweeter, more complexly flavored honey in lieu of granulated sugar, plus a pinch of cinnamon, helped to balance and round out the flavors.

Buckwheat Blueberry Pancakes
MAKES SIXTEEN 3-INCH PANCAKES; SERVES 6

7	ounces (1⅓ cups plus ¼ cup) ATK Gluten-Free Flour Blend (page 13)
3½	ounces (¾ cup) buckwheat flour
2	teaspoons baking powder (see page 20)
1	teaspoon salt
½	teaspoon ground cinnamon
1¾	cups whole milk
3	large eggs, separated
4	tablespoons unsalted butter, melted and cooled
2	tablespoons honey
1–2	teaspoons vegetable oil
5	ounces (1 cup) blueberries

1. Adjust oven rack to middle position and heat oven to 200 degrees. Spray wire rack set inside rimmed baking sheet with vegetable oil spray; place in oven. Whisk flour blend, buckwheat flour, baking powder, salt, and cinnamon together in large bowl. In separate bowl, whisk milk, egg yolks, melted butter, and honey until combined.

2. Using stand mixer fitted with whisk, whip egg whites on medium-low speed until foamy, about 1 minute. Increase speed to medium-high and whip until stiff peaks form, 3 to 4 minutes.

3. Whisk milk mixture into flour mixture until batter has thickened and no lumps remain, about 1 minute. Gently fold in whipped egg whites until just combined and few streaks remain.

4. Heat 1 teaspoon oil in 12-inch nonstick skillet over medium heat until shimmering, 3 to 5 minutes. Using paper towels, carefully wipe out oil, leaving thin film of oil on bottom and sides of pan. Using ¼ cup batter per pancake, portion batter into skillet and sprinkle 1 tablespoon blueberries over each pancake. Cook until bottoms of pancakes are brown and top surfaces start to bubble, 2 to 3 minutes. Flip pancakes and cook until second side has browned, 1 to 2 minutes longer. Serve immediately or transfer pancakes to wire rack in preheated oven (don't overlap). Repeat with remaining batter, using remaining oil as necessary.

SMART SHOPPING **Buckwheat Flour**

Buckwheat, despite its name, is not related to wheat. It is actually an herb, and its seeds are ground to make flour (the kernels can also be hulled and crushed to make groats; kasha is simply toasted buckwheat groats). Buckwheat is native to Russia, where it is used to make that country's traditional small yeast-raised pancakes known as blini. Buckwheat has a strong, earthy flavor, so here we use buckwheat flour in combination with our gluten-free flour blend. Buckwheat products can be found in natural food stores and well-stocked supermarkets. For information on buckwheat groats and kasha, see page 28.

Lemon Ricotta Pancakes

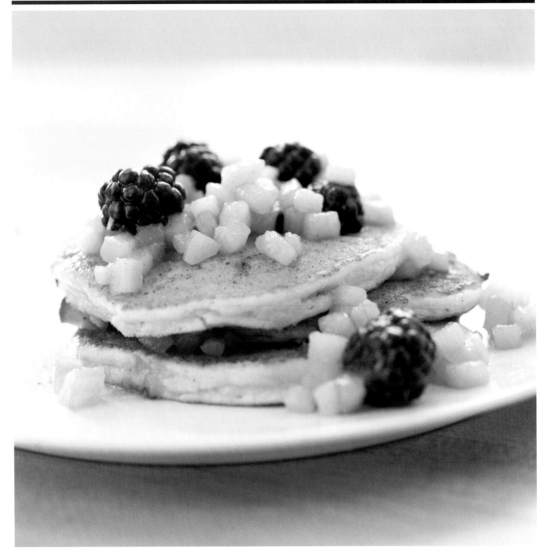

G-F TESTING LAB

FLOUR SUBSTITUTION	King Arthur Gluten-Free Multi-Purpose Flour 3½ ounces = ½ **cup plus 2 tablespoons**	Bob's Red Mill GF All-Purpose Baking Flour 3½ ounces = ⅔ **cup**

Note that pancakes made with Bob's Red Mill will be heavier and not as delicate as they should be, and they will have a distinct bean flavor.

Lemon ricotta pancakes stand apart from the classic versions with their light and creamy interior that is almost soufflé-like, and a subtle milky flavor. While ricotta adds creamy flavor and texture to these pancakes, it also adds weight. To keep the pancakes light, we folded four whipped egg whites into the batter. We also used a combination of baking soda and lemon juice for an extra boost not only to ensure the right ethereal rise, but also to provide a clean, bright flavor that balanced the milky richness of the ricotta. Still, these pancakes seemed a little heavier than we wanted, so we minimized the amount of flour blend, getting it down to just 3½ ounces. We like these pancakes plain or with a drizzle of honey, but we also threw together a quick fruit topping.

Lemon Ricotta Pancakes
MAKES TWELVE 4-INCH PANCAKES; SERVES 4

3½	ounces (¾ cup) ATK Gluten-Free Flour Blend (page 13)
½	teaspoon baking soda
½	teaspoon salt
9	ounces (1 cup) whole-milk ricotta cheese
2	large eggs, separated, plus 2 large egg whites
⅓	cup milk
1	teaspoon grated lemon zest plus 4 teaspoons juice
½	teaspoon vanilla extract
2	tablespoons unsalted butter, melted and cooled
	Pinch cream of tartar
1¾	ounces (¼ cup) sugar
1–2	teaspoons vegetable oil

1. Adjust oven rack to middle position and heat oven to 200 degrees. Spray wire rack set inside rimmed baking sheet with vegetable oil spray; place in oven. Whisk flour blend, baking soda, and salt together in medium bowl, and make well in center. Add ricotta, egg yolks, milk, lemon zest and juice, and vanilla and whisk until combined. Stir in melted butter.

2. Using stand mixer fitted with whisk, whip egg whites and cream of tartar on medium-low speed until foamy, about 1 minute. Increase speed to medium-high and whip whites to soft, billowy mounds, about 1 minute. Gradually add sugar and whip until glossy, soft peaks form, 1 to 2 minutes. Transfer ⅓ of whipped egg whites to batter and whisk gently until mixture is lightened. Using rubber spatula, gently fold remaining egg whites into batter.

3. Heat 1 teaspoon oil in 12-inch nonstick skillet over medium heat until shimmering, 3 to 5 minutes. Using paper towels, carefully wipe out oil, leaving thin film of oil on bottom and sides of pan. Using ladle or ¼ cup measure, portion batter, leaving 2 inches between each portion. Using back of ladle (or spoon, if using measuring cup), gently spread each portion into 4-inch round. Cook until edges are set and first side is deep golden brown, about 2½ minutes. Flip pancakes and continue to cook until second side is golden brown, about 2½ minutes longer. Serve immediately or transfer to wire rack in preheated oven (don't overlap). Repeat with remaining batter, using remaining oil as necessary.

Pear-Blackberry Pancake Topping
MAKES 3 CUPS

3	ripe pears, peeled, cored, halved, and cut into ¼-inch pieces
1	tablespoon sugar
1	teaspoon cornstarch
	Pinch salt
	Pinch ground cardamom
5	ounces (1 cup) blackberries, berries halved crosswise if large

Combine pears, sugar, cornstarch, salt, and cardamom in bowl and microwave until pears are softened but not mushy and juices are slightly thickened, 4 to 6 minutes, stirring once halfway through microwaving. Stir in blackberries and serve.

Sweet Crêpes

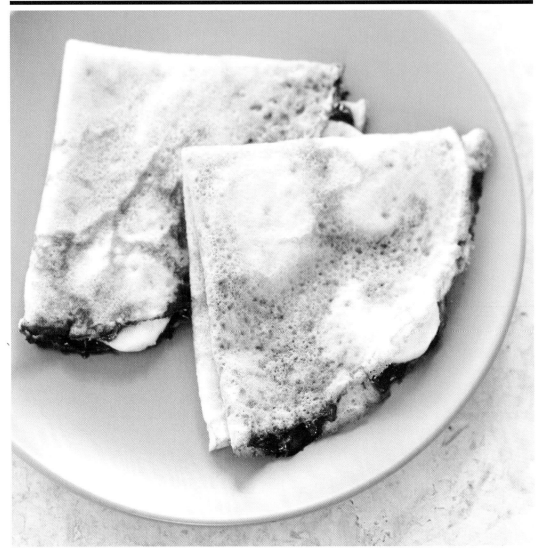

G-F TESTING LAB

FLOUR SUBSTITUTION	King Arthur Gluten-Free Multi-Purpose Flour 5½ ounces = **1 cup**	Bob's Red Mill GF All-Purpose Baking Flour 5½ ounces = **1 cup plus 2 tablespoons**

Note that crêpes made with Bob's Red Mill will be slightly gummier and have a distinct bean flavor.

✓ WHY THIS RECIPE WORKS

A traditional crêpe batter relies on 1 cup of flour, 1½ cups of milk, 3 eggs, and 2 tablespoons of butter (plus salt and sugar), so we swapped in our gluten-free flour blend and cooked up a batch. The results were close, but a bit rubbery. Reducing the number of eggs to two made the crêpes more tender and delicate. As with traditional crêpes, it was crucial to heat the pan properly—if it was too hot, the batter set up before it evenly coated the surface, yielding a crêpe marred by thick, spongy patches and holes; if too cool, the crêpe was pale (read: bland) and too flimsy to flip without tearing. To ensure steady, even cooking, we slowly heated the oiled skillet over low heat for at least 10 minutes. (Crêpes give off steam as they cook, but if at any point the skillet begins to smoke, remove it from the heat immediately and turn down the heat.) Adding just enough batter to coat the pan's bottom, and using the tilt-and-shake method to distribute the batter, ensured browned, flavorful crêpes that were perfectly thin and easy to flip without tearing. To allow for practice, the recipe yields 10 crêpes; only eight are needed for the filling.

Crêpes with Lemon and Sugar
SERVES 4

- ½ teaspoon vegetable oil
- 5½ ounces (1¼ cups) ATK Gluten-Free Flour Blend (page 13)
- 3 tablespoons plus ½ teaspoon sugar
- ¼ teaspoon salt
- 1½ cups whole milk
- 2 large eggs
- 2 tablespoons unsalted butter, melted and cooled
  Lemon wedges

1. Place oil in 10-inch nonstick skillet and heat over low heat for at least 10 minutes. While skillet is heating, whisk flour blend, 1½ teaspoons sugar, and salt together in medium bowl. In separate bowl, whisk together milk and eggs. Add half of milk mixture to dry ingredients and whisk until smooth. Add melted butter and whisk until incorporated. Whisk in remaining milk mixture until smooth.

2. Using paper towel, wipe out skillet, leaving thin film of oil on bottom and sides of pan. Increase heat to medium and let skillet heat for 1 minute. After 1 minute, test heat of skillet by placing 1 teaspoon batter in center and cook for 20 seconds. If mini test crêpe is golden brown on bottom, skillet is properly heated; if too light or too dark, adjust heat accordingly and retest.

3. Whisk batter to recombine and pour scant ¼ cup batter into far side of pan and tilt and shake gently until batter evenly covers bottom of pan. Cook crêpe without moving it until top surface is dry and crêpe starts to brown at edges, loosening crêpe from side of pan with rubber spatula, about 25 seconds. Gently slide spatula underneath edge of crêpe, grasp edge with fingertips, and flip crêpe. Cook until second side is lightly spotted, about 20 seconds. Transfer cooked crêpe to wire rack, inverting so spotted side is facing up. Return pan to heat and heat for 10 seconds before repeating with remaining batter, whisking batter often to recombine. As crêpes are done, stack on wire rack.

4. Sprinkle upper half of 1 crêpe with 1 teaspoon sugar. Fold unsugared bottom half over sugared half, then fold into quarters. Transfer sugared crêpe to serving plate. Continue with remaining crêpes and sugar. Serve immediately, passing lemon wedges separately.

VARIATIONS

Crêpes with Bananas and Nutella
Omit sugar and lemon wedge in step 4. Spread 1 teaspoon Nutella over half of each crêpe, then distribute three to four ¼-inch-thick banana slices atop the Nutella. Fold crêpes into quarters.

Crêpes with Honey and Toasted Almonds
Omit sugar and lemon wedge in step 4. Drizzle 1 teaspoon honey over half of each crêpe and sprinkle with 2 teaspoons finely chopped toasted sliced almonds and pinch salt. Fold crêpes into quarters.

Buttermilk Waffles

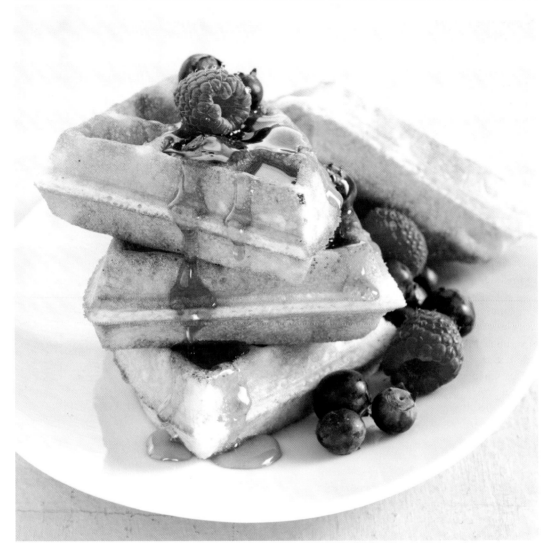

G-F TESTING LAB

FLOUR SUBSTITUTION	King Arthur Gluten-Free Multi-Purpose Flour 12 ounces = **1⅔ cups plus ½ cup**	Bob's Red Mill GF All-Purpose Baking Flour 12 ounces = **2¼ cups plus 2 tablespoons**

Note that waffles made with Bob's Red Mill will be somewhat darker and have a slight bean flavor.

✅ WHY THIS RECIPE WORKS

People often think waffle and pancake batters are interchangeable, and while we don't agree with that in the test kitchen, we thought our gluten-free pancake batter (page 34) would at least serve as a good jumping off point for a waffle recipe. Waffles made with this batter—which includes two whipped egg whites and multiple leaveners—came off of the waffle iron with a crisp shell and a hollow interior. Clearly we had too much lift, so we eliminated the baking powder and stopped separating the eggs and whipping the whites. For more structure, we increased the amount of flour. While these waffles were better, they were a little on the heavy side. Increasing the number of eggs from two to three fixed the problem, giving the batter the heft, volume, and richness it needed without making the waffles leaden. This batter baked up into waffles with a crisp exterior and a substantial interior that was moist, with just the right amount of chew. Buttermilk gives these waffles a nice tang and helps ensure a light texture. We prefer the crisper texture of these waffles when made in a Belgian waffle iron, but a classic iron will also work, though it will make more waffles.

Buttermilk Waffles
MAKES FIVE 7-INCH BELGIAN WAFFLES

12	ounces (2⅔ cups) ATK Gluten-Free Flour Blend (page 13)
2	tablespoons sugar
½	teaspoon salt
½	teaspoon baking soda
1¾	cups buttermilk
3	large eggs
4	tablespoons unsalted butter, melted and cooled

1. Heat waffle iron according to manufacturer's instructions.

2. Whisk flour blend, sugar, salt, and baking soda together in medium bowl. In separate bowl, whisk buttermilk, eggs, and melted butter until combined. Whisk buttermilk mixture into flour mixture thoroughly until batter has thickened and no lumps remain, about 1 minute (batter will be thick).

3. Bake waffles according to manufacturer's instructions (use about ⅓ cup batter for 7-inch round iron and generous ¾ cup for Belgian waffle iron). Repeat with remaining batter. Serve immediately.

TEST KITCHEN TIP **Buttermilk Substitutes**

If you do not have buttermilk on hand, that's not a problem. There are a couple of options for making buttermilk substitutions. For our waffles and Buttermilk Pancakes (page 35), both of which call for 1¾ cups buttermilk, mix ½ cup milk with 1¼ cups yogurt and substitute this mixture for the 1¾ cups buttermilk in the recipe. Both whole-milk and low-fat yogurt will work.

While too thin to use in our waffle and pancake batters, a mixture of lemon juice and milk is often used as a buttermilk substitute in other recipes. For 1 cup buttermilk, mix 1 cup whole milk with 1 tablespoon white vinegar or lemon juice.

Blueberry Muffins

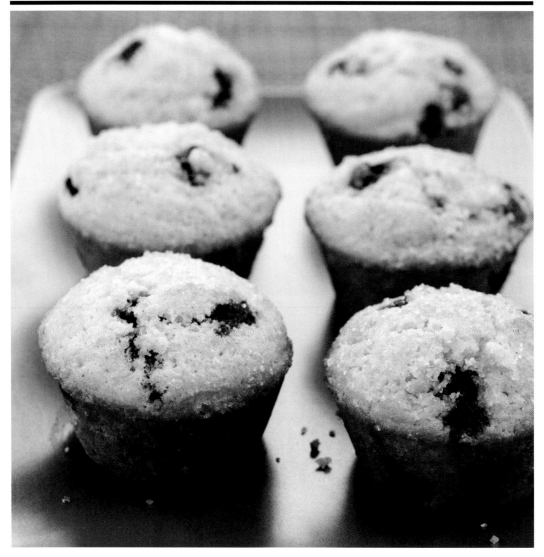

G-F TESTING LAB

FLOUR SUBSTITUTION	King Arthur Gluten-Free Multi-Purpose Flour 11 ounces = **2 cups**	Bob's Red Mill GF All-Purpose Baking Flour 11 ounces = **1⅔ cups plus ½ cup**
	Note that muffins made with King Arthur will have a slightly starchy aftertaste and gritty texture; muffins made with Bob's Red Mill will be somewhat darker and have a distinct bean flavor.	
XANTHAN GUM	The xanthan gum can be omitted, but the muffins will be more crumbly, with slightly less structure, and they will be a little more difficult to get out of the pan.	
RESTING TIME	Do not shortchange the 30-minute rest for the batter; if you do, the muffins will be gritty.	

Even the best traditional bakeshops often come up short when they attempt to make gluten-free muffins—the results are usually gritty, crumbly, and pale. We set out to make a golden-domed gluten-free muffin that also had a tender, delicate interior. To fix the grittiness, we found that resting the batter before baking hydrated the flour and softened its texture—but we had to be careful because the longer we let the batter sit, the more dense the muffins were and the less they rose. While we typically use two eggs in a muffin recipe, this thick batter needed three to achieve the proper richness and structure. For the liquid component, we were after something that would help create a moist crumb and also lend some flavor. A few tests with various dairy options proved plain whole-milk yogurt was the answer (you can use low-fat yogurt, but the muffins will be a little drier). Finally, sprinkling the muffins with turbinado sugar before they went into the oven helped create the browned tops we were after. You can substitute an equal amount of fresh raspberries or chopped strawberries for the blueberries. Frozen berries, rinsed well and blotted dry with paper towels, will also work; however, the berries will bleed slightly into the batter. See page 46 for tips on portioning the muffin batter into the prepared tin.

Blueberry Muffins
MAKES 12 MUFFINS

- 11 ounces (1¾ cups plus ⅔ cup) ATK Gluten-Free Flour Blend (page 13)
- 1 tablespoon baking powder (see page 20)
- ½ teaspoon salt
- ¼ teaspoon ground cinnamon
- ¼ teaspoon xanthan gum
- 5¼ ounces (¾ cup) granulated sugar
- 8 tablespoons unsalted butter, melted and cooled
- ½ cup plain whole-milk yogurt
- 3 large eggs
- 1 teaspoon vanilla extract
- 7½ ounces (1½ cups) blueberries
- 2 tablespoons turbinado sugar

1. Whisk flour blend, baking powder, salt, cinnamon, and xanthan gum together in large bowl. In separate bowl, whisk granulated sugar, melted butter, yogurt, eggs, and vanilla together until well combined. Using rubber spatula, stir egg mixture into flour mixture until thoroughly combined and no lumps remain, about 1 minute. Gently fold in blueberries until evenly distributed (batter will be thick and stiff). Cover bowl with plastic wrap and let batter rest at room temperature for 30 minutes.

2. Adjust oven rack to middle position and heat oven to 375 degrees. Spray 12-cup muffin tin with vegetable oil spray. Using ice cream scoop or large spoon, portion batter evenly into prepared muffin tin. Sprinkle turbinado sugar over top. Bake until muffins are golden and toothpick inserted in center comes out clean, 16 to 20 minutes, rotating pan halfway through baking.

3. Let muffins cool in muffin tin on wire rack for 10 minutes. Remove muffins from tin and let cool for 10 minutes before serving. (Muffins are best eaten warm on day they are made, but they can be cooled, then immediately transferred to zipper-lock bag and stored at room temperature for up to 1 day. To serve, warm in 300-degree oven for 10 minutes. Muffins can also be wrapped individually in plastic wrap, transferred to zipper-lock bag, and frozen for up to 3 weeks. To serve, remove plastic and microwave muffin for 20 to 30 seconds, then warm in 350-degree oven for 10 minutes.)

Cooling and Storing Gluten-Free Quick Breads

Like their traditional counterparts, our gluten-free muffins, quick breads, and coffee cake should be cooled in the tin or pan for a short stint once they come out of the oven. This gives them time to set up, reducing the chance they'll break when you remove them. Then let them cool further, as directed in the recipe, before serving.

However, don't let them sit out for an extended time—our gluten-free muffins, quick breads, and coffee cake may taste as good as versions made with all-purpose flour, but their shelf life is shorter. The high starch content in gluten-free flour absorbs moisture much more quickly than traditional all-purpose flour does, making these baked goods dry and crumbly fairly quickly. Consequently, we highly recommend eating them as soon as they are cooled. Letting them sit out even a couple of hours beyond our recommended times makes a big difference in quality.

If you want to store leftovers, we found that they will all keep acceptably well for a day or two at room temperature (don't refrigerate them, as this only makes them drier). Quick breads and coffee cake don't freeze well, but muffins freeze quite nicely (and you can conveniently thaw them individually as needed). To avoid a starchy aftertaste, we also learned that reheating leftover muffins and quick breads is a must.

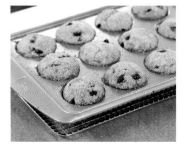 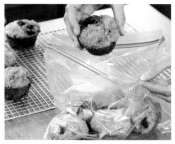 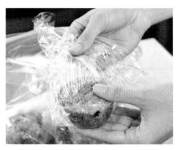

1. Once baked, cool in tin/pan on wire rack for time noted in recipe, then remove and let cool as directed. Serve or store immediately.

2. To store muffins for up to 1 day, immediately transfer cooled muffins to zipper-lock bag and store at room temperature. To store quick breads for up to 2 days, immediately wrap in plastic wrap and store at room temperature. To serve, warm in 300-degree oven for 10 to 15 minutes.

3. To store muffins for up to 3 weeks, wrap each muffin individually in plastic wrap, transfer to zipper-lock bag, and freeze. To serve, remove plastic and microwave muffin for 20 to 30 seconds, then warm in 350-degree oven for 10 minutes.

Pay Attention to Portioning

Not only does portioning the muffin batter haphazardly result in muffins that are of various sizes—some may overflow the cups while others look awkwardly small—but it also means the muffins may cook unevenly. We like to use a ⅓-cup dry measuring cup, large spoon, or spring-loaded #16 ice cream scoop. Whichever tool you use to portion the batter, spray it with vegetable oil spray so that the batter slides off easily.

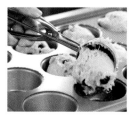

For neat, evenly sized muffins, portion ⅓ cup batter into each cup using measuring cup or ice cream scoop, then circle back and evenly distribute remaining batter with spoon.

Muffins

Muffins are one of the first things many people learn to bake because they're quick (no waiting for yeast to do its job), the ingredients are usually straightforward, and you don't need any special equipment. But as simple as they seem, bad muffins, and bad muffin recipes, abound. Try to make them gluten-free and you've got a host of new problems on your hands. Here's how we made gluten-free muffins that can hold their own against the best of the traditional versions.

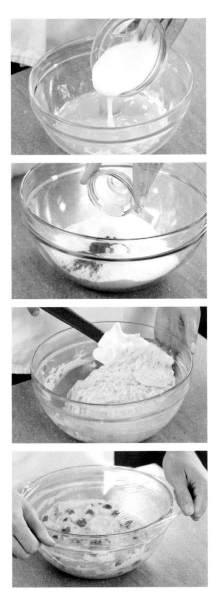

1. ADD AN EXTRA EGG AND YOGURT: We typically use two eggs in a traditional muffin recipe, but for various reasons this gluten-free batter needed three. First, the extra egg boosted the flavor and richness, which was a must because the starch granules in gluten-free flour absorb a lot of flavor. Second, the egg provided more moisture and structure, which our thick batter required for the proper rise and a moist, tender crumb. When it came to the liquid component, whole-milk yogurt, like the egg, provided a flavor boost and helped add moisture.

2. ADD XANTHAN GUM: Xanthan gum acts as a binding agent, providing the structure and stability that traditional baked goods usually get from the gluten protein (see page 16 for more about xanthan gum). While our muffins will work without it, they will be a little more crumbly and harder to get out of the pan. We think adding just ¼ teaspoon delivers a superior muffin.

3. STIR, STIR, STIR: The most common pitfall in traditional muffin making is overmixing because it works the gluten in the flour, and this leads to a tough, tunneled interior rather than a uniform, fluffy texture. Overworking the gluten was obviously not a concern with our gluten-free muffins. In fact, we discovered we needed to be more worried about undermixing. All that starch in the gluten-free flour blend made the muffin batter dense and thick. We had to stir the mixture for a full minute to ensure the leaveners and xanthan gum were evenly distributed.

4. LET THE BATTER SIT: Our early versions had a gritty texture—the result of gluten-free flour's higher starch content. Starch is very slow to absorb water, so if the batter goes straight into the oven right after it's mixed, the starch granules clump together and absorb water only on their surface. The result is a muffin with a noticeably gritty texture. Letting the batter sit at room temperature allowed those granules to hydrate and soften uniformly before baking. But you can overhydrate the starches, making the muffins denser and squat. Don't let the batter rest for more than 30 minutes.

Cranberry-Orange Pecan Muffins

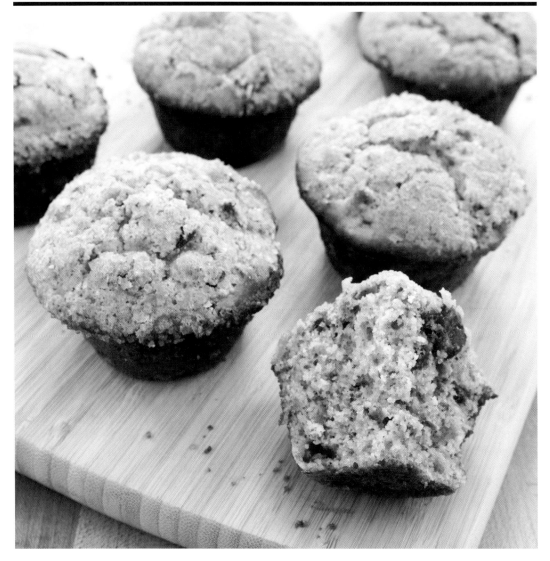

G-F TESTING LAB

FLOUR SUBSTITUTION	King Arthur Gluten-Free Multi-Purpose Flour 11 ounces = **2 cups**	Bob's Red Mill GF All-Purpose Baking Flour 11 ounces = **1⅔ cups plus ½ cup**
	Note that muffins made with King Arthur will have a slightly starchy aftertaste and gritty texture; muffins made with Bob's Red Mill will be somewhat darker and have a distinct bean flavor.	
XANTHAN GUM	The xanthan gum can be omitted, but the muffins will be more crumbly, with slightly less structure, and they will be a little more difficult to get out of the pan.	
RESTING TIME	Do not shortchange the 30-minute rest for the batter; if you do, the muffins will be gritty.	

✓ WHY THIS RECIPE WORKS

With a successful gluten-free Blueberry Muffin recipe (page 44) under our belts, we decided to try a different take using a similar base. We swapped whole cranberries in for the blueberries, and added pecans for nutty flavor and texture. The tartness of whole cranberries overwhelmed some bites (and was absent in others), so we pulsed the cranberries in the food processor to temper their punch and ensure they were more evenly distributed. We started testing with 1 cup of pecans, but this amount made our muffins too dense and heavy. But cutting back to ½ cup wasn't enough. We didn't want to sacrifice any more pecan flavor, so we ground the pecans in the food processor. This gave us a nut flour that we could add to the flour blend. And since we already had the food processor out, we decided to see if we could streamline things and prepare the batter in it rather than combining ingredients by hand in mixing bowls. The results were great: The muffins were perfectly tender and light and had a nutty flavor throughout. Because the nuts made our batter a bit denser and added fat, we needed to increase the oven temperature from 375 to 400 degrees to ensure the rise and nicely domed tops. Finally, a touch of orange zest added sweetness and brightness that complemented the cranberries. If fresh cranberries aren't available, substitute frozen: Microwave them in a bowl until they're partially but not fully thawed, 30 to 45 seconds. Plain low-fat yogurt will work just fine in this recipe, although the muffins will be a bit drier.

Cranberry-Orange Pecan Muffins
MAKES 12 MUFFINS

- 8 ounces (2 cups) cranberries
- 5¼ ounces (¾ cup) granulated sugar
- ½ cup pecans, toasted
- 2 teaspoons grated orange zest
- 11 ounces (1¾ cups plus ⅔ cup) ATK Gluten-Free Flour Blend (page 13)
- 1 tablespoon baking powder (see page 20)
- ½ teaspoon salt
- ¼ teaspoon xanthan gum
- 8 tablespoons unsalted butter, melted and cooled
- ½ cup plain whole-milk yogurt
- 3 large eggs
- 2 tablespoons turbinado sugar

1. Pulse cranberries in food processor until very coarsely chopped, 4 to 5 pulses. Transfer to bowl and set aside. Process granulated sugar, pecans, and orange zest in now-empty food processor to coarse sand, 10 to 15 seconds. Add flour blend, baking powder, salt, and xanthan gum and pulse until well combined, 5 to 10 pulses.

2. Whisk melted butter, yogurt, and eggs together in large bowl until well combined. Add to food processor and process until thoroughly combined and no lumps remain, about 30 seconds. Transfer to now-empty bowl and fold in chopped cranberries (batter will be thick and stiff). Cover bowl with plastic wrap and let batter rest at room temperature for 30 minutes.

3. Adjust oven rack to middle position and heat oven to 400 degrees. Spray 12-cup muffin tin with vegetable oil spray. Using ice cream scoop or large spoon, portion batter evenly into prepared muffin tin. Sprinkle turbinado sugar over top. Bake until muffins are golden and toothpick inserted in center comes out clean, 16 to 20 minutes, rotating pan halfway through baking.

4. Let muffins cool in muffin tin on wire rack for 10 minutes. Remove muffins from tin and let cool for 10 minutes before serving. (Muffins are best eaten warm on day they are made, but they can be cooled, then immediately transferred to zipper-lock bag and stored at room temperature for up to 1 day. To serve, warm in 300-degree oven for 10 minutes. Muffins can also be wrapped individually in plastic wrap, transferred to zipper-lock bag, and frozen for up to 3 weeks. To serve, remove plastic and microwave muffin for 20 to 30 seconds, then warm in 350-degree oven for 10 minutes.)

Millet-Cherry Almond Muffins

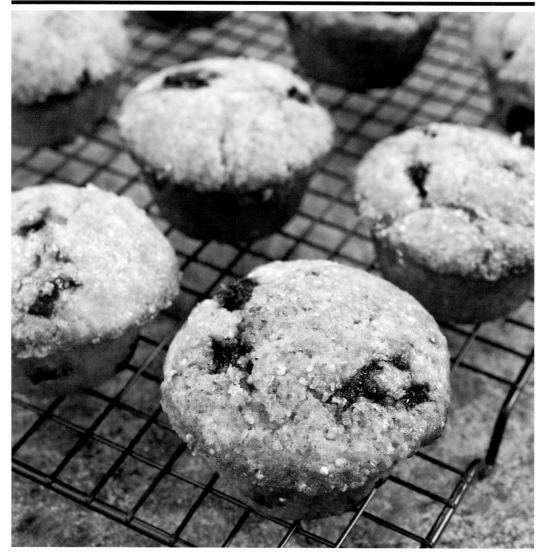

FLOUR SUBSTITUTION	King Arthur Gluten-Free Multi-Purpose Flour 11 ounces = **2 cups**	Bob's Red Mill GF All-Purpose Baking Flour 11 ounces = **1⅔ cups plus ½ cup**
	Note that muffins made with King Arthur will have a slightly starchy aftertaste and gritty texture; muffins made with Bob's Red Mill will be somewhat darker and have a distinct bean flavor.	
XANTHAN GUM	The xanthan gum can be omitted, but the muffins will be more crumbly and will have slightly less structure, and they will be a little more difficult to get out of the pan.	
RESTING TIME	Do not shortchange the 30-minute rest for the batter; if you do, the muffins will be gritty.	

After developing a couple of muffin recipes with a classic profile—blueberry and cranberry-nut (see pages 44 and 48)—we set out to make one with a more rustic profile. Incorporating a gluten-free grain plus some dried fruit into our batter seemed like a good route to take. We started with our blueberry muffin batter, then stirred in millet seeds and dried cherries. We quickly discovered a little millet went a long way—too much created a crunchy, distracting texture. Just ¼ cup of millet lent the right nutty flavor and crunch. When it came to the fruit, the muffins clearly needed the plump, juicy bursts of fresh or frozen fruit because the dried cherries turned out hard and chewy. Six ounces of frozen cherries gave the muffins the right sweet-tart punch. Almond extract was just the right finishing flavor touch that complemented the cherries and the millet. Do not thaw the cherries or your batter will turn purple. When fresh cherries are in season, you can substitute 6 ounces fresh sweet cherries, pitted and chopped coarse, for the frozen cherries. Plain low-fat yogurt will work just fine in this recipe, although the muffins will be a bit drier

Millet-Cherry Almond Muffins
MAKES 12 MUFFINS

11	ounces (1¾ cups plus ⅔ cup) ATK Gluten-Free Flour Blend (page 13)
1	tablespoon baking powder (see page 20)
½	teaspoon salt
¼	teaspoon xanthan gum
5¼	ounces (¾ cup) granulated sugar
8	tablespoons unsalted butter, melted and cooled
½	cup plain whole-milk yogurt
3	large eggs
½	teaspoon almond extract
6	ounces frozen sweet cherries, chopped coarse
¼	cup millet, rinsed
2	tablespoons turbinado sugar

1. Whisk flour blend, baking powder, salt, and xanthan gum together in large bowl. In separate bowl, whisk granulated sugar, melted butter, yogurt, eggs, and almond extract together until well combined. Using rubber spatula, stir egg mixture into flour mixture until thoroughly combined and no lumps remain, about 1 minute. Gently fold in cherries and millet until evenly distributed (batter will be thick and stiff). Cover bowl with plastic wrap and let batter rest at room temperature for 30 minutes.

2. Adjust oven rack to middle position and heat oven to 375 degrees. Spray 12-cup muffin tin with vegetable oil spray. Using ice cream scoop or large spoon, portion batter evenly into prepared muffin tin. Sprinkle turbinado sugar over top. Bake until muffins are golden and toothpick inserted in center comes out clean, 16 to 20 minutes, rotating pan halfway through baking.

3. Let muffins cool in muffin tin on wire rack for 10 minutes. Remove muffins from tin and let cool for 10 minutes before serving. (Muffins are best eaten warm on day they are made, but they can be cooled, then immediately transferred to zipper-lock bag and stored at room temperature for up to 1 day. To serve, warm in 300-degree oven for 10 minutes. Muffins can also be wrapped individually in plastic wrap, transferred to zipper-lock bag, and frozen for up to 3 weeks. To serve, remove plastic and microwave muffin for 20 to 30 seconds, then warm in 350-degree oven for 10 minutes.)

Pumpkin Bread

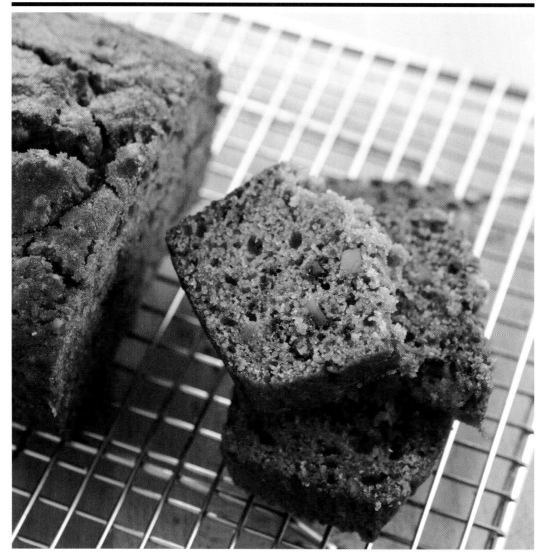

G-F TESTING LAB

FLOUR SUBSTITUTION	King Arthur Gluten-Free Multi-Purpose Flour 5½ ounces = **1 cup**	Bob's Red Mill GF All-Purpose Baking Flour 5½ ounces = **1 cup plus 2 tablespoons**

Note that bread made with King Arthur will be slightly denser; bread made with Bob's Red Mill will be denser and darker, and will have a slight bean flavor.

WHY THIS RECIPE WORKS

Pumpkin bread is usually boring. No loaf is remarkably bad, but none is remarkably good. We wanted a pumpkin bread that not only was gluten-free but also had just the right texture—neither too dense nor too cakey—and that had a rich pumpkin flavor tempered by sweetness and enhanced (not obscured) by spices. Our first task was to improve the raw metallic flavor of canned pumpkin puree. Cooking it (along with the spices) on the stovetop gave it a richer, fuller flavor. The only problem was that this process also drove off some of the moisture and increased its sweetness—the flavors were out of balance. Adding buttermilk solved the dryness problem, and incorporating cream cheese into the mix regained some of the tanginess that the sweetness was overpowering. Since we had to melt the cream cheese, we just added it to the pan of hot puree, achieving the dual goals of melting it and cooling the puree. Once the puree was cool, we were able to use the pot as the mixing bowl. After adding the flour blend and leaveners to our puree mixture, we continued stirring for a full minute to ensure they were thoroughly incorporated into the thick pumpkin puree mixture. Stirring for this amount of time also guaranteed the batter was properly aerated, giving our bread a good rise. Unlike our muffin recipes, this wetter batter did not need to be rested to hydrate the flour; the extra moisture plus the longer baking time prevented any grittiness. A handful of toasted and chopped walnuts gave the loaf some textural contrast and nice flavor. The test kitchen's preferred loaf pan measures 8½ by 4½ inches; if you use a 9 by 5-inch loaf pan, start checking for doneness 5 minutes earlier than advised in the recipe. You can substitute milk for the buttermilk if you don't have buttermilk.

Pumpkin Bread

MAKES 1 LOAF

- 5½ ounces (1¼ cups) ATK Gluten-Free Flour Blend (page 13)
- ¾ teaspoon baking powder (see page 20)
- ¼ teaspoon baking soda
- 7½ ounces canned pumpkin puree (¾ cup)
- ¾ teaspoon ground cinnamon
- ½ teaspoon salt
- ⅛ teaspoon ground nutmeg
  Pinch ground cloves
- 3½ ounces (½ cup) granulated sugar
- 3½ ounces (½ cup packed) light brown sugar
- ¼ cup vegetable oil
- 2 ounces cream cheese
- 2 large eggs
- 2 tablespoons buttermilk
- ½ cup walnuts, toasted and chopped fine

1. Adjust oven rack to middle position and heat oven to 350 degrees. Grease 8½ by 4½-inch loaf pan. Whisk flour blend, baking powder, and baking soda together in bowl.

2. Combine pumpkin puree, cinnamon, salt, nutmeg, and cloves in medium saucepan over medium heat. Cook, stirring constantly, until mixture is reduced to ¾ cup, 2 to 4 minutes.

3. Off heat, stir in granulated sugar, brown sugar, oil, and cream cheese until combined. Let mixture stand for 5 minutes. Whisk until no visible pieces of cream cheese remain and mixture is homogeneous.

4. Whisk together eggs and buttermilk in separate bowl. Add egg mixture to pumpkin mixture and whisk to combine. Stir flour mixture into pumpkin mixture until thoroughly combined and no lumps remain, about 1 minute. Fold walnuts into batter.

5. Scrape batter into prepared pan. Bake until toothpick inserted in center comes out clean, 45 to 50 minutes. Let bread cool in pan on wire rack for 20 minutes. Remove bread from pan and let cool for at least 1½ hours before serving. (Pumpkin bread is best eaten on day it is baked, but bread can be cooled, immediately wrapped in plastic wrap, and stored at room temperature for up to 2 days. To serve, warm in 300-degree oven for 10 to 15 minutes.)

Banana Bread

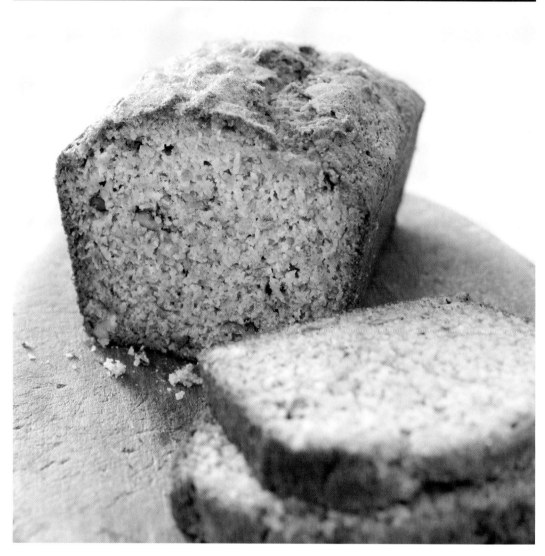

G-F TESTING LAB

FLOUR SUBSTITUTION	King Arthur Gluten-Free Multi-Purpose Flour 9½ ounces = **1¾ cups**	Bob's Red Mill GF All-Purpose Baking Flour 9½ ounces = **1¾ cups plus 2 tablespoons**
	Note that bread made with King Arthur will be slightly denser; bread made with Bob's Red Mill will be denser and darker, and will have a distinct bean flavor.	
XANTHAN GUM	The xanthan gum can be omitted, but the banana bread will be more crumbly and have less structure.	

✔ WHY THIS RECIPE WORKS

For the ultimate banana bread, we wanted to pack in as much banana flavor as possible without turning out a mushy loaf. We found we could smash five bananas into a single loaf. The key was eliminating some of their moisture. We microwaved the bananas until they started to break down, then moved them to a fine-mesh strainer to drain. Reducing the released liquid gave us an intense syrup that we could mix into the batter without adding excess water. To ensure the dense batter rose properly, we found we had to add a full tablespoon of baking powder plus baking soda. Xanthan gum ensured that our loaf had enough structure and stability. Stirring the batter for 1 minute before transferring it to the loaf pan ensured that all the ingredients were thoroughly incorporated and that the thick batter was properly aerated. Unlike our muffin recipes, this wetter batter did not need to be rested to hydrate the flour; the extra moisture plus the longer baking time prevented any grittiness. The test kitchen's preferred loaf pan measures 8½ by 4½ inches; if you use a 9 by 5-inch loaf pan, start checking for doneness 5 minutes early.

Banana Bread
MAKES 1 LOAF

9½	ounces (2 cups plus 2 tablespoons) ATK Gluten-Free Flour Blend (page 13)
1	tablespoon baking powder (see page 20)
1	teaspoon baking soda
½	teaspoon salt
¼	teaspoon xanthan gum
5	large very ripe bananas (about 1¾ pounds), peeled
8	tablespoons unsalted butter, melted and cooled
2	large eggs
5¼	ounces (¾ cup packed) light brown sugar
1	teaspoon vanilla extract
½	cup walnuts, toasted and chopped (optional)
2	teaspoons granulated sugar

1. Adjust oven rack to middle position and heat oven to 350 degrees. Grease 8½ by 4½-inch loaf pan. Whisk flour blend, baking powder, baking soda, salt, and xanthan gum together in large bowl.

2. Microwave bananas in separate bowl, covered, until they have softened and released liquid, about 5 minutes. Transfer bananas to fine-mesh strainer placed over medium bowl and let drain, stirring occasionally, about 15 minutes (you should have ½ to ¾ cup liquid).

3. Transfer banana juice to medium saucepan and cook over medium-high heat until reduced to ¼ cup, about 5 minutes. Return reduced juice to bowl, add bananas, and mash with potato masher until mostly smooth. Whisk in melted butter, eggs, brown sugar, and vanilla.

4. Using rubber spatula, stir banana mixture into flour mixture until thoroughly combined and no lumps remain, about 1 minute. Gently fold in walnuts, if using. Scrape batter into prepared pan and sprinkle granulated sugar evenly over loaf.

5. Bake until toothpick inserted in center comes out clean, 55 to 75 minutes. Let bread cool in pan on wire rack for 15 minutes. Remove bread from pan and let cool for at least 1 hour before serving. (Banana bread is best eaten on day it is baked, but bread can be cooled, immediately wrapped in plastic wrap, and stored at room temperature for up to 2 days. To serve, warm in 300-degree oven for 10 to 15 minutes.)

TEST KITCHEN TIP
Top Bananas Are Black Bananas

For maximum flavor, be sure to use very ripe, heavily speckled (or even black) bananas. If you like, you can freeze overly ripe bananas, one at a time, and save them expressly for use in this recipe. Thawed frozen bananas will release their liquid without the need for microwaving, so you can skip that step and put them directly into the fine-mesh strainer, then continue as directed.

Coffee Cake

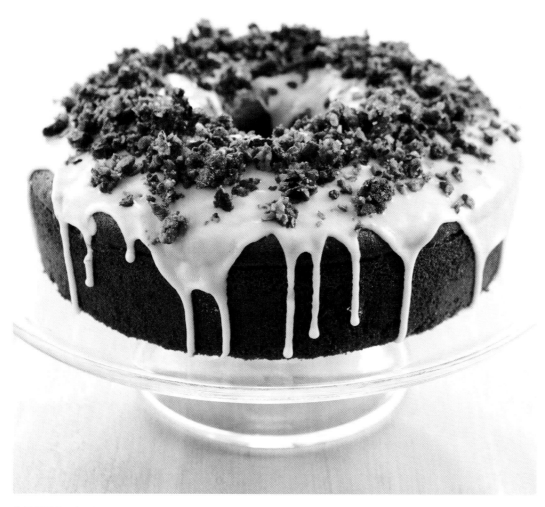

G-F TESTING LAB

FLOUR SUBSTITUTION	King Arthur Gluten-Free Multi-Purpose Flour 12 ounces = **1⅔ cups plus ½ cup**	Bob's Red Mill GF All-Purpose Baking Flour 12 ounces = **2¼ cups plus 2 tablespoons**
	Note that cake made with Bob's Red Mill will be slightly denser and darker, and will have a slight bean flavor.	
XANTHAN GUM	The xanthan gum can be omitted, but the coffee cake will be more crumbly and slightly more dense and it will not rise as well.	

✓ WHY THIS RECIPE WORKS

A coffee cake that feeds a crowd is perfect for Sunday brunches or holiday breakfasts. Most cake recipes cream butter and sugar, beat in eggs, and then alternate additions of dry ingredients and wet. While that method is great for producing a fluffy yellow cake, we wanted a coffee cake with a dense, rich crumb. Adding the butter with a portion of the sour cream to the dry ingredients, mixing for a few minutes, then adding the rest of the liquid was the key: It ensured the fat was evenly distributed (the flour clumped when we added butter and all the liquid at once), and because this approach reduced the mixing time—which meant less air was beaten into the batter—it delivered exactly the crumb we wanted. To avoid a greasy cake we found it essential to use less butter than you'd find in a traditional coffee cake; unlike the proteins in all-purpose flour, the starches in our gluten-free flour blend can't absorb as much fat. For the baking pan, we liked the simplicity of a round cake pan (rather than a tube or Bundt pan), but our cake sank in the middle and didn't cook through. A tube pan was essential, as the center tube, which conducts heat, ensured an even rise and a cake that cooked through evenly. The biggest hurdle was figuring out the streusel filling and topping. A classic streusel was too heavy for our cake—the high-starch gluten-free flour blend didn't offer the same structure or stability of all-purpose flour—and it sank as it baked. Instead, we took a portion of the batter, added cinnamon and nutmeg, then swirled this spiced batter into the plain batter in the pan. For a topping, a simple glaze plus candied nuts added texture and visual appeal the cake needed.

Coffee Cake
SERVES 12 TO 16

CAKE
- 4   **large eggs**
- 1½ **cups sour cream**
- 3½ **teaspoons vanilla extract**
- 12 **ounces (2⅔ cups) ATK Gluten-Free Flour Blend (page 13)**
- 8¾ **ounces (1¼ cups) granulated sugar**
- 1   **tablespoon baking powder (see page 20)**
- 1   **teaspoon salt**
- ¾ **teaspoon baking soda**
- ¼ **teaspoon xanthan gum**
- 8   **tablespoons unsalted butter, cut into ½-inch pieces and softened**
- 1   **tablespoon ground cinnamon**
- ¼ **teaspoon ground nutmeg**

TOPPING AND GLAZE
- ½ **cup pecans, chopped fine**
- 2   **tablespoons granulated sugar**
- ½ **teaspoon ground cinnamon**
-    **Pinch salt**
- 2   **tablespoons unsalted butter, melted and cooled**
- 4   **ounces (1 cup) confectioners' sugar**
- 5   **teaspoons milk**
- 1   **teaspoon vanilla extract**

1. FOR THE CAKE: Adjust oven rack to lowest position and heat oven to 350 degrees. Grease 16-cup tube pan. Whisk eggs, 1 cup sour cream, and 1 tablespoon vanilla together in bowl.

2. Using stand mixer fitted with paddle, mix flour blend, granulated sugar, baking powder, salt, baking soda, and xanthan gum on low speed until combined. Add remaining ½ cup sour cream and butter and mix until dry ingredients are moistened and few large butter pieces remain, about 1½ minutes. Gradually add egg mixture in 3 additions, beating for 20 seconds after each addition, scraping down bowl as needed. Increase speed to medium-high and beat until batter is light and fluffy, about 1 minute. Give batter final stir by hand (batter will be thick).

3. Measure 1 cup batter into bowl and whisk in remaining ½ teaspoon vanilla, cinnamon, and nutmeg. Pour remaining batter into prepared pan. Drop spoonfuls of spiced batter over top. Using butter knife, and working once around pan, gently fold batters together to make large swirls of spice inside cake; do not overmix.

4. Bake until cake feels firm to touch and skewer inserted in center comes out clean, 45 to 55 minutes. Let cake cool in pan on wire rack for 30 minutes. Run thin knife around edge of cake to loosen. Remove cake from pan and let cool on rack, about 1 hour. (Do not turn off oven.)

5. FOR THE TOPPING AND GLAZE: Meanwhile, line rimmed baking sheet with parchment paper. Combine pecans, granulated sugar, cinnamon, and salt in small bowl. Stir in melted butter until well combined. Transfer pecan mixture to prepared sheet and bake until golden, about 15 minutes. Let pecan mixture cool, then break into small pieces. In separate bowl, whisk confectioners' sugar, milk, and vanilla together until smooth. Pour glaze evenly over top of cooled cake, then sprinkle with pecan topping. Let glaze set for 20 minutes before serving. (Coffee cake is best eaten on day it is baked, but cake can be cooled, immediately wrapped in plastic wrap, and stored at room temperature for up to 2 days.)

TEST KITCHEN TIP **Making Coffee Cake**

Our recipe rethinks the usual streusel filling and topping. Here are the key steps.

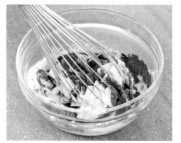

1. Transfer 1 cup batter to separate bowl and whisk in vanilla, cinnamon, and nutmeg.

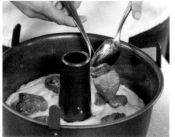

2. Pour remaining batter evenly into greased 16-cup tube pan. Using 2 spoons, drop spoonfuls of spiced batter on top.

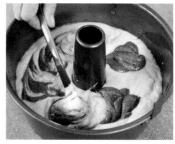

3. Using butter knife and working around pan only once, gently fold batters together to make large swirls of spice inside cake; do not overmix.

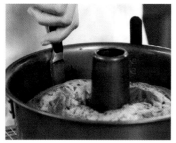

4. After baking cake and letting it cool for 30 minutes in pan on wire rack, run paring knife around edge of cake to loosen, then flip out onto wire rack.

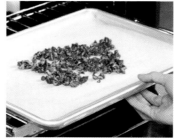

5. After preparing nut mixture, spread mixture over parchment-lined rimmed baking sheet and bake until golden. Let cool, then break into small pieces.

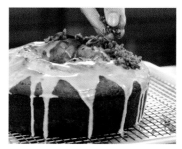

6. Whisk together glaze, then drizzle over cooled cake and sprinkle with topping. Let glaze set 20 minutes before serving.

Putting the Streusel in Coffee Cake

THE PROBLEM The test kitchen's traditional sour cream coffee cake starts with a rich, ultra-moist cake as its base. A streusel made with flour, brown and granulated sugars, cold butter, cinnamon, and chopped pecans gets swirled into this rich batter, and more gets sprinkled over the top. The result is a decadent, pleasantly rich and dense cake with crisp, crunchy, melt-in-your-mouth streusel inside and on top. At the outset, we thought the biggest challenge to making a gluten-free coffee cake would be the cake itself. We quickly discovered that the cake was the easy part. Incorporating the warm spices, sugar, and nuts—as a streusel or otherwise—turned out to be the main hurdle.

A SINKING FEELING We started with the same streusel ingredients as our traditional recipe and simply swapped in our gluten-free flour blend for all-purpose flour. Once baked, this cake had a layer of streusel that had sunk to the bottom of the pan, and the topping portion had caved into the middle. Clearly our gluten-free cake batter didn't have the same stability as our traditional version. We learned that this is because of the abundance of starch and limited amount of protein in the blend. In a cake made with all-purpose flour, the gluten begins to form a strong structure as it heats in the oven and at a certain temperature the structure becomes rigid, even when hot. But for starch to form a rigid structure, the granules have to absorb water and swell when heated, then cool to form a fairly strong gel—while hot, the starch gel is not strong enough to hold much weight. We wondered, How much weight could our gluten-free version take? Testing a slew of options was the only way to find out.

LIGHTENING UP To retain all the flavor and texture but lessen the weight, we omitted the flour (about 4 ounces) from the streusel for our next test. This helped, but the mixture still sank. Next we tried cutting back on the butter. Our traditional streusel calls for 2 tablespoons; it's not much, but we wondered if it was making our mixture too wet, thus causing it to sink into the cake and take the spices, sugar, and nuts with it. But the mixture sank again, both in the middle of the cake and on top. As a final resort, suspecting the nuts were too heavy, we decided to try swapping them out for oats, an ingredient often used in gluten-free streusels. We hoped that they would add nuttiness and texture but not much weight. But they likewise sank—and also were unappealingly chewy—so they didn't make the cut.

SPICE SWIRL It was time to come at the problem from a new angle. We abandoned the streusel entirely and instead took a cue from marble-style cakes. We prepared the coffee cake batter as usual, then took a portion of it and stirred in plenty of cinnamon, as well as nutmeg and vanilla. We spooned the spiced batter over the plain and ran a knife through it in a zigzag motion around the pan. But this led to overmixing—we ended up with a nearly homogeneous cake that lacked the visual appeal a swirl of spice would provide, and the spice flavor was faintly distributed throughout instead of being a swirl with a potent punch. Next we tried a circular folding motion to gently swirl the spiced batter into the plain batter. Success—this technique left a thin but distinct trail that was visually appealing and packed plenty of flavor.

TACKLING THE TOPPING Our spiced batter swirl delivered a cake with the right warm-spice flavor and some great visual appeal, but we still needed a solution for the topping. We wondered if we could make a sugar-centric topping that could lock a handful of nuts in place in the heat of the oven. A mixture of butter, granulated sugar, cinnamon, and nuts was a failure—a dusty, dry mix that didn't adhere to the baked cake at all. We then switched to turbinado sugar instead of the granulated because it melts more readily and contains a small amount of moisture not present in granulated sugar, but one test proved this alternative to be equally unsuccessful.

THE SOLUTION THAT STUCK After a lot of flops, we landed on a two-part approach that applied the topping after baking, when the cake would have enough structure not to collapse. While the cake cooled, we made a candied nut topping by baking a mix of pecans, sugar, cinnamon, salt, and melted butter. Then we drizzled the baked, cooled cake with a simple confectioners' sugar–based glaze and sprinkled our candied spiced pecans over the top. Once the glaze set, it locked the nuts in place. Together with our swirl of spiced cake, we had a coffee cake with the visual appeal, texture, and flavor—inside and out—that we were after.

Almond Granola with Dried Fruit

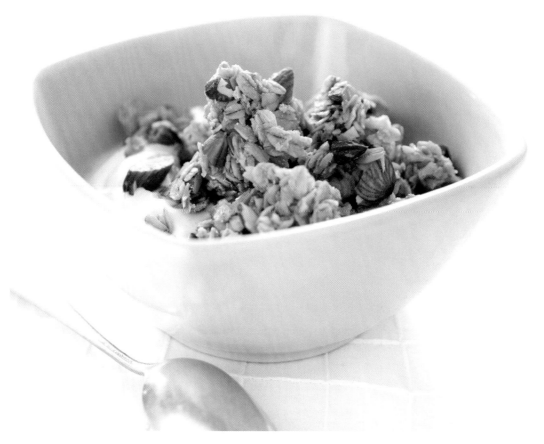

WHY THIS RECIPE WORKS

Granola is a great staple in the gluten-free pantry, ideal not just as an energy-packed breakfast cereal, but also for topping yogurt or serving as a satisfying afternoon snack. Store-bought granola is often loose and gravelly, and/or infuriatingly expensive. We wanted to make our own granola at home, with big, satisfying clusters and a crisp texture. The secret was to pack the granola mixture firmly into a rimmed baking sheet before baking. Once it was baked, we had a granola "bark" that we could break into crunchy clumps of any size. Chopping the almonds by hand is the first choice for superior texture and crunch. If you prefer not to hand-chop, substitute an equal quantity of slivered or sliced almonds. (A food processor does a lousy job of chopping whole nuts evenly.) Use either a single type of your favorite dried fruit or a combination.

Almond Granola with Dried Fruit
MAKES ABOUT 9 CUPS

⅓   **cup maple syrup**
2⅓   **ounces (⅓ cup packed) light brown sugar**
4   **teaspoons vanilla extract**
½   **teaspoon salt**
½   **cup vegetable oil**
5   **cups gluten-free old-fashioned rolled oats**
2   **cups whole almonds, chopped coarse**
2   **cups raisins or other dried fruit, chopped**

1. Adjust oven rack to upper-middle position and heat oven to 325 degrees. Line rimmed baking sheet with parchment paper.

2. Whisk maple syrup, sugar, vanilla, and salt together in large bowl. Whisk in oil. Fold in oats and almonds until thoroughly coated.

3. Transfer oat mixture to prepared sheet and spread across sheet into thin, even layer (about ⅜ inch thick). Using stiff metal spatula, compress oat mixture until very compact. Bake until lightly browned, 40 to 45 minutes, rotating pan halfway through baking.

4. Remove granola from oven and cool on wire rack to room temperature, about 1 hour. Break cooled granola into pieces of desired size. Stir in raisins. (Granola can be stored in airtight container for up to 2 weeks.)

TEST KITCHEN TIP **Making Chunky Granola**

For granola with nice substantial chunks, we found it was key to pack it into the baking sheet and to avoid stirring.

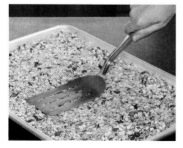

1. Spread oat mixture onto parchment-lined baking sheet, then press down firmly with spatula to create compact layer.

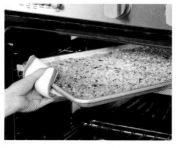

2. Bake granola at 325 degrees for 40 to 45 minutes, rotating pan halfway through baking; do not stir.

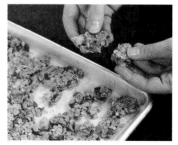

3. Let granola cool, then break into pieces.

10-Minute Steel-Cut Oatmeal

WHY THIS RECIPE WORKS
Oats are a great gluten-free option, and most oatmeal fans agree that the steel-cut style offers the best flavor and texture. However, many balk at the 40-minute cooking time, especially when all you want is a quick breakfast. We decreased the morning-of cooking time to only 10 minutes by stirring our steel-cut oats into boiling water the night before. This allowed the grains to hydrate and soften overnight. In the morning, all we had to do was add more water (fruit juice or milk would also work) and simmer the mixture for about 5 minutes. A brief rest off the heat ensured it had the perfect consistency. Whether eaten plain or with a handful of our favorite toppings, this recipe finally made great oatmeal a weekday option. The oatmeal will continue to thicken as it cools; if you prefer a looser consistency, thin the oatmeal with boiling water. Customize your oatmeal with toppings such as brown sugar, toasted nuts, maple syrup, or dried fruit.

10-Minute Steel-Cut Oatmeal
SERVES 4

- 4 **cups water**
- 1 **cup gluten-free steel-cut oats**
- ¼ **teaspoon salt**

1. Bring 3 cups water to boil in large saucepan over high heat. Remove pan from heat; stir in oats and salt. Cover pan and let stand overnight.

2. Stir remaining 1 cup water into oats and bring to boil over medium-high heat. Reduce heat to medium and cook, stirring occasionally, until oats are softened but still retain some chew and mixture thickens and resembles warm pudding, 4 to 6 minutes. Remove pan from heat and let stand for 5 minutes. Stir and serve, passing desired toppings separately.

VARIATIONS
Apple-Cinnamon 10-Minute Steel-Cut Oatmeal
Increase salt to ½ teaspoon. Substitute ½ cup apple cider and ½ cup whole milk for water in step 2. Stir ½ cup peeled, grated sweet apple, 2 tablespoons packed dark brown sugar, and ½ teaspoon ground cinnamon into oatmeal with cider and milk. Sprinkle each serving with 2 tablespoons coarsely chopped toasted walnuts.

Cranberry-Orange 10-Minute Steel-Cut Oatmeal
Increase salt to ½ teaspoon. Substitute ½ cup orange juice and ½ cup whole milk for water in step 2. Stir ½ cup dried cranberries, 3 tablespoons packed dark brown sugar, and ⅛ teaspoon ground cardamom into oatmeal with orange juice and milk. Sprinkle each serving with 2 tablespoons toasted sliced almonds.

Carrot Spice 10-Minute Steel-Cut Oatmeal
Increase salt to ¾ teaspoon. Substitute ½ cup carrot juice and ½ cup whole milk for water in step 2. Stir ½ cup finely grated carrot, ¼ cup packed dark brown sugar, ⅓ cup dried currants, and ½ teaspoon ground cinnamon into oatmeal with carrot juice and milk. Sprinkle each serving with 2 tablespoons coarsely chopped toasted pecans.

SMART SHOPPING **Know Your Oats**

Yes, oats are a gluten-free grain, but they're often processed in facilities that also process wheat, which creates cross-contamination issues. It's critical to make sure you are buying oats that are processed in a gluten-free facility; check the label when shopping. Once you've narrowed the oats field to gluten-free, you'll find there are a variety of options—but not all of them make for a good bowl of oatmeal. Groats are whole oats that have been hulled and cleaned. They are the least processed oat product, but we find them too coarse for oatmeal. Steel-cut oats are groats that have been cut crosswise into coarse bits. They're our preference for making oatmeal; they cook up creamy yet chewy, with a rich, nutty flavor. Rolled oats (often labeled "old-fashioned") are groats steamed and pressed into flat flakes. Rolled oats cook faster than steel-cut but make for a gummy, lackluster bowl of oatmeal; they are best saved for granola and baking.

Millet Porridge with Maple Syrup

WHY THIS RECIPE WORKS

The mellow corn flavor and fine texture of tiny millet seeds make them extremely versatile in both savory and sweet applications. We'd already discovered a small amount could add appealing texture to baked goods (see Millet-Cherry Almond Muffins on page 50), but a little research revealed it could be used in myriad other types of dishes. Going through its long history (as far back as the Stone Age!), we made a short list of the breakfast options and settled on developing a sweet millet porridge, a traditional staple for Germans and Russians. We started by cooking the seeds in plenty of liquid until they turned tender, then added more liquid (in the form of milk) and continued to cook the millet, uncovered, to encourage the swollen seeds to burst and release their starch. This delivered a porridge with just the right creamy consistency. We settled on cooking the millet in 3 cups of water until it was almost tender, then added milk to the pot to finish cooking it through and add richness. Simple flavorings of maple syrup and cinnamon, plus a little salt, were all our porridge needed to turn it into an appealing morning meal. We prefer this porridge made with whole milk, but low-fat or skim milk can be substituted. For more information on millet, see page 87.

Millet Porridge with Maple Syrup
SERVES 4

- 3 cups water
- 1 cup millet, rinsed (see page 31)
- ⅛ teaspoon ground cinnamon
- ⅛ teaspoon salt
- 1 cup whole milk
- 3 tablespoons maple syrup

1. Bring water, millet, cinnamon, and salt to boil in medium saucepan over high heat. Reduce heat to low, cover, and cook until millet has absorbed all water and is almost tender, about 20 minutes.

2. Uncover and increase heat to medium, add milk, and simmer, stirring frequently, until millet is fully tender and mixture is thickened, about 10 minutes. Stir in maple syrup and serve.

VARIATIONS

Millet Porridge with Dried Cherries and Pecans
Substitute 2 tablespoons packed brown sugar for maple syrup. Stir in ½ cup dried cherries and ½ cup chopped, toasted pecans along with brown sugar in step 2.

Millet Porridge with Coconut and Bananas
Omit cinnamon and maple syrup. Substitute coconut milk for whole milk. Stir in 2 sliced bananas, ½ cup shredded, toasted coconut, and ½ teaspoon vanilla just before serving.

Hot Quinoa Breakfast Cereal

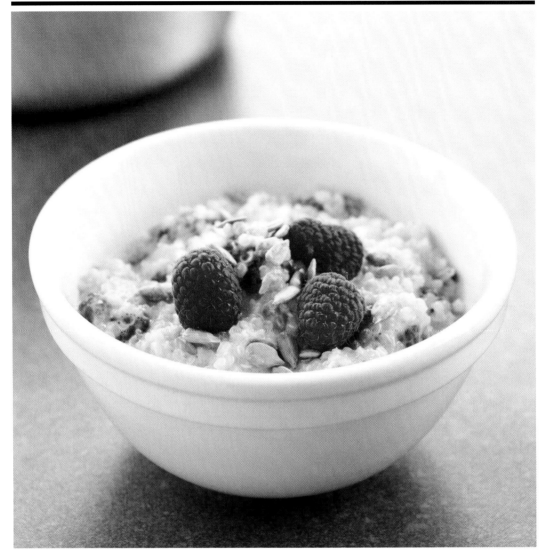

G-F TESTING LAB

QUINOA   We like the convenience of prewashed quinoa. If you buy unwashed quinoa (or if you are unsure if it's washed), quinoa should be rinsed before cooking to remove its bitter protective coating (called saponin); see page 31. We developed this recipe using white quinoa; we don't recommend using red or black quinoa here.

WHY THIS RECIPE WORKS

Given quinoa's availability, great nutritional profile, appealing nutty flavor, and quick cooking time, it seemed like a shoo-in for a great breakfast. We skipped toasting the quinoa to keep the flavor profile on the neutral side so that it could work with a variety of stir-ins, and also because we wanted to keep this morning recipe simple. To deliver the consistency we were after, we used a 2:1 ratio of liquid to quinoa and then cooked the quinoa until it partially broke down. We started by cooking it with 1 cup of water until it was almost done, then we added a cup of almond milk (for a little richness and flavor boost) and continued to cook until the milk was mostly absorbed and the quinoa had the consistency of porridge. With the technique down, we looked at flavorings. Honey, almonds, and blueberries were a good trio, and we used almond milk to reinforce the nut flavor. Sweet-tart raspberries paired well with mildly nutty sunflower seeds and maple syrup, while golden raisins, brown sugar, pistachios, and cardamom gave us an appealing version with a slightly Indian profile. If you prefer, replace almond milk with an equal amount of whole milk.

Hot Quinoa Breakfast Cereal with Blueberries and Almonds
SERVES 6

- 1 **cup prewashed white quinoa**
- 1 **cup water**
- ⅛ **teaspoon salt**
- 1 **cup almond milk, plus extra for serving**
- 5 **ounces (1 cup) fresh blueberries**
- ½ **cup whole almonds, toasted and chopped**
- 1 **tablespoon honey**

1. Bring quinoa, water, and salt to simmer in medium saucepan. Reduce heat to low, cover, and continue to simmer until quinoa is just tender, 15 to 17 minutes.

2. Uncover, stir in milk, and cook, stirring often, until milk is mostly absorbed and quinoa has consistency of porridge, about 10 minutes. Stir in blueberries, almonds, and honey. Serve, adding additional milk as needed to adjust consistency.

VARIATIONS

Hot Quinoa Breakfast Cereal with Raspberries and Sunflower Seeds
Substitute whole milk for almond milk. Substitute raspberries for blueberries, toasted sunflower seeds for almonds, and maple syrup for honey.

Hot Quinoa Breakfast Cereal with Golden Raisins and Pistachios
Substitute whole milk for almond milk. Substitute ½ cup golden raisins for blueberries, shelled pistachios for almonds, and 2 tablespoons packed brown sugar for honey. Add pinch ground cardamom along with raisins in step 2.

TEST KITCHEN TIP **Toasting Nuts and Seeds**

Toasting nuts and seeds maximizes their flavor and takes only a few minutes. To toast a small amount (1 cup or less) of nuts or seeds, put them in a dry skillet over medium heat. Shake the skillet occasionally to prevent scorching and toast until they are lightly browned and fragrant, 3 to 8 minutes. Watch the nuts closely because they can go from golden to burnt very quickly. To toast a large quantity of nuts, spread the nuts in a single layer on a rimmed baking sheet and toast in a 350-degree oven. To promote even toasting, shake the baking sheet every few minutes, and toast until the nuts are lightly browned and fragrant, 5 to 10 minutes.

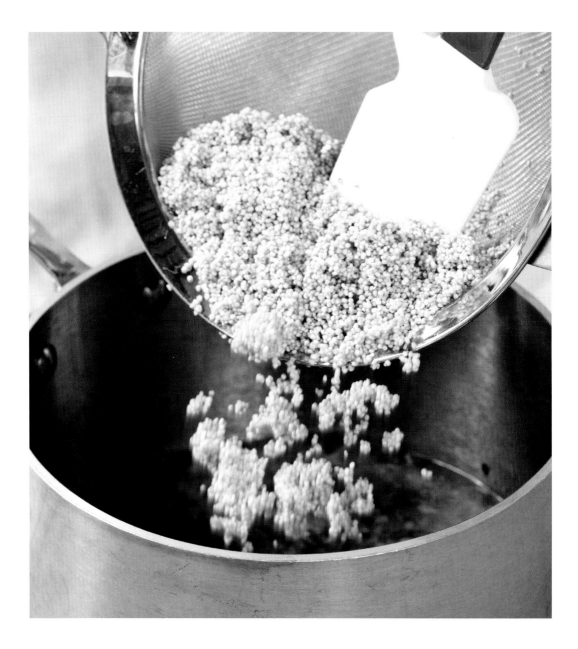

GRAINS

Basmati Rice Pilaf

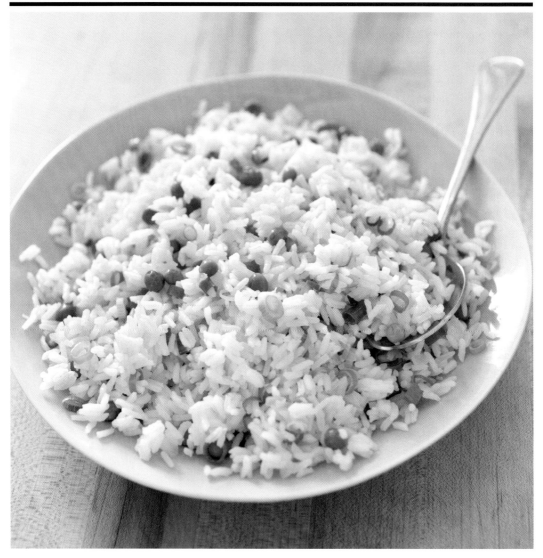

G-F TESTING LAB

RICE   Because of its nutty flavor and fluffy texture, basmati rice is our first choice for pilaf. That said, long-grain white, jasmine, or Texmati rice can be substituted with good results. For more details about basmati rice, see page 27.

✔ WHY THIS RECIPE WORKS

Rice is a staple in any gluten-free pantry, but no one wants plain rice or, worse, rice that's improperly cooked, night after night. Though simple, rice pilaf—fragrant and fluffy, perfectly steamed and tender—takes plain rice to the next level. Recipes for pilaf abound, but none seem to agree on the best method for guaranteeing these results; many espouse rinsing the rice and soaking it overnight to maximize grain elongation and prevent the grains from breaking, but we wondered if this extra work was really necessary for a simple rice dish. Rinsing the rice removed excess starch, ensuring separate rather than clumpy grains, but soaking was a failure—it actually resulted in mushy rice and unevenly sized and broken grains. Sautéed onion, cooked in the pot before adding the rice, lent sweetness. We then added the rice, sautéed it for a few minutes to give it a toasted, extra-nutty flavor; this step also helped to produce more discrete grains. And when it came to the liquid, instead of following the traditional 1:2 ratio of rice to water, we found using a little less water delivered better results.

Basmati Rice Pilaf
SERVES 4 TO 6

1	tablespoon olive oil
1	small onion, chopped fine
	Salt and pepper
1½	cups basmati rice, rinsed (see page 31)
2¼	cups water

1. Heat oil in large saucepan over medium heat until shimmering. Add onion and ¼ teaspoon salt and cook, stirring occasionally, until onion is softened, about 5 minutes.

2. Stir in rice and cook, stirring often, until grain edges begin to turn translucent, about 3 minutes. Stir in water and bring to simmer. Reduce heat to low, cover, and continue to simmer until rice is tender and water is absorbed, 16 to 18 minutes.

3. Remove pot from heat and lay clean folded dish towel underneath lid. Let sit for 10 minutes. Fluff rice with fork, season with salt and pepper to taste, and serve.

VARIATIONS

Herbed Basmati Rice Pilaf
Add 2 minced garlic cloves and 1 teaspoon minced fresh thyme to pot with rice. Before covering rice with kitchen towel in step 3, sprinkle ¼ cup minced fresh parsley and 2 tablespoons minced fresh chives over top.

Basmati Rice Pilaf with Peas, Scallions, and Lemon
Add 2 minced garlic cloves, 1 teaspoon grated lemon zest, and ⅛ teaspoon red pepper flakes to pot with rice. Before covering rice with kitchen towel in step 3, sprinkle ½ cup thawed frozen peas over top. When fluffing rice, stir in 2 thinly sliced scallions and 1 tablespoon lemon juice.

Basmati Rice Pilaf with Currants and Toasted Almonds
Add 2 minced garlic cloves, ½ teaspoon turmeric, and ¼ teaspoon ground cinnamon to pot with rice. Before covering rice with kitchen towel in step 3, sprinkle ¼ cup currants over top. When fluffing rice, stir in ¼ cup toasted sliced almonds.

TEST KITCHEN TIP
Ensuring Fluffy Rice Pilaf

The first key steps to getting fluffy rice pilaf are selecting basmati rice, which cooks up particularly fluffy, and then rinsing the rice to remove excess starch. We also place a towel under the pan lid while the rice rests to absorb excess moisture,

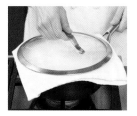

Remove pot from heat and lay clean, folded dish towel under lid. Let rice sit for 10 minutes, then fluff with fork.

Hearty Baked Brown Rice

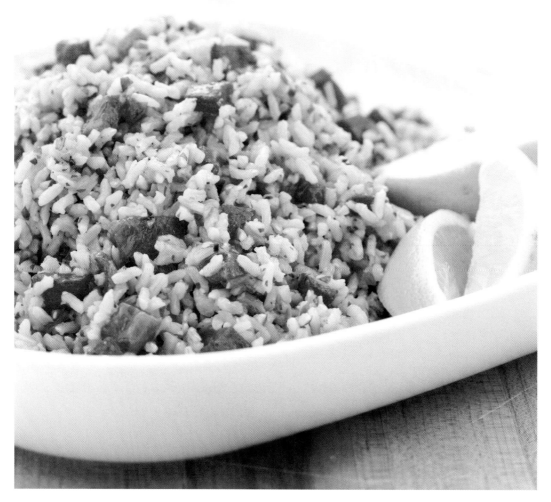

G-F TESTING LAB

RICE   You can substitute short- or medium-grain brown rice for the long-grain if desired, but the results will be a little more sticky. For more details about brown rice, see page 27.

✓ WHY THIS RECIPE WORKS

All too often brown rice cooks unevenly, with the grains on the bottom of the pot (near the burner) scorching while the grains at the top of the pot are underdone. We found that moving from the stovetop to the oven, an environment that mimics the even heat of the rice cooker, delivered perfectly cooked grains. For our foolproof approach, we brought the liquid (a combination of broth and water) to a boil on the stovetop, stirred in our rice, then transferred the pot to the oven. To add heartiness, we turned to several flavorful combinations of add-ins: red peppers and onions, black beans and cilantro, peas and feta. But after adding these ingredients to the pot with our rice, we found that we needed to tinker with the liquid-to-rice ratio a bit more. Increasing the amount of liquid ensured that the rice cooked through perfectly every time. Fresh herbs, added just before serving, brightened the dish and balanced the earthiness of the rice. To make this vegetarian, substitute vegetable broth for chicken broth.

Hearty Baked Brown Rice with Onions and Roasted Red Peppers
SERVES 4 TO 6

4	teaspoons olive oil
2	onions, chopped fine
2¼	cups water
1	cup chicken broth
1½	cups long-grain brown rice
	Salt and pepper
¾	cup chopped jarred roasted red peppers
½	cup minced fresh parsley
1	ounce Parmesan cheese, grated (½ cup)
	Lemon wedges

1. Adjust oven rack to middle position and heat oven to 375 degrees. Heat oil in Dutch oven over medium heat until shimmering. Add onions and cook, stirring occasionally, until well browned, 12 to 14 minutes.

2. Add water and broth, cover, and bring to boil. Off heat, stir in rice and 1 teaspoon salt. Cover, transfer pot to oven, and bake rice until tender, 65 to 70 minutes.

3. Remove pot from oven and uncover. Fluff rice with fork, stir in roasted red peppers, and replace lid; let sit for 5 minutes. Stir in parsley and ¼ teaspoon pepper. Serve, passing Parmesan and lemon wedges separately.

VARIATIONS

Hearty Baked Brown Rice with Black Beans and Cilantro
Substitute 1 finely chopped green bell pepper for 1 onion. Once vegetables are well browned in step 1, stir in 3 minced garlic cloves and cook until fragrant, about 30 seconds. Substitute 1 (15-ounce) can black beans for roasted red peppers and ¼ cup minced fresh cilantro for parsley. Omit Parmesan and substitute lime wedges for lemon wedges.

Hearty Baked Brown Rice with Peas, Feta, and Mint
Reduce amount of olive oil to 1 tablespoon and omit 1 onion. Substitute 1 cup thawed frozen peas for roasted red peppers, ¼ cup minced fresh mint for parsley, and ½ teaspoon grated lemon zest for pepper. Omit Parmesan and sprinkle with ½ cup crumbled feta before serving.

SMART SHOPPING **Long-Grain Brown Rice**

Brown rice is essentially a less-processed version of white rice. For a product with so little processing, we wondered if the brand of brown rice really mattered. We tasted five brands of long-grain brown rice prepared two ways: steamed in a rice cooker and baked in the oven. While most were fairly neutral in flavor, one brand boasted distinct nutty and toasty flavors. In both taste tests, Goya Brown Rice Natural Long Grain Rice came out on top—though by a slim margin. What separated it from the rest of the group was a bolder, more distinct flavor.

Wild Rice Pilaf

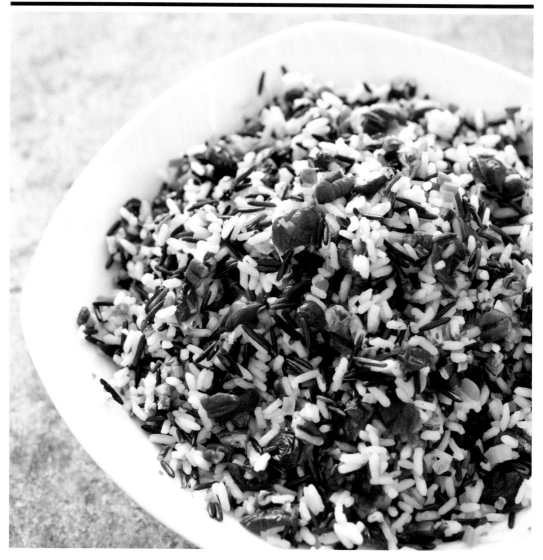

✔ WHY THIS RECIPE WORKS

Properly cooked wild rice is chewy yet tender, and pleasingly rustic—not crunchy or gluey, like the wild rice so many recipes produce. We wanted to figure out how to turn out properly cooked wild rice with fluffy pilaf-style results every time. In the end, we found that simmering the wild rice in plenty of liquid and then draining off any excess was the most reliable method. Cooking times from batch to batch were variable, so we started checking for doneness after 35 minutes. For the liquid, using water alone resulted in a muddy flavor. A combination of water and chicken broth performed much better. Mild yet rich, the broth tempered the rice's muddiness and brought out its earthy, nutty flavors. We also added some white rice to balance the wild rice's strong flavor profile.

Wild Rice Pilaf with Pecans and Cranberries
SERVES 6 TO 8

1¾	cups chicken broth
2½	cups water
2	bay leaves
8	sprigs fresh thyme, divided into 2 bundles, each tied together with kitchen twine
1	cup wild rice, picked over and rinsed
3	tablespoons unsalted butter
1	onion, chopped fine
1	large carrot, peeled and chopped fine
	Salt and pepper
1½	cups long-grain white rice, rinsed
¾	cup dried cranberries
¾	cup pecans, toasted and chopped coarse
4½	teaspoons minced fresh parsley

1. Bring broth, ¼ cup water, bay leaves, and 1 bundle thyme to boil in medium saucepan over medium-high heat. Add wild rice, cover, and reduce heat to low; simmer until rice is plump and tender and has absorbed most of liquid, 35 to 45 minutes. Drain rice in fine-mesh strainer to remove excess liquid. Remove bay leaves and thyme. Return rice to now-empty saucepan, cover, and set aside.

2. Meanwhile, melt butter in medium saucepan over medium-high heat. Add onion, carrot, and 1 teaspoon salt and cook, stirring frequently, until vegetables are softened but not browned, about 4 minutes. Add white rice and stir to coat grains with butter; cook, stirring frequently, until grains begin to turn translucent, about 3 minutes. Meanwhile, bring remaining 2¼ cups water to boil in small saucepan or in microwave. Add boiling water and second thyme bundle to rice and return to boil. Reduce heat to low, sprinkle cranberries evenly over rice, and cover. Simmer until all liquid is absorbed, 16 to 18 minutes. Off heat, remove thyme and fluff rice with fork.

3. Combine wild rice, white rice mixture, pecans, and parsley in large bowl and toss with rubber spatula. Season with salt and pepper to taste; serve immediately.

VARIATION

Wild Rice Pilaf with Scallions, Cilantro, and Almonds
Omit dried cranberries. Substitute ¾ cup toasted sliced almonds for pecans and 2 tablespoons minced fresh cilantro for parsley. Add 2 thinly sliced scallions and 1 teaspoon lime juice with almonds.

SMART SHOPPING **Wild Rice**

When we tasted five brands, textural differences stood out the most. Some cooked up springy and firm, while others blew out. The differences come from the way the rice is processed. To create a shelf-stable product, manufacturers heat the grains by either parching or parboiling, which gelatinizes their starches and drives out moisture. To parch, manufacturers load the rice into cylinders that spin over a fire, but this is an inexact process that produces "crumbly" results. Parboiling, however, steams the grains for more uniform gelatinization, which translates into rice that cooks more evenly. The top three brands, including our winner, Goose Valley Wild Rice, were all parboiled.

Almost Hands-Free Risotto

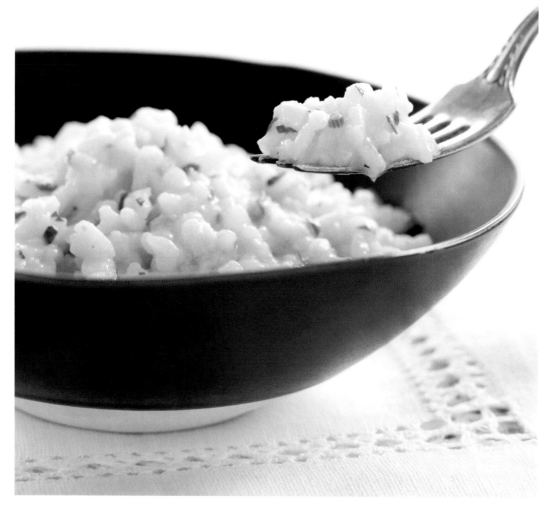

ARBORIO	Carnaroli rice can be substituted for the Arborio; the risotto will be softer and creamier. For more details on Arborio rice, see page 28.

✅ WHY THIS RECIPE WORKS

Classic risotto can demand half an hour of stovetop tedium for the best creamy results. Our goal was 5 minutes of stirring, tops. First, we swapped out the saucepan for a Dutch oven, which has a thick, heavy bottom, deep sides, and a tight-fitting lid—perfect for trapping and distributing heat as evenly as possible. Typical recipes dictate adding the broth in small increments (and stirring constantly after each addition), but we added most of the broth at once and covered the pot, allowing the rice to simmer until almost all the broth had been absorbed (stirring just twice). Cooking the rice in a large amount of liquid actually agitated the grains much like stirring. After adding the second and final addition of broth, we stirred the pot to ensure the bottom didn't cook more quickly than the top and then turned off the heat and let the rice finish cooking by residual heat. To finish, we simply stirred in butter, herbs, and a squeeze of lemon juice to brighten the flavors. This more hands-off method requires precise timing, so we strongly recommend using a timer.

Almost Hands-Free Risotto with Parmesan and Herbs
SERVES 6

- 5 cups chicken broth
- 1½ cups water
- 4 tablespoons unsalted butter
- 1 large onion, chopped fine
  Salt and pepper
- 1 garlic clove, minced
- 2 cups Arborio rice
- 1 cup dry white wine
- 2 ounces Parmesan cheese, grated (1 cup)
- 2 tablespoons minced fresh parsley
- 2 tablespoons minced fresh chives
- 1 teaspoon lemon juice

1. Bring broth and water to boil in large saucepan over high heat. Reduce heat to medium-low to maintain gentle simmer.

2. Melt 2 tablespoons butter in Dutch oven over medium heat. Add onion and ¾ teaspoon salt and cook, stirring frequently, until onion is softened, 4 to 5 minutes. Add garlic and cook until fragrant, about 30 seconds. Add rice and cook, stirring frequently, until grains are translucent around edges, about 3 minutes.

3. Add wine and cook, stirring constantly, until fully absorbed, 2 to 3 minutes. Stir 5 cups hot broth mixture into rice; reduce heat to medium-low, cover, and simmer until almost all liquid has been absorbed and rice is just al dente, 16 to 18 minutes, stirring twice during cooking.

4. Add ¾ cup hot broth mixture and stir constantly until risotto becomes creamy, about 3 minutes. Stir in Parmesan. Remove pot from heat, cover, and let stand for 5 minutes. Stir in remaining 2 tablespoons butter, herbs, and lemon juice. To loosen risotto, add up to ½ cup remaining broth mixture. Season with salt and pepper to taste and serve immediately.

Almost Hands-Free Risotto with Chicken and Herbs
SERVES 6

The thinner ends of the chicken breasts may be fully cooked by the time the broth is added to the rice, with the thicker ends finishing about 5 minutes later.

- 5 cups chicken broth
- 2 cups water
- 1 tablespoon olive oil
- 2 (12-ounce) bone-in split chicken breasts, trimmed and cut in half crosswise
- 4 tablespoons unsalted butter
- 1 large onion, chopped fine
  Salt and pepper
- 1 garlic clove, minced
- 2 cups Arborio rice
- 1 cup dry white wine
- 2 ounces Parmesan cheese, grated (1 cup)
- 2 tablespoons minced fresh parsley
- 2 tablespoons minced fresh chives
- 1 teaspoon lemon juice

1. Bring broth and water to boil in large saucepan over high heat. Reduce heat to medium-low to maintain gentle simmer.

2. Heat oil in Dutch oven over medium heat until just starting to smoke. Add chicken skin side down and cook without moving until golden brown, 4 to 6 minutes. Flip chicken and cook second side until lightly browned, about 2 minutes. Transfer chicken to saucepan of simmering broth and cook until chicken registers 165 degrees, 10 to 15 minutes. Transfer to large plate.

3. Melt 2 tablespoons butter in now-empty Dutch oven over medium heat. Add onion and ¾ teaspoon salt and cook, stirring frequently, until onion is softened, 4 to 5 minutes. Add garlic and cook until fragrant, about 30 seconds. Add rice and cook, stirring frequently, until grains are translucent around edges, about 3 minutes.

4. Add wine and cook, stirring constantly, until fully absorbed, 2 to 3 minutes. Stir 5 cups hot broth mixture into rice; reduce heat to medium-low, cover, and simmer until almost all liquid has been absorbed and rice is just al dente, 16 to 18 minutes, stirring twice during cooking.

5. Add ¾ cup hot broth mixture to risotto and stir constantly until risotto becomes creamy, about 3 minutes. Stir in Parmesan. Remove pot from heat, cover, and let stand for 5 minutes.

6. Meanwhile, remove and discard skin and bones from chicken and shred meat into bite-size pieces. Gently stir shredded chicken, remaining 2 tablespoons butter, herbs, and lemon juice into risotto. To loosen risotto, add up to ½ cup remaining broth mixture. Season with salt and pepper to taste and serve immediately.

SMART SHOPPING **Arborio Rice**

The stubby, milky grains of Arborio rice, once grown exclusively in Italy, are valued for their high starch content and the creaminess they bring to risotto. But does the best Arborio have to come from Italy? To find out, we cooked up batches of Parmesan risotto with two domestically grown brands of Arborio rice and four Italian imports. To our surprise, the winning rice, RiceSelect Arborio Rice, hails from Texas. Tasters were won over by its "creamy, smooth" grains with their "good bite."

TEST KITCHEN TIP **Easier Risotto**

We achieve the same creamy, evenly cooked risotto as that produced in traditional recipes—but with far less stirring—by adding more liquid at the outset and cooking the grains in a covered Dutch oven. A brief stir followed by a 5-minute rest provides additional insurance that the rice will be perfectly al dente.

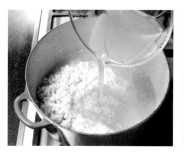
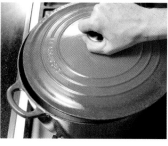
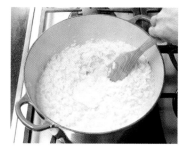

1. After rice has absorbed wine, add portion of hot broth mixture.

2. Reduce heat to medium-low, cover pot with lid, and simmer until almost all liquid has been absorbed, stirring twice.

3. After adding more broth and stirring for 3 minutes, stir in Parmesan and let pot sit, off heat and covered, for 5 minutes.

Creamy Parmesan Polenta

WHY THIS RECIPE WORKS

Polenta is a great option for a wintry, satisfying side that's also gluten-free; however, if you don't stir polenta almost constantly to ensure even cooking, it forms intractable lumps, and it can take up to an hour to cook. We wanted to get creamy, smooth polenta with rich corn flavor—but without the fussy process. From the outset, we knew that the right type of cornmeal was essential. Coarse-ground degerminated cornmeal gave us the soft but hearty texture and nutty flavor we were looking for. Taking a cue from dried bean recipes, which use baking soda to help break down the tough bean skins and accelerate cooking, we added a pinch of baking soda to our polenta. As we had hoped, the baking soda helped to soften the cornmeal's endosperm, which cut the cooking time. Baking soda also helped the granules break down and release their starch in a uniform way, so we could virtually eliminate the stirring time if we covered the pot and kept the heat on low. If the polenta bubbles or sputters even slightly after the first 10 minutes, the heat is too high and you may need a flame tamer (see page 79). Parmesan cheese and butter, stirred in at the last minute, ensured a satisfying, rich side dish. Instead of serving our polenta with a meaty ragu or grilled sausages (as is the custom in Italy), we opted to create a few hearty vegetable-based main course toppings, which can be prepared while the polenta cooks.

Creamy Parmesan Polenta
SERVES 4

- 7½ cups water
  - Salt and pepper
  - Pinch baking soda
- 1½ cups coarse-ground cornmeal (see page 78)
- 4 ounces Parmesan cheese, grated (2 cups), plus extra for serving
- 2 tablespoons unsalted butter

1. Bring water to boil in large saucepan over medium-high heat. Stir in 1½ teaspoons salt and baking soda. Slowly pour cornmeal into water in steady stream while stirring back and forth with wooden spoon or rubber spatula. Bring mixture to boil, stirring constantly, about 1 minute. Reduce heat to lowest possible setting and cover.

2. After 5 minutes, whisk polenta to smooth out any lumps that may have formed, about 15 seconds. (Make sure to scrape down sides and bottom of pan.) Cover and continue to cook, without stirring, until polenta grains are tender but slightly al dente, about 25 minutes longer. (Polenta should be loose and barely hold its shape; it will continue to thicken as it cools.)

3. Remove from heat, stir in Parmesan and butter, and season with pepper to taste. Let stand, covered, for 5 minutes. Serve, passing extra Parmesan separately.

Sautéed Cherry Tomato and Fresh Mozzarella Topping
MAKES ENOUGH FOR 4 SERVINGS

Don't stir the cheese into the sautéed tomatoes or it will melt prematurely and turn rubbery.

- 3 tablespoons extra-virgin olive oil
- 2 garlic cloves, peeled and sliced thin
  - Pinch red pepper flakes
  - Pinch sugar
- 1½ pounds cherry tomatoes, halved
  - Salt and pepper
- 6 ounces fresh mozzarella cheese, cut into ½-inch cubes (1 cup)
- 2 tablespoons shredded fresh basil

Heat oil, garlic, pepper flakes, and sugar in 12-inch nonstick skillet over medium-high heat until fragrant and sizzling, about 1 minute. Stir in tomatoes and cook until just beginning to soften, about 1 minute. Season with salt and pepper to taste and remove from heat. Spoon tomato mixture over individual portions of polenta, top with mozzarella, sprinkle with basil, and serve.

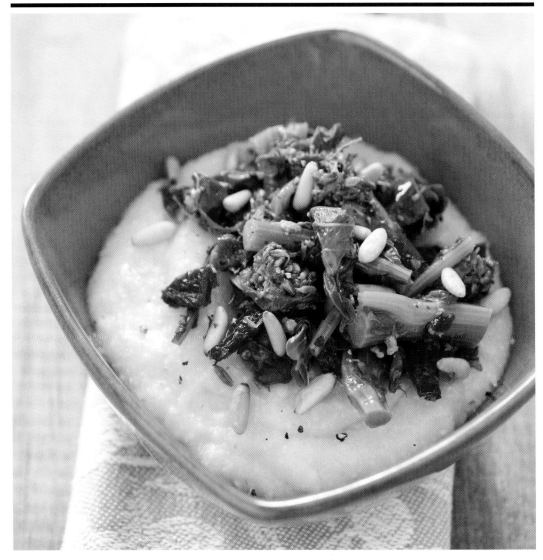

G-F TESTING LAB

CORNMEAL   Coarse-ground degerminated cornmeal such as yellow grits (with grains the size of couscous) works best in this recipe. Avoid instant and quick-cooking products, as well as whole grain, stone-ground, and regular cornmeal. Not all brands of cornmeal are processed in a gluten-free facility; make sure to read the label. For more details on cornmeal, see page 149.

Broccoli Rabe, Sun-Dried Tomato, and Pine Nut Topping

MAKES ENOUGH FOR 4 SERVINGS

- ½ cup oil-packed sun-dried tomatoes, chopped coarse
- 3 tablespoons extra-virgin olive oil
- 6 garlic cloves, minced
- ½ teaspoon red pepper flakes
  Salt
- 1 pound broccoli rabe, trimmed and cut into 1½-inch pieces
- ¼ cup chicken broth
- 3 tablespoons pine nuts, toasted

Heat sun-dried tomatoes, oil, garlic, pepper flakes, and ½ teaspoon salt in 12-inch nonstick skillet over medium-high heat, stirring frequently, until garlic is fragrant and slightly toasted, about 1½ minutes. Add broccoli rabe and broth, cover, and cook until rabe turns bright green, about 2 minutes. Uncover and cook, stirring frequently, until most of broth has evaporated and rabe is just tender, 2 to 3 minutes. Season with salt to taste. Spoon broccoli rabe mixture over individual portions of polenta, sprinkle with pine nuts, and serve.

Wild Mushroom and Rosemary Topping

MAKES ENOUGH FOR 4 SERVINGS

If you use shiitake mushrooms, they should be stemmed. To make this topping vegetarian, replace the chicken broth with an equal amount of vegetable broth.

- 2 tablespoons unsalted butter
- 2 tablespoons olive oil
- 1 small onion, chopped fine
- 2 garlic cloves, minced
- 2 teaspoons minced fresh rosemary
- 1 pound wild mushrooms (such as cremini, shiitake, or oyster), trimmed and sliced thin
- ⅓ cup chicken broth
  Salt and pepper

1. Heat butter and oil in 12-inch nonstick skillet over medium-high heat until shimmering. Add onion and cook, stirring frequently, until onion softens and begins to brown, 5 to 7 minutes. Stir in garlic and rosemary and cook until fragrant, about 30 seconds.

2. Add mushrooms and cook, stirring occasionally, until juices release, about 6 minutes. Add broth and salt and pepper to taste; simmer briskly until sauce thickens, about 8 minutes. Spoon mushroom mixture over individual portions of polenta and serve.

TEST KITCHEN TIP **Making a Flame Tamer**

To ensure even cooking, it's important to cook polenta over very gentle heat. If your stove runs hot, use a flame tamer (a metal disk that fits on top of the burner and helps regulate heat output) to keep the polenta from simmering too briskly. If you don't have a flame tamer, you can easily make one.

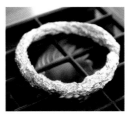

Take long sheet of heavy-duty aluminum foil and shape it into 1-inch-thick ring that will fit on your burner. The ring should be even thickness so that pot will rest flat on it.

TEST KITCHEN TIP **Making Polenta**

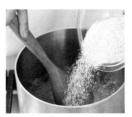

Slowly pour cornmeal into water in steady stream while stirring back and forth with wooden spoon or rubber spatula to prevent cornmeal from clumping.

Quinoa Pilaf

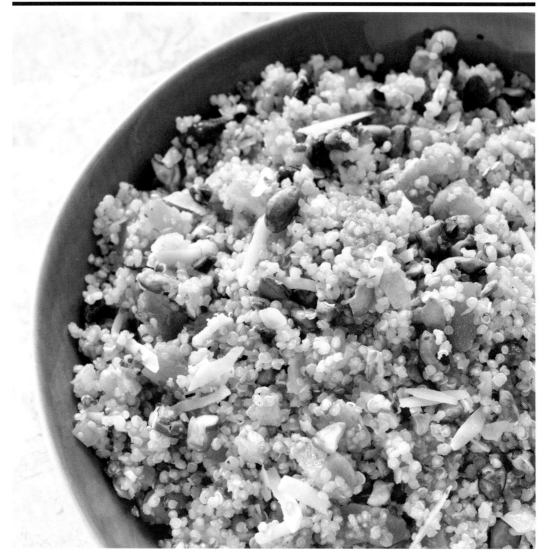

G-F TESTING LAB

QUINOA We like the convenience of prewashed quinoa. If you buy unwashed quinoa (or if you are unsure if it's washed), quinoa should be rinsed before cooking to remove its bitter protective coating (called saponin) and dried on a towel; see page 31. We developed this recipe using white quinoa. Red quinoa will work, but because its seed coat is thicker, the grains have a crunchier texture. Black quinoa's seed coat is even thicker than that of red quinoa; we don't recommend it for this recipe.

✔ WHY THIS RECIPE WORKS

Quinoa, often called a "supergrain" because of its great nutritional profile, has an appealingly firm bite and a nutty flavor, and it is easy to prepare, generally requiring 15 to 20 minutes of hands-off cooking. For a pilaf-style side dish, we toasted the quinoa prior to adding liquid; this ensured plump individual grains and also brought out its nutty flavor. Next, we considered the cooking liquid. Water was passable, but chicken broth better complemented the quinoa's flavor. After the quinoa had simmered, we pulled the pan off the heat and let it sit, covered, to allow the grains to steam. The result was evenly cooked, fluffy quinoa with just the right bite. We particularly like a combination of thyme and parsley in this recipe, but mint, tarragon, chives, or cilantro are also good choices.

Quinoa Pilaf with Herbs and Lemon
SERVES 4 TO 6

- 1½ cups prewashed quinoa
- 2 tablespoons unsalted butter, cut into 2 pieces
- 1 small onion, minced
- ¾ teaspoon salt
- 1¾ cups water
- 3 tablespoons chopped fresh herbs
- 1 tablespoon lemon juice

1. Toast quinoa in medium saucepan over medium-high heat, stirring frequently, until quinoa is very fragrant and makes continuous popping sound, 5 to 7 minutes. Transfer quinoa to bowl and set aside.

2. Return now-empty saucepan to medium-low heat and melt butter. Add onion and salt; cook, stirring frequently, until onion is softened and light golden, 5 to 7 minutes.

3. Increase heat to medium-high, stir in water and quinoa, and bring to simmer. Cover, reduce heat to low, and simmer until grains are just tender and liquid is absorbed, 18 to 20 minutes, stirring once halfway through cooking. Remove pot from heat and let sit, covered, for 10 minutes. Fluff quinoa with fork, stir in herbs and lemon juice, and serve.

VARIATIONS

Quinoa Pilaf with Chile, Queso Fresco, and Peanuts

Add 1 teaspoon chipotle powder and ¼ teaspoon ground cumin with onion. Substitute ½ cup crumbled queso fresco, 2 scallions, sliced thin, and ½ cup roasted unsalted peanuts, chopped coarse, for herbs. Substitute 4 teaspoons lime juice for lemon juice.

Quinoa Pilaf with Apricots, Pistachios, and Aged Gouda

Add ½ teaspoon ground coriander, ½ teaspoon grated lemon zest, ¼ teaspoon ground cumin, and ⅛ teaspoon black pepper with onion. Stir in ½ cup dried apricots, chopped coarse, before letting quinoa sit for 10 minutes in step 3. Substitute ½ cup shelled pistachios, chopped coarse, 2 ounces aged Gouda, shredded, and 2 tablespoons chopped fresh mint for herbs.

Quinoa Pilaf with Olives, Raisins, and Cilantro

Add ¼ teaspoon ground cumin, ¼ teaspoon dried oregano, and ⅛ teaspoon ground cinnamon with onion. Add ¼ cup golden raisins when stirring halfway through cooking in step 3. Substitute ⅓ cup pimento-stuffed green olives, chopped coarse, and 3 tablespoons minced fresh cilantro for herbs. Substitute 4 teaspoons red wine vinegar for lemon juice.

Quinoa Pilaf with Shiitakes, Edamame, and Ginger

Substitute 2 tablespoons vegetable oil for butter. Substitute whites of 4 scallions, minced, 4 ounces shiitake mushrooms, stemmed and sliced thin, and 2 teaspoons grated fresh ginger for onion. Stir in ½ cup cooked shelled edamame before letting quinoa sit for 10 minutes in step 3. Substitute 4 scallion greens, sliced thin, for herbs. Substitute 4 teaspoons rice vinegar and 1 tablespoon mirin for lemon juice.

Quinoa Salad with Bell Pepper and Cilantro

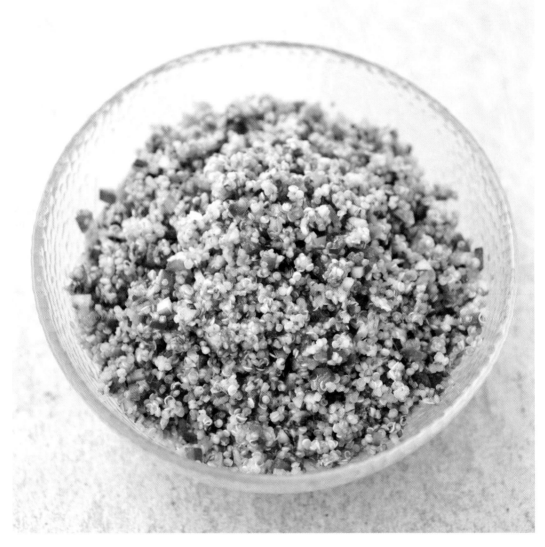

G-F TESTING LAB

QUINOA We like the convenience of prewashed quinoa. If you buy unwashed quinoa (or if you are unsure if it's washed), quinoa should be rinsed before cooking to remove its bitter protective coating (called saponin) and dried on a towel; see page 31. We used white quinoa to develop this recipe. Red quinoa will work, but because its seed coat is thicker, the grains have a crunchier texture. Black quinoa's seed coat is even thicker than that of red quinoa; we don't recommend it for this recipe.

WHY THIS RECIPE WORKS

Easy to prepare in advance and quick to assemble, quinoa salad makes a great fresh-tasting weekday lunch or picnic food. But too often the grains are either overcooked or unevenly cooked, and the resulting salad is clumpy or gritty. Toasting the quinoa in a dry pot helped to deepen its flavor. The liquid then went into the pot and the quinoa was covered and simmered gently until it was nearly tender, then spread over a rimmed baking sheet to cool. This ensured the grains (quinoa is actually a seed, but it is treated as a grain) didn't overcook and stayed fluffy and separate. Inspired by quinoa's Peruvian roots, we decided to give our salad a Latin flavor profile. Red bell pepper, jalapeño, and cilantro provided fresh flavors as well as color, sweetness, and some heat, and adding lime juice and cumin to the dressing brought it all together. After the 12-minute simmer in step 1, there will still be a little bit of water in the pan; it will be absorbed as the quinoa cools. To make this dish spicier, add the chile seeds.

Quinoa Salad with Red Bell Pepper and Cilantro
SERVES 4

1	cup prewashed quinoa
1½	cups water
	Salt and pepper
½	red bell pepper, stemmed, seeded, and chopped fine
½	jalapeño chile, stemmed, seeded, and minced
2	tablespoons finely chopped red onion
1	tablespoon minced fresh cilantro
2	tablespoons lime juice
1	tablespoon extra-virgin olive oil
2	teaspoons Dijon mustard
1	garlic clove, minced
½	teaspoon ground cumin

1. Toast quinoa in medium saucepan over medium-high heat, stirring frequently, until quinoa is lightly toasted and aromatic, about 5 minutes. Stir in water and ¼ teaspoon salt and bring to simmer. Reduce heat to low, cover, and continue to simmer until quinoa has absorbed most of water and is nearly tender, about 12 minutes. Spread quinoa out over rimmed baking sheet and set aside until tender and cool, about 20 minutes.

2. When quinoa is cool, transfer to large bowl. Stir in bell pepper, jalapeño, onion, and cilantro. In separate bowl, whisk lime juice, oil, mustard, garlic, and cumin together, then pour over quinoa mixture and toss to coat. Season with salt and pepper to taste and serve. (Quinoa salad can be refrigerated for up 1 day.)

SMART SHOPPING
The Many Colors of Quinoa

In just the past few years, quinoa has moved beyond the shelves of natural food stores and can be found at most supermarkets. And while at one time you typically saw only white (or golden) quinoa, you'll notice that red and black (or a mixture of the three) are also increasingly available. White quinoa has the largest seeds of the three varieties. It has a nutty, vegetal flavor with a hint of bitternesss; white quinoa is also the softest of the three types. Medium-sized red quinoa offers a heartier crunch and more prominent nuttiness. (Some of our tasters called it the "brown rice" of the quinoa world.) Black quinoa is the smallest of the three and has the thickest seed coat. As a result, black quinoa retains its shape during cooking and is very crunchy. Our tasters found the texture a bit sandy, although they liked the mild flavor that has hints of molasses. Red and white quinoa can be used interchangeably in pilaf and salad recipes. However, for our quinoa patties (see page 84), use white quinoa since only the softer white grains hold together enough to make a cohesive patty. We think black quinoa is best used in recipes tailored for its distinctive texture and flavor.

Quinoa Patties

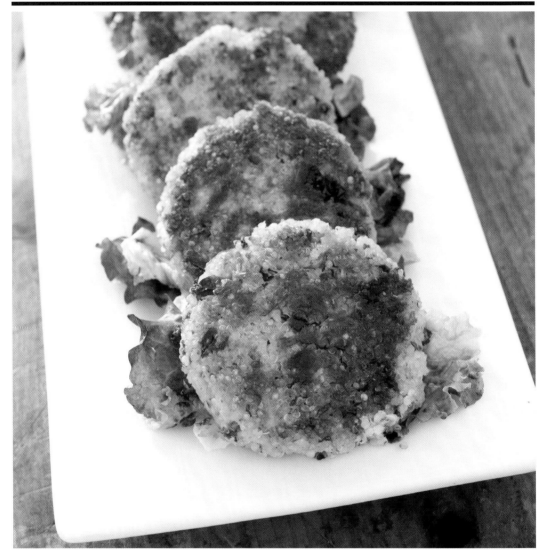

G-F TESTING LAB

QUINOA	We like the convenience of prewashed quinoa. If you buy unwashed quinoa (or if you are unsure if it's washed), quinoa should be rinsed before cooking to remove its bitter protective coating (called saponin) and dried on a towel; see page 31. White quinoa was used to develop this recipe. Do not substitute red or black quinoa; the patties will not hold together.

☑ WHY THIS RECIPE WORKS

We set out to develop a recipe for quinoa patties with bright, fresh flavors and enough add-ins to make them hearty and satisfying. While we liked the earthy flavor of red quinoa, no matter how long we cooked it, it simply didn't soften enough to form cohesive patties. Classic white (or golden) quinoa performed much better, and upping the amount of cooking liquid delivered even more cohesive patties since the quinoa cooked up extra-moist. We skipped the usual toasting step, which encourages the individual grains to separate rather than stick together. As for the binders, we tried mashed beans and potatoes, a variety of cheeses, bread, and processing some of the quinoa itself—but only the duo of a whole egg plus one yolk and cheese were successful. Chilling the formed patties for 30 minutes further ensured that they stayed together. Baking was an appealing hands-off cooking method, but the heat of the oven dried them out. It was much easier on the stovetop to create a crust on the exterior while maintaining a moist interior. Because the patties needed at least 8 minutes on each side to set up and cook through, cooking them over medium heat prevented burning but still resulted in a nice crust.

Quinoa Patties with Spinach and Sun-Dried Tomatoes
SERVES 4

- ½ cup oil-packed sun-dried tomatoes, chopped coarse, plus 1 tablespoon oil
- 4 scallions, chopped fine
- 4 garlic cloves, minced
- 2 cups water
- 1 cup prewashed white quinoa
- 1 teaspoon salt
- 1 large egg plus 1 large yolk, lightly beaten
- 2 ounces baby spinach, chopped (2 cups)
- 2 ounces Monterey Jack cheese, shredded (½ cup)
- ½ teaspoon grated lemon zest plus 2 teaspoons juice
- 2 tablespoons olive oil

1. Line rimmed baking sheet with parchment paper. Heat tomato oil in large saucepan over medium heat until shimmering. Add scallions and cook until softened, 3 to 5 minutes. Stir in garlic and cook until fragrant, about 30 seconds. Stir in water, quinoa, and salt and bring to simmer. Reduce heat to medium-low, cover, and continue to simmer until quinoa is tender, 18 to 20 minutes. Remove pot from heat and let sit, covered, until liquid is fully absorbed, about 10 minutes. Transfer to large bowl and let cool for 15 minutes.

2. Add sun-dried tomatoes, egg, egg yolk, spinach, Monterey Jack, lemon zest, and lemon juice to cooled quinoa and mix until uniform. Divide mixture into 8 equal portions (about ½ cup each), pack firmly into ½-inch-thick patties (about 3½ inches wide), and place on prepared sheet. Refrigerate, uncovered, until patties are chilled and firm, about 30 minutes.

3. Heat 1 tablespoon olive oil in 12-inch non-stick skillet over medium heat until shimmering. Carefully lay 4 patties in skillet and cook until well browned on first side, 8 to 10 minutes. Gently flip patties and continue to cook until golden on second side, 8 to 10 minutes.

4. Transfer patties to plate and tent loosely with aluminum foil. Return now-empty skillet to medium heat and repeat with remaining 1 tablespoon olive oil and remaining 4 patties. Serve.

TEST KITCHEN TIP **Cooking Quinoa Patties**

To keep patties from falling apart, wait until they are well browned before attempting to flip them.

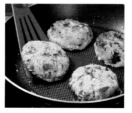

Carefully lay 4 chilled patties in hot skillet. Cook until set up and well browned on first side, 8 to 10 minutes. Gently flip patties. Cook until golden on second side, 8 to 10 minutes.

Kasha Pilaf with Caramelized Onions

✔ WHY THIS RECIPE WORKS

Kasha (buckwheat groats that have been roasted) has a deep, earthy flavor and a tender bite that make it a great fall or wintertime side dish for pairing with chicken or beef roasts. But we quickly learned that these kernels cook to an unappealing mush when simply simmered in liquid. Some research revealed that kasha kernels are often cooked with a beaten egg or egg white before the liquid is added to keep the kernels separate and firm. We wondered if vinegar, which we often add to the pot with dried lentils and beans to keep them from blowing out, would do the same thing (and keep things simpler). We gave it a shot; it made a big step in the right direction. But white vinegar's flavor was far too strong here. A couple tablespoons of milder, bright lemon juice worked perfectly. However, some grains were still breaking down too much, so we evaluated the cooking method next. Up to this point, we were bringing the kasha and liquid to a boil together, then reducing the heat and simmering until the kasha was cooked through—just as we do when we prepare a pilaf. In the end, waiting to add the kasha until the liquid was already at a boil solved the issue with blowouts. To balance the kasha's strong grassy flavor, we added plenty of sweet caramelized onions (which we cooked in the pan before preparing the kasha), along with garlic, parsley, and pine nuts. Use a gentle hand when stirring in the add-ins at the end, as the kasha will become pasty if mixed too vigorously.

Kasha Pilaf with Caramelized Onions
SERVES 4 TO 6

- 3 tablespoons extra-virgin olive oil
- 2 onions, chopped
  Salt and pepper
- 3 garlic cloves, minced
- 3 cups water
- 1½ cups kasha, rinsed (see page 31)
- 2 tablespoons lemon juice
- ¼ cup pine nuts, toasted
- 2 tablespoons minced fresh parsley

1. Heat 1 tablespoon oil in large saucepan over medium heat until shimmering. Add onions and ¼ teaspoon salt and cook, stirring occasionally, until browned, 10 to 15 minutes. Add garlic and cook until fragrant, about 30 seconds. Stir in ¼ cup water, scraping up any browned bits; transfer onion mixture to bowl.

2. Add remaining 2¾ cups water to now-empty pan and bring to boil. Stir in kasha, lemon juice, and 1 teaspoon salt and return to simmer. Reduce heat to low, cover, and simmer until liquid is absorbed, about 10 minutes. Remove pot from heat and lay clean folded kitchen towel underneath lid. Let sit for 10 minutes.

3. Fluff kasha with fork and gently stir in onion mixture, pine nuts, parsley, and remaining 2 tablespoons oil until just combined. Season with salt and pepper to taste. Serve.

SMART SHOPPING Kasha

Buckwheat, despite its name, is not related to wheat. It is actually an herb. In addition to being ground to make buckwheat flour, the kernels of its triangular seeds can be hulled and crushed to make groats (see pages 37 and 28 for more on flour and groats). Kasha is buckwheat groats that have been roasted to bring out their flavor and aroma. Kasha is often used in blintzes, knishes, and varnitchkes, or to make pilaf and hot cereal. Because kasha, unlike groats, has a fairly bold flavor and a distinctly earthy smell, we find that it pairs best with fall- and winter-inspired dishes like roasted meats. Buckwheat products can be found in natural food stores and well-stocked supermarkets.

Creamy Cheesy Millet

✓ WHY THIS RECIPE WORKS

After turning millet into a satisfying breakfast porridge (see our recipe on page 63), we realized it wasn't a far leap to use these tiny seeds to prepare a rustic, savory side dish similar to a creamy polenta. However, it wasn't just a matter of making some savory ingredient additions to a stripped-down version of the porridge. The porridge had a texture that was slightly set up, like oatmeal, and we wanted looser results for this dish. While we'd cooked our porridge in 3 cups of water and then simply stirred in 1 cup of milk at the end for some richness, we found the millet broke down only so much, even with additional cooking. To get looser results, we had to start the millet in 5 cups of liquid (we settled on 4 cups of water and 1 cup of milk). This made all the difference. We slightly overcooked the millet, just as we had done for our porridge, so that the seeds burst and released their starch, creating the right creamy consistency. Since millet is very mild, we stirred in a good amount of Parmesan and basil to ensure this dish had plenty of flavor.

Creamy Cheesy Millet
SERVES 4 TO 6

- 1 tablespoon olive oil
- 1 shallot, minced
- 2 garlic cloves, minced
- 1 cup millet, rinsed and dried on a towel (see page 31)
- 4 cups water
- 1 cup whole milk
  Salt and pepper
- 2 ounces Parmesan cheese, grated (1 cup)
- 2 tablespoons shredded fresh basil

1. Heat oil in large saucepan over medium heat until shimmering. Stir in shallot and cook until softened, about 2 minutes. Add garlic and cook until fragrant, about 30 seconds. Stir in millet and cook, stirring often, until fragrant and lightly browned, about 2 minutes.

2. Stir in water, milk, and 1 teaspoon salt and bring to boil. Reduce heat to low, cover, and simmer, stirring occasionally, until thick and porridgy, about 20 minutes. Uncover and continue to cook, stirring frequently, until millet is mostly broken down, 8 to 10 minutes.

3. Off heat, stir in Parmesan until melted. Sprinkle with basil and season with salt and pepper to taste. Serve.

SMART SHOPPING **Millet**

Believed to be the first domesticated cereal grain, this tiny cereal grass seed has a long history and is still a staple in a large part of the world, particularly Asia and Africa. The seeds can be ground into flour or used whole. Millet has a mellow corn flavor that makes it work well in both savory and sweet applications, including flatbreads, puddings, and pan-fried cakes. It can be cooked pilaf-style or turned into a creamy breakfast porridge or polenta-like dish (as in the recipe on this page) by slightly overcooking the seeds, which causes the seeds to burst and release starch.

Curried Millet Pilaf

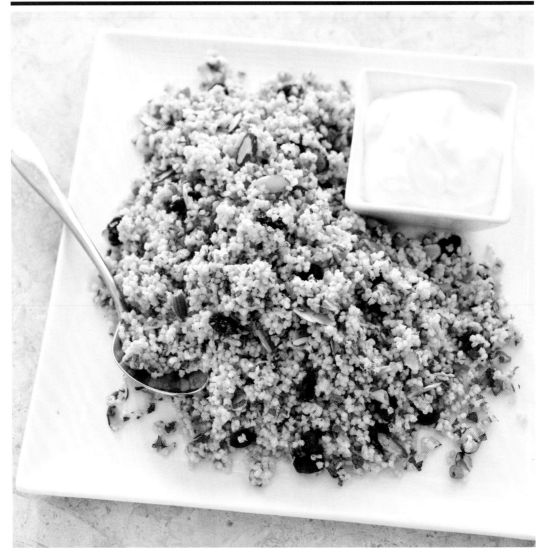

MILLET See page 87 for more details on millet.

☑ WHY THIS RECIPE WORKS

Now that we had two creamier millet dishes in our arsenal (see Millet Porridge with Maple Syrup, page 63, and Creamy Cheesy Millet, page 87), we set out to feature the tiny seeds in a pilaf-style dish. Toasting the millet before simmering the seeds in water gave them some nutty depth, and, after some testing, we landed on a 2:1 ratio of liquid to millet, which ensured evenly cooked, fluffy seeds. Since millet is a staple in Middle Eastern and Indian cuisines, we turned to that part of the world to inspire the flavor profile of our pilaf, adding basil, mint, raisins, almonds, and curry powder. To finish, we served it with a dollop of yogurt for richness and an appealing cooling counterpoint to the heat of the curry. We prefer whole-milk yogurt in this recipe but low-fat yogurt can be substituted if desired. Unlike other grains, we have found that millet can become gluey if allowed to steam off heat. Once all the liquid has been absorbed, use a gentle hand to stir in the basil, raisins, almonds, and scallion greens, and then immediately serve this pilaf.

Curried Millet Pilaf
SERVES 4 TO 6

1	tablespoon extra-virgin olive oil
3	scallions, white and green parts separated, sliced thin
1	teaspoon curry powder
1½	cups millet, rinsed and dried on a towel (see page 31)
3	cups water
	Salt and pepper
½	cup chopped fresh basil and/or mint
¼	cup raisins
¼	cup sliced almonds, toasted
½	cup plain yogurt

1. Heat oil in large saucepan over medium heat until shimmering. Add scallion whites and curry and cook until fragrant, about 1 minute. Stir in millet and cook, stirring often, until lightly browned, about 2 minutes.

2. Stir in water and ¾ teaspoon salt and bring to boil. Reduce heat to low, cover, and simmer until liquid is absorbed, 15 to 20 minutes.

3. Off heat, using fork, gently stir in basil, raisins, almonds, and scallion greens until just combined. Season with salt and pepper to taste. Serve, dolloping individual portions with yogurt.

SMART SHOPPING **Curry Powder**

Though blends can vary dramatically, sweet curry powder (also known as mild) combines as many as 20 different ground spices, herbs, and seeds, the staples being turmeric, coriander, cumin, black and red pepper, cinnamon, cloves, fennel seeds, cardamom, ginger, and fenugreek. Neither too sweet nor too hot, our winning blend is Penzeys Sweet Curry Powder, which sets the standard for a balanced yet complex curry powder.

Buckwheat Tabbouleh

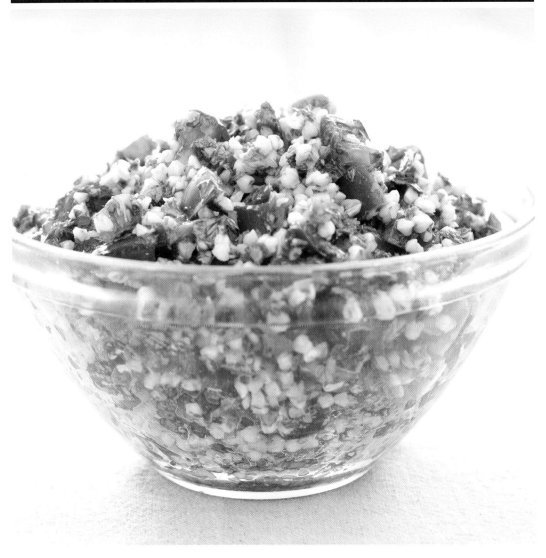

BUCKWHEAT   Mild-tasting buckwheat groats work better in this recipe than kasha (roasted buckwheat groats). See page 86 for more information on kasha.

☑ WHY THIS RECIPE WORKS

Featuring parsley, bulgur (a product of the wheat berry), mint, and chopped tomatoes tossed in a bright lemon vinaigrette, classic Mediterranean tabbouleh has a refreshing flavor profile that makes it a great light side. All we had to do was find a gluten-free substitute with a clean flavor to use in lieu of the bulgur. In the end, we landed on buckwheat groats. Millet, though similar in appearance to bulgur, was too starchy and clumpy. Kasha, which is roasted buckwheat groats, added a deep earthiness that overwhelmed the delicate flavor profile of tabbouleh. The buckwheat groats (the same kernels as kasha but raw rather than roasted) lent a mild, appealing earthiness to our salad that didn't dominate. As for the cooking method, the pilaf approach seemed like the best option at first, but it produced groats that were too starchy and gummy. Boiling the kernels in plenty of water was a much better solution. Some of the starch washed away in the cooking water, giving us separate, evenly cooked kernels. For the herbs, we wanted plenty of fresh, peppery parsley; 1½ cups made just enough of a presence and balanced well with ½ cup of fresh mint. To ensure undiluted, bright flavor in the final tabbouleh, we salted the tomatoes to rid them of excess moisture before tossing them into the salad.

Buckwheat Tabbouleh
SERVES 4

- ¾ **cup buckwheat groats, rinsed (see page 31)**
- **Salt and pepper**
- 3 **tomatoes, cored and cut into ½-inch pieces**
- 2 **tablespoons lemon juice**
- **Pinch cayenne pepper**
- ¼ **cup extra-virgin olive oil**
- 1½ **cups minced fresh parsley**
- ½ **cup minced fresh mint**
- 2 **scallions, sliced thin**

1. Bring 2 quarts water to boil in large saucepan. Stir in buckwheat and 1 teaspoon salt. Return to boil, then reduce to simmer and cook until tender, 10 to 12 minutes. Drain buckwheat, transfer to bowl, and let cool 15 minutes.

2. Meanwhile, toss tomatoes and ¼ teaspoon salt in bowl. Transfer to fine-mesh strainer, set strainer in bowl, and let stand for 30 minutes, tossing occasionally.

3. Whisk lemon juice, cayenne, and ¼ teaspoon salt together in large bowl. Whisking constantly, drizzle in oil.

4. Add drained tomatoes, cooled buckwheat, parsley, mint, and scallions; toss gently to combine. Cover and let sit at room temperature until flavors blend, about 30 minutes or up to 2 hours. Toss to recombine and season with salt and pepper to taste. Serve.

SMART SHOPPING **Buckwheat Groats**

Buckwheat, despite its name, is not related to wheat. It is actually an herb. In addition to being ground to make buckwheat flour, which is often used in pancakes (see our recipe for Buckwheat Blueberry Pancakes, page 36), the kernels of its triangular seeds can be hulled and crushed to make groats. These groats have a relatively mild, grassy flavor, making them a good side dish to a variety of entrées. Buckwheat groats cook relatively quickly, making them a good option for weeknight meals. Buckwheat products can be found in natural food stores and well-stocked supermarkets.

Oat Berry Pilaf

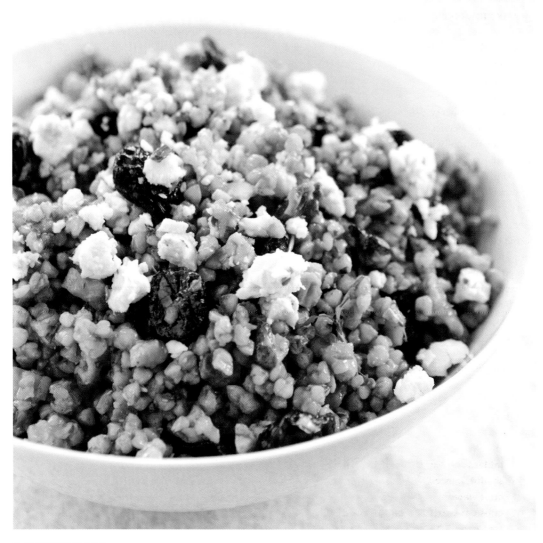

G-F TESTING LAB

OAT BERRIES   Oat berries may also be labeled oat groats. Not all oat berries are processed in a gluten-free facility, so make sure to read the label.

✓ WHY THIS RECIPE WORKS

While we think of oats mostly as part of a wholesome breakfast, oat berries—whole oats that have been hulled and cleaned but not processed—have a pleasant chew and are the perfect gluten-free replacement for farro or wheat berries. We wanted a satisfying oat berry pilaf with hearty add-ins. To cook the oat berries, we opted not to toast them since they naturally have a nutty flavor, and instead added the water and oat berries to the pan after sautéing some shallot. After testing various ratios of water to oat berries, we settled on 4:3 (2 cups water to 1½ cups oat berries). Creamy, pungent Gorgonzola seemed like it would be a nice balance to the earthy oat berries' nutty flavor, so we started there for our add-ins. First we tried stirring the Gorgonzola into the oat berries once they were cooked, but the result was a thick, gluey mixture. It was better to wait and simply sprinkle the cheese over the oat berries just before serving. The addition of tart cherries and tangy balsamic vinegar cut through the richness and strong flavors, while parsley gave our pilaf the freshness it needed.

Oat Berry Pilaf with Walnuts and Gorgonzola
SERVES 4 TO 6

1	tablespoon extra-virgin olive oil
1	shallot, minced
2	cups water
1½	cups oat berries (groats), rinsed (see page 31)
	Salt and pepper
¾	cup walnuts, toasted and chopped
½	cup dried cherries
2	tablespoons minced fresh parsley
1	tablespoon balsamic vinegar
2	ounces Gorgonzola cheese, crumbled (½ cup)

1. Heat oil in large saucepan over medium heat until shimmering. Add shallot and cook, stirring occasionally, until softened, about 2 minutes. Stir in water, oat berries, and ¼ teaspoon salt and bring to simmer. Reduce heat to low, cover, and continue to simmer until oat berries are tender but still slightly chewy, 30 to 40 minutes.

2. Remove pot from heat and lay clean folded dish towel underneath lid. Let sit for 10 minutes. Fluff oat berries with fork and fold in walnuts, cherries, and parsley. Drizzle with vinegar. Transfer pilaf to serving bowl. Sprinkle Gorgonzola over top and season with salt and pepper to taste. Serve.

SMART SHOPPING **Oat Berries**

Labeled either oat berries or oat groats, this gluten-free whole grain is simply whole oats that have been hulled and cleaned. They are the least processed oat product (other forms are processed further, such as being rolled flat, cut, or ground). Because they haven't been processed, they retain a high nutritional value. They have an appealing chewy texture and mildly nutty flavor. Oats are usually thought of as a breakfast cereal, but oat berries make a great savory side dish cooked pilaf-style.

Oat Berry Salad

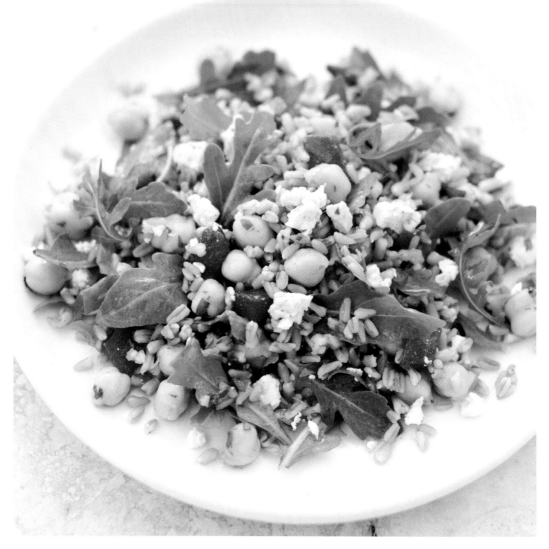

G-F TESTING LAB

OAT BERRIES   Oat berries may also be labeled oat groats. Not all oat berries are processed in a gluten-free facility, so make sure to read the label. See page 93 for more information on oat berries.

WHY THIS RECIPE WORKS

Chewy, nutty oat berries make a great side dish (see our pilaf recipe, page 92), but we also thought these qualities were worth highlighting in a main-course salad. Cooking the oat berries in a large amount of water, pasta style, then draining and rinsing them under cold water to stop the cooking, gave us the chewy, tender berries we were after. For the leafy component of our dinner salad, peppery arugula paired well with the nutty oat berries, and we added chickpeas for a little more heft and complementary nutty flavor and creamy-firm texture. Roasted red peppers added sweetness, and creamy feta lent the right richness and salty bite. A simple lemon and cilantro vinaigrette spiked with cumin, paprika, and cayenne provided the perfect amount of spice and brightness.

Oat Berry, Chickpea, and Arugula Salad
SERVES 4 TO 6

  2 **tablespoons lemon juice**
  2 **tablespoons minced fresh cilantro**
  1 **teaspoon honey**
  1 **garlic clove, minced**
  ¼ **teaspoon ground cumin**
     Salt and pepper
  ⅛ **teaspoon paprika**
     Pinch cayenne pepper
  3 **tablespoons extra-virgin olive oil**
  1 **cup oat berries (groats), rinsed (see page 31)**
  1 **(15-ounce) can chickpeas, rinsed**
  ½ **cup jarred roasted red peppers, drained, patted dry, and chopped**
  2 **ounces feta cheese, crumbled (½ cup)**
  6 **ounces (6 cups) baby arugula**

1. Whisk lemon juice, cilantro, honey, garlic, cumin, ¼ teaspoon salt, paprika, and cayenne together in bowl. Whisking constantly, drizzle in oil; set aside.

2. Bring 2 quarts water to boil in large saucepan. Add oat berries and ½ teaspoon salt, partially cover, and cook, stirring often, until tender but still chewy, 45 to 50 minutes. Drain oat berries and rinse under cold running water until cool. Transfer oat berries to large bowl.

3. Stir in chickpeas, roasted red peppers, and feta. Whisk vinaigrette to re-emulsify, then drizzle dressing over oat berry mixture and toss to combine. (Oat berry mixture can be refrigerated overnight; bring to room temperature before proceeding.) Add arugula and gently toss to combine. Season with salt and pepper to taste. Serve.

SMART SHOPPING **Chickpeas**

Popular particularly in Mediterranean, Middle Eastern, and Indian cuisines, canned chickpeas are a favorite among canned beans in the test kitchen because they hold up well to cooking. However, our tasters found that many brands are bland or have bitter and metallic flavors. They preferred those that were well seasoned and had a creamy yet "al dente" texture. Pastene Chickpeas came out on top.

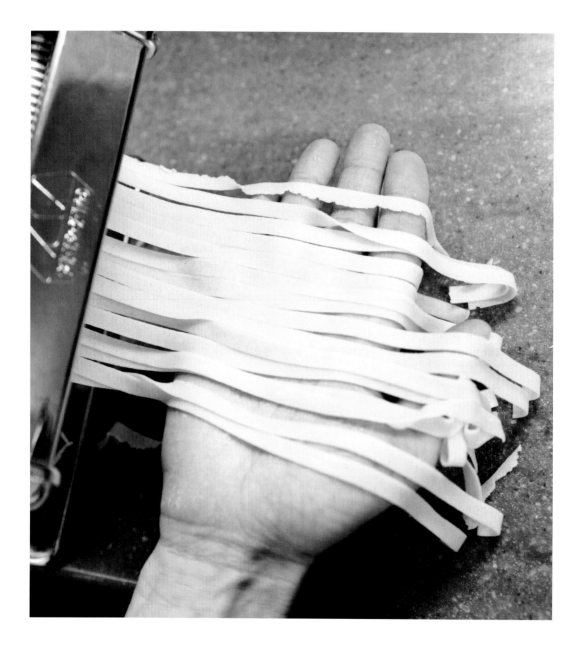

PASTA

Fresh Pasta

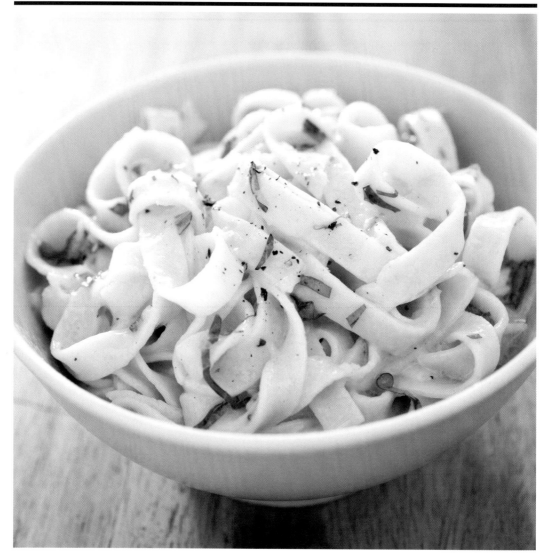

BROWN RICE FLOUR	Not all brands of brown rice flour are milled the same way. We strongly recommend using a finely ground flour such as Bob's Red Mill. See page 19 for details on buying brown rice flour.
TAPIOCA STARCH	Tapioca starch is often labeled tapioca flour. See page 20 for more details on this ingredient.
XANTHAN GUM	Do not omit the xanthan gum; it is crucial to the structure of the pasta dough. For more information, see page 16.

✔ WHY THIS RECIPE WORKS

Dried pasta (made with or without wheat) isn't always the best choice, especially for refined cream and butter sauces. So how do you make great fresh pasta without wheat flour—one of only two ingredients in the classic recipe (the other is eggs)? We started by testing as many different flours as possible. In the end we settled on a combination of brown rice flour for structure and tapioca starch for elasticity. Our traditional pasta recipe uses three whole eggs. However, since gluten-free pasta is more brittle, we found we needed to add a fourth egg to ensure the noodles set up properly once cooked. Xanthan gum was a must for structure, while a little oil made the dough easier to roll out. We developed a few sauces (see page 102) that could be put together quickly and offered good flavor but didn't outshine our fresh noodles. It takes just seconds to make pasta dough in the food processor, but you can use a stand mixer if you prefer. Combine the dry ingredients on low speed, then add the eggs and oil and mix on medium-low until the dough comes together in a rough ball, about 10 seconds. You will need a manual pasta machine to make this recipe. Do not attempt to roll this pasta with just a rolling pin; it will be too difficult to get the pasta thin enough, and the dough will be much more likely to tear. We make fettuccine here, but you can also follow the recipe through step 4 and shape the pasta sheets into farfalle or garganelli following the steps on page 103.

Fresh Pasta
MAKES ABOUT 1 POUND PASTA; SERVES 4 TO 6

7½	ounces (1⅔ cups) brown rice flour, plus extra for rolling
2½	ounces (½ cup plus 2 tablespoons) tapioca starch
1	tablespoon xanthan gum
½	teaspoon salt
4	large eggs
1	tablespoon olive oil

1. Pulse brown rice flour, tapioca starch, xanthan gum, and salt in food processor until combined. Add eggs and oil and process until dough forms and clears sides of bowl, about 10 seconds.

2. Transfer dough to clean counter and knead until dough comes together, about 30 seconds. (Dough should hold together but won't be smooth.) Shape dough into 6-inch-long cylinder. Cut cylinder into 6 equal pieces and cover with plastic wrap.

3. Working with 1 piece of dough at a time (keeping remaining dough covered), shape into 4-inch square using rolling pin and hands. Using manual pasta machine, run flattened dough through widest setting twice. Fold ends of dough toward middle to re-form 4-inch square, press to seal, and feed open side of dough once more through widest setting. Repeat folding and rolling on widest setting 2 or 3 more times, until edges of dough are even.

4. Narrow setting and continue to run dough through each setting twice, until dough is translucent and thin enough that you can clearly see outline of your hand through dough. (If dough begins to stick and tear, dust sheet with brown rice flour and roll through same setting until smooth. If dough becomes too long to manage, cut in half crosswise.)

5. If not already done, cut sheet in half. Run each piece through cutter for fettuccine, lay pasta on dish towel in baking sheet, and cover with plastic wrap. Repeat steps 3 through 5 with remaining dough. (Noodles can be held for 2 hours before cooking.)

TO COOK PASTA: Bring 4 quarts water to boil in large pot. Add pasta and 1 tablespoon salt and cook, stirring often, until tender but still al dente, about 2 minutes. Reserve 1 cup cooking water. Drain pasta, return to pot, toss with sauce and reserved cooking water as needed, and serve immediately.

TO MAKE AHEAD: Spread pasta out evenly over baking sheet (avoid clumps). Transfer sheet to freezer and chill until pasta is firm, about 1 hour. Transfer pasta to zipper-lock bag and freeze for up to 2 weeks. Cook frozen pasta straight from freezer as directed.

TEST KITCHEN TIP **Making Fresh Gluten-Free Pasta**

The process for making gluten-free pasta is similar to the one used to make fresh pasta with wheat flour, but the dough is softer and tears more easily. Support the dough with one hand while feeding it through the machine. Also, don't let the dough drape over the machine because it can tear from its own weight.

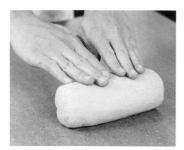

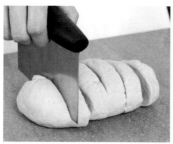

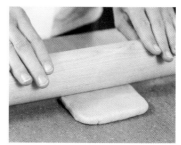

1. After kneading dough briefly, shape it into 6-inch cylinder.

2. Divide into 6 equal pieces. Cover pieces of dough with plastic wrap to prevent drying.

3. Working with 1 piece at a time, shape dough into 4-inch square using rolling pin and your hands.

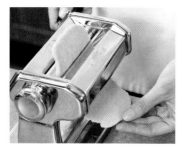

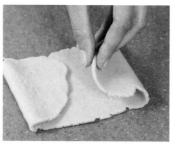

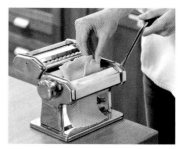

4. Using manual pasta machine, run flattened dough through widest setting twice.

5. Fold ends of dough toward middle to re-form 4-inch square and press to seal.

6. Feed open side of dough through widest setting. Repeat folding and rolling 2 or 3 more times until edges are even.

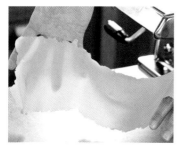

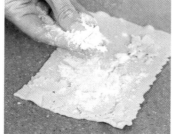

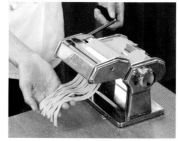

7. Narrow setting and run dough through machine twice. Narrow setting and repeat, continuing to roll dough through each setting twice, until dough is thin enough that you can clearly see outline of your hand through dough.

8. If dough begins to stick and tear, dust sheet with brown rice flour and roll through same setting until smooth. If dough becomes too long to manage, cut in half crosswise and work with each piece individually.

9. If not already done, cut sheet in half crosswise. Make fettuccine noodles by running each sheet of pasta through wide cutter on pasta machine (each noodle will measure $\frac{1}{8}$ to $\frac{1}{4}$ inch across).

Fresh Pasta

Homemade pasta dough has so few ingredients that we knew coming up with a gluten-free alternative with the same delicate flavor and chew would be daunting. Getting the ingredients right as well as developing a reliable rolling method turned out to be trickier than we imagined. Here's what we learned.

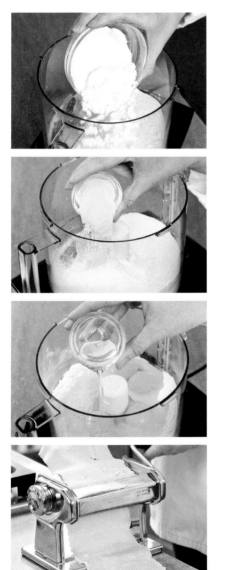

1. TWO FLOURS ARE KEY: Using our flour blend (or commercial gluten-free flour blends) produced pasta that was tough, so we turned to individual flours instead. We knew that tapioca starch (flour) might be a good place to start because we found that it provided elasticity in previous recipes. Tests using all tapioca starch, however, turned out pasta that was rubbery. We needed a flour that had a higher protein content, which would provide some structure for our dough. Brown rice flour complemented the tapioca starch perfectly, and we settled on a ratio of 3 parts brown rice flour to 1 part tapioca starch.

2. ADD XANTHAN GUM: The brown rice flour and tapioca starch created the desired soft but resilient texture, but we still needed xanthan gum to hold our dough together. (Without it, our pasta dough was unworkable.) However, we quickly discovered that too much xanthan gum can be a bad thing; the dough can absorb only so much, and after it has reached that capacity the excess leaches out, coating the outside of the pasta and making it slimy when cooked. In the end, 1 tablespoon of xanthan gum made the dough easy to work with but didn't affect the texture of the cooked noodles.

3. AN ADDITIONAL EGG AND OLIVE OIL: Eggs are traditional in pasta recipes (we use three in our established recipe), and we found that four were necessary for our gluten-free recipe. The eggs provided a rich flavor and texture (without which the dough didn't set up properly once cooked). In addition, the moisture they contributed to the raw dough made it easier to roll out. We noticed, however, that the cut pasta became brittle if we didn't cook it right away. A tablespoon of olive oil solved this problem and made the dough even more pliable and easier to roll out.

4. ROLL AND ROLL AGAIN: Our gluten-free pasta dough was much more likely than traditional pasta dough to tear and stick to the rollers of our manual pasta machine. Sprinkling our sheet of dough with a little brown rice flour helped, but we had real success when we rolled the sheet of dough through each setting on the pasta machine an additional time. This second pass through the machine smoothed out any imperfections and created a more cohesive sheet. We also found that holding the dough while rolling it through, and not letting it drag along the back of the pasta machine, prevented the dough from tearing.

Sauces for Fresh Pasta

Fresh Pasta al Limone
SERVES 4 TO 6

✔ **WHY THIS RECIPE WORKS**

With its clean, simple flavor profile featuring lemon and olive oil, this classic Italian sauce comes together as easily as a vinaigrette and is a great match for fresh pasta. Stirring in grated Parmesan cheese slightly thickened the sauce so that it could coat the pasta properly, while a generous amount of basil lent color and a necessary herbal balance. Finally, we found just a bit of butter helped to round out the flavors.

⅓ cup extra-virgin olive oil
2 teaspoons grated lemon zest plus ¼ cup juice (2 lemons)
1 garlic clove, minced to paste
  Salt and pepper
2 ounces Parmesan cheese, grated (1 cup)
1 recipe Fresh Pasta (page 99)
½ cup shredded fresh basil
2 tablespoons unsalted butter, softened

1. Whisk oil, lemon zest and juice, garlic, and ½ teaspoon salt together in large bowl, then stir in Parmesan until thick and creamy; cover and set aside.

2. Meanwhile bring 4 quarts water to boil in large pot. Add pasta and 1 tablespoon salt and cook, stirring often, until tender but still al dente, about 2 minutes. Reserve 1 cup cooking water, then drain pasta and return it to pot. Add sauce, basil, and butter and toss to combine, adding reserved cooking water as needed to adjust consistency. Season with salt and pepper to taste and serve immediately.

Fresh Pasta with Tomato–Brown Butter Sauce
SERVES 4 TO 6

✔ **WHY THIS RECIPE WORKS**

While most tomato sauces start with olive oil, we put browned butter to work here for a nuttier, just-rich-enough sauce that would work well with our homemade fresh pasta. After browning the butter we added garlic for depth and then our tomatoes; processing whole canned tomatoes before incorporating them delivered a sauce with the proper consistency. Simmering the sauce for less than 10 minutes thickened it just enough, then we finished with sherry vinegar (adding it at the end preserved its bright flavor) and more butter. When browning the butter, make sure to use a skillet with a traditional (not a dark nonstick) finish. Butter can go from brown to burnt quickly, and the light finish of the pan will ensure you can see the color change.

1 (28-ounce) can whole peeled tomatoes
4 tablespoons unsalted butter, cut into 4 pieces
2 garlic cloves, minced
½ teaspoon sugar
  Salt and pepper
2 teaspoons sherry vinegar
1 recipe Fresh Pasta (page 99)
3 tablespoons chopped fresh basil
  Grated Parmesan cheese

1. Process tomatoes and their juice in food processor until smooth, about 30 seconds. Melt 3 tablespoons butter in 12-inch skillet over medium-high heat, swirling occasionally, until butter is dark brown and releases nutty aroma, about 1½ minutes. Stir in garlic and cook for 10 seconds. Stir in processed tomatoes, sugar, and ½ teaspoon salt and simmer until sauce is slightly reduced, about 8 minutes. Off heat, whisk in remaining piece butter and vinegar. Season with salt and pepper to taste; cover to keep warm.

2. Meanwhile bring 4 quarts water to boil in large pot. Add pasta and 1 tablespoon salt and cook, stirring often, until tender but still al dente, about 2 minutes. Reserve 1 cup cooking water, then drain pasta and return it to pot. Add sauce, ¼ cup reserved cooking water, and basil to pot with pasta; toss to combine, adding remaining cooking water as needed to adjust consistency. Season with salt and pepper to taste and serve immediately, passing Parmesan separately.

Fresh Pasta Alfredo
SERVES 4 TO 6

✓ WHY THIS RECIPE WORKS
We wanted an Alfredo sauce that was rich and coated the noodles well but we also wanted one that wasn't too heavy. The challenge is managing the heavy cream, which is usually reduced by half, making the sauce unpalatably thick. We got the best results by reducing only 1 cup of the cream and saving the remaining ½ cup to add at the end. We also used a lighter hand when adding the cheese and butter; just ¾ cup Parmesan and 2 tablespoons butter were sufficient. Try to find cream that has been only pasteurized, not ultrapasteurized. The latter tastes flat since it has been heated to a higher temperature during processing.

1½	cups heavy cream
2	tablespoons unsalted butter
	Salt and pepper
1	recipe Fresh Pasta (page 99)
1½	ounces Parmesan cheese, grated (¾ cup)
⅛	teaspoon ground nutmeg

1. Bring 1 cup cream and butter to simmer in large saucepan. Reduce heat to low and simmer gently until mixture measures ⅔ cup, 12 to 15 minutes. Off heat, stir in remaining ½ cup cream, ½ teaspoon salt, and ½ teaspoon pepper. Cover and set aside.

2. Meanwhile bring 4 quarts water to boil in large pot. Add pasta and 1 tablespoon salt and cook, stirring often, until tender but still al dente, about 2 minutes. Reserve 1 cup cooking water, then drain pasta and return it to pot.

3. Add cream mixture, Parmesan, and nutmeg to pot with pasta and cook over low heat, tossing to combine, until cheese is melted and sauce coats pasta, about 1 minute. Add reserved cooking water as needed to adjust consistency (sauce may look thin but will gradually thicken as pasta is served). Season with salt and pepper to taste and serve immediately.

TEST KITCHEN TIP **Making Shaped Pastas**

Instead of cutting the pasta into fettuccine, you can follow the Fresh Pasta recipe through step 4 and then follow the steps below to make shapes from the rolled sheets. Before you begin, make sure to trim the ragged edges from the pasta sheets to create a straight edge. After shaping each piece of pasta, transfer it to a rimmed baking sheet lined with a clean dish towel. The shaped pasta should be cooked within 2 hours of being shaped. It can also be frozen like fettuccine (see directions on page 99).

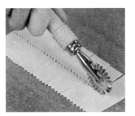

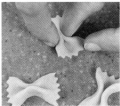

1. FOR FARFALLE: Cut sheet of dough into 1 by 1½-inch rectangles using fluted cutter to cut short sides of rectangle.

2. Place index finger in center of rectangle. Using thumb and index finger of other hand, pinch in long sides until they reach finger in center of pasta. Remove finger and firmly pinch center together.

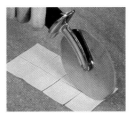

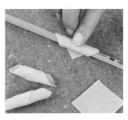

1. FOR GARGANELLI: Cut sheet of dough into 1½-inch squares. Lay square of pasta diagonally on counter or, to create ridges in pasta, on top of clean hair comb or wire rack.

2. Wrap corner of pasta around pencil, and with gentle pressure roll away from you until pasta is completely wrapped around pencil. Slide shaped pasta off pencil and repeat.

Penne with Spiced Butter and Cauliflower

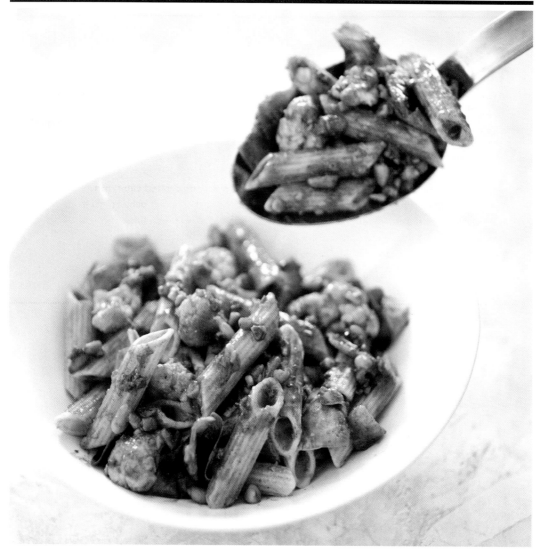

G-F TESTING LAB

PASTA Our favorite brand is Jovial Gluten Free Brown Rice Pasta (see pages 25–26 for complete tasting). Cooking times for gluten-free pasta vary from brand to brand. Make sure to taste the pasta often, as it can overcook quickly.

☑ WHY THIS RECIPE WORKS

Cauliflower is an appealing complement to the nutty flavor and toothsome texture of gluten-free pasta, assuming you treat it right. We found it best to brown the cauliflower in a skillet to bring out its sweet notes, then add water to the pan, set the cover in place, and let the cauliflower steam until tender. We had to use olive oil to sauté the cauliflower because butter burned during this long cooking time. Building a butter sauce separately, and letting the butter brown, complemented the cauliflower with a deeper, nuttier flavor. A selection of warm spices added depth with minimal prep, and blooming the ground spices in the butter mellowed and deepened their flavors. We eventually settled on the combination of coriander, ginger, paprika, and just a hint of cinnamon. We tried to streamline this list but found each was a must to create just the right balance. To give the dish heft and also freshness, we then tested a few more vegetable additions. Asparagus seemed out of place, but baby spinach added the needed burst of color and a balancing earthiness. Pine nuts lent richness as well as texture, and sautéed shallots added another layer of sweetness. To keep our multicomponent sauce to one pan, we set the cauliflower aside after browning it, then used the same pan to toast the nuts and brown our butter. We then added the spices and gave them a minute to cook and mellow. A final squirt of lemon juice brightened the dish just enough and cut through the richness. When browning the butter, make sure to use a skillet with a traditional (not a dark nonstick) finish. Butter can go from brown to burnt quickly, and the light finish of the pan will ensure you can see the color change.

Penne with Spiced Butter, Cauliflower, and Pine Nuts
SERVES 4

- 2 tablespoons olive oil
- 1 small head cauliflower (1½ pounds), cored and cut into 1-inch florets
- 4 shallots, sliced ½ inch thick
   Salt and pepper
- ¼ cup water
- ½ cup pine nuts, chopped
- 6 tablespoons unsalted butter, cut into 6 pieces
- 2 garlic cloves, minced
- ¾ teaspoon ground coriander
- ¾ teaspoon ground ginger
- ¾ teaspoon paprika
- ¼ teaspoon ground cinnamon
- 3 ounces (3 cups) baby spinach
- ¾ teaspoon lemon juice
- 12 ounces gluten-free penne

1. Heat oil in 12-inch skillet over medium-high heat until shimmering. Add cauliflower, shallots, and ¼ teaspoon salt and cook, stirring occasionally, until well browned and nearly tender, 12 to 15 minutes. Add water to skillet, cover, and continue to cook until cauliflower is tender, about 2 minutes. Transfer to bowl and set aside.

2. Wipe out now-empty skillet with paper towels. Add nuts and toast over medium heat, shaking skillet frequently, until fragrant and lightly brown, 3 to 5 minutes. Add butter, increase heat to medium-high, and cook, swirling occasionally, until butter is browned and releases nutty aroma, 1 to 2 minutes. Off heat, stir in garlic, coriander, ginger, paprika, and cinnamon, swirling pan until garlic and spices are fragrant, about 1 minute. Stir in cauliflower-shallot mixture, spinach, lemon juice, and ¼ teaspoon salt, cover, and let sit until spinach is wilted, about 2 minutes.

3. Meanwhile bring 4 quarts water to boil in large pot. Add pasta and 1 tablespoon salt and cook, stirring often, until al dente. Reserve ½ cup cooking water, then drain pasta and return it to pot. Add sauce, toss to combine, and season with salt and pepper to taste. Before serving, add remaining cooking water as needed to adjust consistency.

Fusilli with Basil Pesto

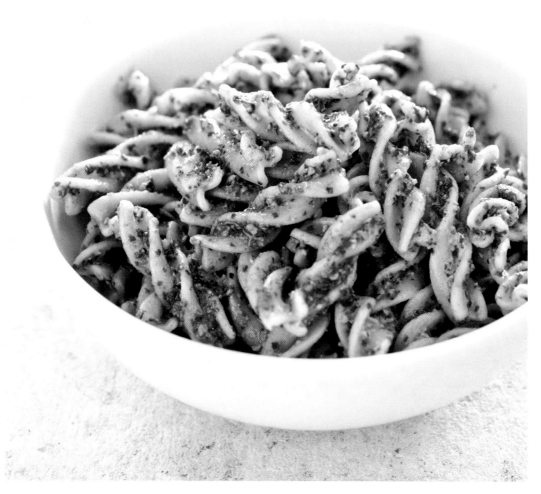

G-F TESTING LAB

PASTA Our favorite brand is Jovial Gluten Free Brown Rice Pasta (see pages 25–26 for complete tasting). Cooking times for gluten-free pasta vary from brand to brand. Make sure to taste the pasta often, as it can overcook quickly.

The ultimate no-cook sauce, basil pesto is simple in that it requires only a few ingredients, but its simplicity also makes it a bit trickier to perfect. A great pesto should balance the flavors of each component: fresh basil, spicy garlic, nutty Parmesan, rich pine nuts, and fruity-peppery extra-virgin olive oil. To tame the raw garlic flavor, we toasted the cloves in a skillet, and while the skillet was out we toasted the nuts as well to deepen their flavor. Because the basil usually turns dark green in homemade pesto and gives the sauce a muddy appearance, we added some parsley to lend a bright green color boost. Processing everything together in the food processor delivered a sauce that retained some texture, and since we were cooking our pasta at the same time, we thinned the sauce with some reserved pasta cooking water so it would coat the pasta evenly. The pesto tended to clump when we tossed it with strand pasta; short shapes like fusilli made it easier to ensure even coverage. For sharper flavor, use Pecorino Romano cheese in place of the Parmesan. Toasting the pine nuts brings out their flavor, but don't walk away from the skillet, as pine nuts can burn rather quickly. An equal amount of another nut, such as walnuts or almonds, can be used if you prefer.

Fusilli with Basil Pesto
SERVES 4

- 3 garlic cloves, unpeeled
- ¼ cup pine nuts
- 2 cups packed fresh basil leaves
- 2 tablespoons fresh parsley leaves
- ⅓ cup extra-virgin olive oil
- ¼ cup grated Parmesan or Pecorino Romano cheese, plus extra for serving
- Salt and pepper
- 12 ounces gluten-free fusilli

1. Toast garlic in 8-inch skillet over medium heat, shaking pan occasionally, until garlic is softened and spotty brown, about 8 minutes. When cool enough to handle, remove and discard skin. While garlic cools, toast pine nuts in now-empty skillet over medium heat, stirring often, until golden and fragrant, 4 to 5 minutes.

2. Process garlic, pine nuts, basil, parsley, oil, Parmesan, and ¼ teaspoon salt in food processor until smooth, 30 to 60 seconds, scraping down bowl as needed. Transfer to medium bowl and season with salt and pepper to taste.

3. Meanwhile, bring 4 quarts water to boil in large pot. Add pasta and 1 tablespoon salt and cook, stirring often, until al dente. Reserve ¾ cup cooking water, then drain pasta and return it to pot.

4. Add sauce and ¼ cup reserved cooking water to pasta, toss to combine, and season with salt and pepper to taste. Add remaining cooking water as needed to adjust consistency. Serve, passing Parmesan separately.

VARIATIONS

Fusilli with Kale–Sunflower Seed Pesto
Reduce garlic to 1 clove and substitute ⅓ cup sunflower seeds for pine nuts. Reduce basil to ¾ cup and replace parsley with 1½ cups chopped kale leaves. Add ½ teaspoon red pepper flakes to processor in step 2, and increase Parmesan to ½ cup.

Fusilli with Roasted Red Pepper Pesto
Reduce garlic to 2 cloves. Omit pine nuts and basil. Add 1 cup patted dry jarred roasted red peppers, 2 tablespoons parsley, and 1 small chopped shallot to processor in step 2, and increase salt added to processor to ½ teaspoon.

Fusilli with Spring Vegetable Cream Sauce

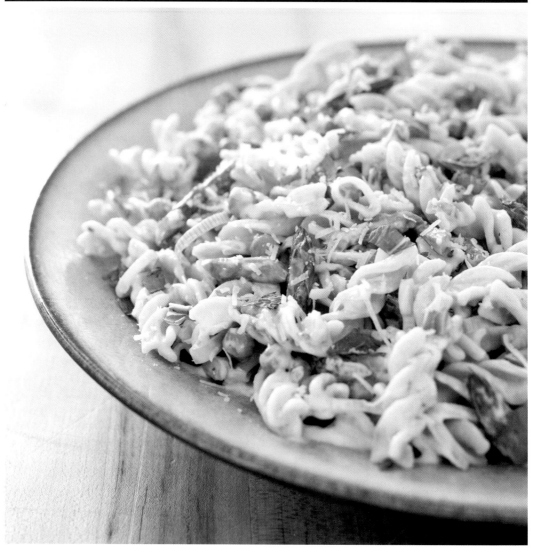

G-F TESTING LAB

PASTA   Our favorite brand is Jovial Gluten Free Brown Rice Pasta (see pages 25–26 for complete tasting). Cooking times for gluten-free pasta vary from brand to brand. Make sure to taste the pasta often, as it can overcook quickly.

✓ WHY THIS RECIPE WORKS

For a vegetarian springtime pasta that could be whipped together on a weeknight, quick-cooking peas and asparagus were a good start. Leeks added sweetness, while fresh mint and thyme plus lemon zest and a splash of white wine added brightness. We started out by using vegetable broth as the base for our sauce, but while we liked the light profile it created, the broth added a slightly tinny flavor. Our dish also seemed unfinished. Using 1 cup of heavy cream instead as the base, plus a good dose of Parmesan, brought it all together into a cohesive whole and provided the richness and elegant finish the recipe needed.

Fusilli with Spring Vegetable Cream Sauce
SERVES 4

- 2 tablespoons olive oil
- 1 pound leeks, white and light green parts only, halved lengthwise, sliced thin, and washed thoroughly
- 3 garlic cloves, minced
- 1 teaspoon grated lemon zest
- 1½ teaspoons minced fresh thyme or ¾ teaspoon dried
- 1 pound asparagus, trimmed and cut on bias into 1-inch lengths
- ½ cup dry white wine
- 1 cup heavy cream
  Salt and pepper
- ¾ cup frozen peas
- 1 ounce Parmesan cheese, grated (½ cup), plus extra for serving
- 12 ounces gluten-free fusilli
- 2 tablespoons chopped fresh mint

1. Heat oil in 12-inch nonstick skillet over medium heat until shimmering. Add leeks and cook until softened, 5 to 7 minutes. Stir in garlic, lemon zest, and thyme and cook until fragrant, about 30 seconds.

2. Stir in asparagus and wine, bring to simmer, and cook until asparagus is crisp-tender, about 3 minutes. Add cream and 1 teaspoon salt and bring to simmer. Cook until sauce is slightly thickened, about 2 minutes. Off heat, stir in peas and Parmesan and let sit, covered, until peas are heated through.

3. Meanwhile, bring 4 quarts water to boil in large pot. Add pasta and 1 tablespoon salt and cook, stirring often, until al dente. Reserve ½ cup cooking water, then drain pasta and return it to pot. Add sauce, toss to combine, and season with salt and pepper to taste. Add reserved cooking water as needed to adjust consistency. Sprinkle with mint and serve, passing Parmesan separately.

TEST KITCHEN TIP **Preparing Leeks**

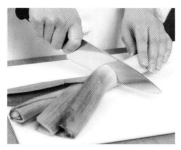

1. Trim and discard root and dark green leaves.

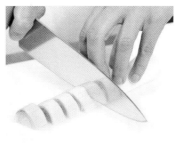

2. Cut trimmed leek in half lengthwise, then slice it crosswise as directed in recipe.

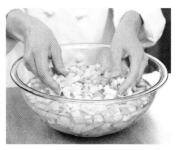

3. Rinse cut leeks thoroughly to remove all dirt and sand using either salad spinner or bowl of water.

Spaghetti with Puttanesca Sauce

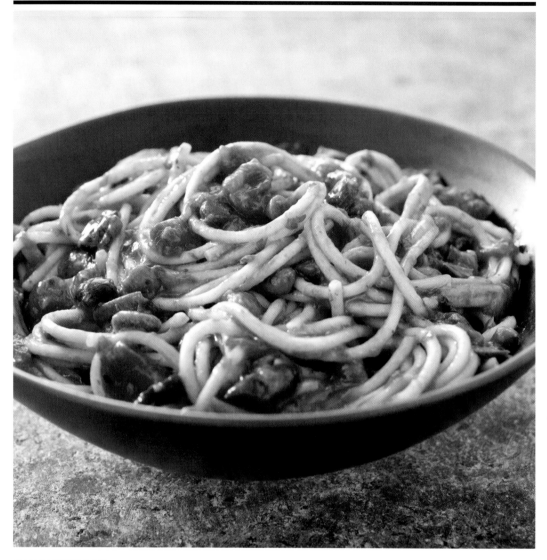

G-F TESTING LAB

PASTA	Our favorite brand is Jovial Gluten Free Brown Rice Pasta (see pages 25–26 for complete tasting). Cooking times for gluten-free pasta vary from brand to brand. Make sure to taste the pasta often, as it can overcook quickly.

✓ WHY THIS RECIPE WORKS

A spicy profile and minimal prep make this Neapolitan classic a quick pasta dinner that's beyond the everyday. And the strong flavors in this tomato sauce work well with the nutty notes in gluten-free pasta. That said, with a number of bold ingredients—garlic, anchovies, olives, and capers—the key to making a great Puttanesca is finding balance; a little too much of one ingredient will completely overpower the others. We found that blooming the garlic, anchovies, and red pepper flakes in olive oil helped to develop, mellow, and blend their flavors. To avoid burning the garlic, it was important to add it (and the other two ingredients) to the pan at the same time as the oil; the garlic burned when we heated the oil first. After adding the tomatoes (diced plus crushed delivered the right consistency), we simmered the sauce long enough to infuse it with flavor and thicken it slightly, but not too long because we wanted to preserve the tomatoes' sweetness and texture. Waiting to add the olives, capers, and parsley until the end kept them from disintegrating into the sauce and also ensured the sauce retained the right amount of piquant flavor. For a bit more richness, we drizzled olive oil over each bowl of pasta before serving. This dish is fairly spicy; to make it milder, reduce the amount of red pepper flakes.

Spaghetti with Puttanesca Sauce
SERVES 4

- 2 tablespoons extra-virgin olive oil, plus extra for serving
- 6 anchovy fillets, rinsed and minced
- 3 garlic cloves, minced
- ¼ teaspoon red pepper flakes
- 1 (28-ounce) can crushed tomatoes
- 1 (14.5-ounce) can diced tomatoes
- ½ cup pitted kalamata olives, chopped coarse
- 3 tablespoons minced fresh parsley
- 2 tablespoons capers, rinsed
- Salt and pepper
- 12 ounces gluten-free spaghetti

1. Cook oil, anchovies, garlic, and pepper flakes together in 12-inch skillet over medium heat, stirring often, until garlic turns golden but not brown, 1 to 2 minutes.

2. Stir in crushed tomatoes and diced tomatoes and their juice. Bring to simmer and cook until thickened slightly, 15 to 20 minutes. Off heat, stir in olives, parsley, and capers, and season with salt and pepper to taste.

3. Meanwhile, bring 4 quarts water to boil in large pot. Add pasta and 1 tablespoon salt and cook, stirring often, until al dente. Reserve ½ cup cooking water, then drain pasta and return it to pot. Add sauce and toss to combine. Add reserved cooking water as needed to adjust consistency. Drizzle individual portions with additional oil to taste. Serve.

SMART SHOPPING
Anchovy Fillets versus Paste

Because most recipes call for only a small amount of anchovies, we wondered whether a tube of anchovy paste might be a more convenient option. Made from pulverized anchovies, vinegar, salt, and water, anchovy paste promises all the flavor of oil-packed anchovies without the mess. When we tested the paste and jarred or canned anchovies side by side in recipes calling for an anchovy or two, we found little difference, though a few astute tasters felt that the paste had a "saltier" and "slightly more fishy" flavor. You can substitute ¼ teaspoon of the paste for each fillet. However, when a recipe calls for more than a couple of anchovies, stick with jarred or canned, as the paste's more intense flavor will be overwhelming. Our favorite brand of anchovies is Ortiz Oil-Packed Anchovies.

Spaghetti and Meatballs

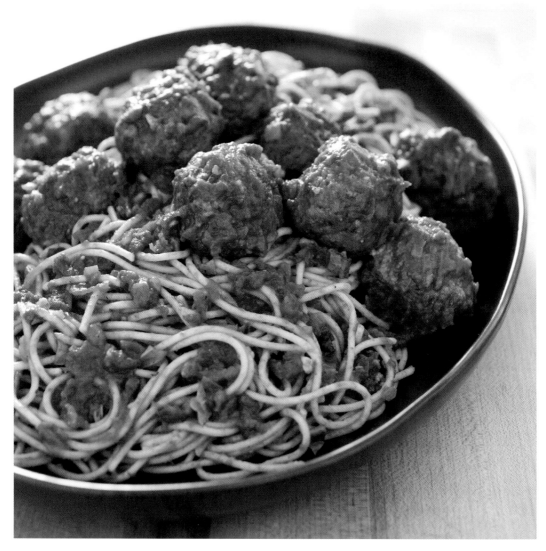

G-F TESTING LAB

PASTA	Our favorite brand is Jovial Gluten Free Brown Rice Pasta (see pages 25–26 for complete tasting). Cooking times for gluten-free pasta vary from brand to brand. Make sure to taste the pasta often, as it can overcook quickly.
POTATO FLAKES	Make sure to buy potato flakes, not potato granules, which have a slightly metallic taste.

Traditional spaghetti and meatballs is off-limits to the gluten-free crowd, and not just because of the noodles. Classic meatballs rely on a panade—a paste made by mashing sandwich bread into milk—to keep the ground meat from becoming tough and dry. And while we didn't want to settle for substandard meatballs, we knew the fix wasn't as simple as swapping in a few slices of gluten-free bread. We'd recently tried to make a panade using gluten-free bread for meatloaf, but rather than breaking down into a paste, the gluten-free bread turned into spongy bits and delivered a meat mixture that was tough and chewy. However, we'd discovered a surprising ingredient—potato flakes—could provide just the right tenderizing effect (see page 144 for more detail on our meatloaf recipe) and keep our mixture gluten-free. One test proved that along with buttermilk and an egg yolk for moisture and rich flavor, the potato flakes worked perfectly in our meatball recipe. To ensure meatballs with good flavor, we used a combination of ground pork (for a hint of sweetness) and ground beef. Since overworked ground beef makes tough meatballs, we waited to add it to the mixture until after we'd mixed the other ingredients together with the pork. Browning the meatballs added flavor and ensured they stayed together, while cooking them through in the sauce gave both the sauce and the meatballs a boost. We like the tang that buttermilk adds, but you can use regular milk; substitute ½ cup whole milk combined with 1½ teaspoons lemon juice or distilled white vinegar. See page 43 for more about buttermilk substitutes. Potato flakes are an instant mashed potato product made by cooking, processing, and dehydrating potatoes. Unlike potato flour, dehydrated potato flakes are less likely to clump when combined with liquid. Avoid potato granules, which have a slightly metallic taste. We find that 85 percent lean ground beef is the best option here. Fattier options (like 80 percent lean ground beef) can be a bit greasy. Leaner options will make fairly dry meatballs.

Spaghetti and Meatballs
SERVES 4

MEATBALLS
- ½ cup buttermilk
- 1 large egg yolk
- 4 ounces ground pork
- 1 ounce Parmesan cheese, grated (½ cup)
- ¼ cup instant potato flakes
- 3 tablespoons minced fresh parsley
- 2 garlic cloves, minced
- ½ teaspoon salt
- ¼ teaspoon pepper
- 12 ounces 85 percent lean ground beef
- 2 tablespoons olive oil

PASTA AND SAUCE
- 1 onion, chopped fine
- 4 garlic cloves, minced
- ⅛ teaspoon red pepper flakes
- 1 (28-ounce) can crushed tomatoes
- 1 (14.5-ounce) can diced tomatoes
  Salt and pepper
- 12 ounces gluten-free spaghetti
- 3 tablespoons chopped fresh basil
  Grated Parmesan cheese

1. FOR THE MEATBALLS: Whisk together buttermilk and egg yolk in large bowl. Add ground pork, Parmesan, potato flakes, parsley, garlic, salt, and pepper, and knead with hands until mixture is thoroughly combined. Add beef and continue to knead until uniform. Gently form mixture into 1½-inch round meatballs (about 12 meatballs).

2. Heat oil in 12-inch nonstick skillet over medium heat until just smoking. Brown meatballs on all sides, about 10 minutes. Transfer meatballs to paper towel–lined plate. Pour off all but 1 tablespoon fat left in skillet.

3. FOR THE PASTA AND SAUCE: Add onion to fat left in skillet and cook over medium heat until softened, about 5 minutes. Stir in garlic and red pepper flakes and cook until fragrant, about 30 seconds. Stir in crushed tomatoes and diced tomatoes and their juice. Bring to simmer and cook until sauce has thickened slightly, about 20 minutes.

4. Add meatballs to sauce and simmer, turning meatballs occasionally, until cooked through, about 10 minutes. Season sauce with salt and pepper to taste.

5. Meanwhile, bring 4 quarts water to boil in large pot. Add pasta and 1 tablespoon salt and cook, stirring often, until al dente. Reserve ½ cup cooking water, then drain pasta and return it to pot.

6. Add basil and several large spoonfuls of sauce (without meatballs) to pasta and toss to combine. Add reserved cooking water as needed to adjust consistency. Divide pasta among individual bowls and top each with tomato sauce and meatballs. Serve, passing Parmesan separately.

TEST KITCHEN TIP **Making Tender Gluten-Free Meatballs**

For traditional meatballs, we usually rely on the addition of a panade (a paste made with bread and milk). For our gluten-free version, we found a surprising ingredient—potato flakes—was the best stand-in for the bread-based mixture. Overworked ground beef makes for dense, rubbery meatballs, so adding it last during the mixing step helps prevent overkneading. Browning the meatballs adds meaty depth and also helps them hold together, while simmering them in the sauce boosts the flavor of both the meatballs and the sauce.

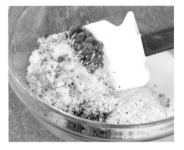

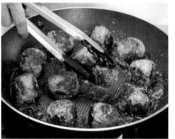

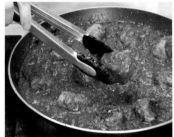

1. Add ground pork, Parmesan, potato flakes, parsley, garlic, salt, and pepper to buttermilk and egg yolk, and mix until thoroughly combined. Then add ground beef and mix just until thoroughly combined.

2. After forming meatballs, brown on all sides, about 10 minutes, using tongs to gently turn meatballs as necessary. Transfer meatballs to paper towel–lined plate to drain briefly.

3. After sauce has cooked and thickened slightly, add meatballs and simmer, turning occasionally, until meatballs are cooked through, about 10 minutes.

Penne with Sausage and Red Pepper Ragu

✓ WHY THIS RECIPE WORKS

For a kid-friendly weeknight pasta dinner that would be equally satisfying to adults, we started by pairing rich Italian sausage with sweet red peppers. A can of crushed tomatoes worked well as the base and coated the pasta fairly well, but the sauce was a bit on the thin side and one-dimensional. Wine added depth without making it too boozy, while a few tablespoons of tomato paste helped to thicken it and also gave it a deeper tomato flavor. Incorporating garlic, oregano, and onion complemented the sausage and boosted the overall flavor of the sauce. Tossing in some parsley at the end gave it a little color and freshness. Make sure not to overcook the sausage in step 1. You want to cook it until it is just no longer pink; overbrowning the sausage will make it dry and tough. Our favorite brand is Jovial Gluten Free Brown Rice Pasta (see pages 25–26 for complete tasting). Cooking times for gluten-free pasta vary from brand to brand. Make sure to taste the pasta often, as it can overcook quickly.

Penne with Sausage and Red Pepper Ragu
SERVES 4

- 1 tablespoon extra-virgin olive oil
- 1 onion, chopped fine
- 1 red bell pepper, stemmed, seeded, and cut into ½-inch pieces
- 2 tablespoons tomato paste
- 3 garlic cloves, minced
- 2 teaspoons minced fresh oregano or 1 teaspoon dried
- 1 pound sweet or hot Italian sausage, casings removed
- ½ cup dry red wine
- 1 (28-ounce) can crushed tomatoes
- 12 ounces gluten-free penne
  Salt and pepper
- 2 tablespoons minced fresh parsley
  Grated Parmesan cheese

1. Heat oil in Dutch oven over medium heat until shimmering. Add onion and bell pepper and cook until softened, about 5 minutes. Stir in tomato paste, garlic, and oregano and cook until fragrant, about 30 seconds. Add sausage and cook, breaking up any large pieces with wooden spoon, until no longer pink, about 5 minutes. Stir in wine, scraping up any browned bits, and simmer until liquid has thickened, about 2 minutes.

2. Stir in crushed tomatoes, bring to simmer, and cook until sauce thickens slightly, about 30 minutes.

3. Meanwhile, bring 4 quarts water to boil in large pot. Add pasta and 1 tablespoon salt and cook, stirring often, until al dente. Reserve ½ cup cooking water, then drain pasta and return it to pot. Add sauce and parsley, toss to combine, and season with salt and pepper to taste. Add reserved cooking water as needed to adjust consistency. Serve, passing Parmesan separately.

TEST KITCHEN TIP
Removing Sausage from Its Casing

Italian sausage is sold in several forms, including links (which is most common), bulk-style tubes, and patties. If using links, remove the meat from the casing before cooking so that it can crumble into small, bite-size pieces.

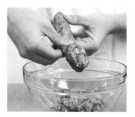

To remove sausage from its casing, hold sausage firmly on one end, and squeeze sausage out of opposite end.

Penne with Weeknight Meat Sauce

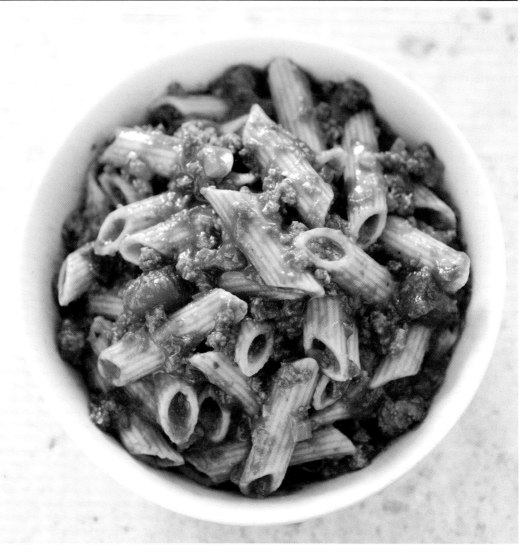

G-F TESTING LAB

PASTA   Our favorite brand is Jovial Gluten Free Brown Rice Pasta (see pages 25–26 for complete tasting). Cooking times for gluten-free pasta vary from brand to brand. Make sure to taste the pasta often, as it can overcook quickly.

✓ WHY THIS RECIPE WORKS

A classic old-fashioned Italian meat sauce depends on hours of cooking to develop rich flavors. At the other end of the spectrum, the typical easy meat sauce turns out rubbery ground beef in a lackluster tomato sauce. We wanted a recipe that had deep flavor and tender meat, but it had to be doable on a weeknight. We started with ground beef because it was still the clear winner in terms of speed, but we ramped up our sauce's meaty flavor by adding umami-packed ingredients like mushrooms and tomato paste. We pulsed the mushrooms in the food processor to get the right texture (larger pieces seemed noticeably spongy), then sautéed them in the pot along with onions to develop plenty of flavorful fond. To keep the meat tender, we knew from test kitchen experience that tossing ground meat with baking soda and a little water, then letting it sit briefly, would help tenderize it. We also knew to skip the browning step since that would only dry the meat out and make it tough. Instead, we added it straight to the pot after adding the tomatoes. After a brief simmer, we had a weeknight meat sauce with deep flavor and tender beef. We use a food processor to make quick work of the mushrooms. If you don't own a food processor you can chop them by hand but make sure to chop them very fine.

Penne with Weeknight Meat Sauce
SERVES 4

- 1 pound 85 percent lean ground beef
- 2 tablespoons water
  Salt and pepper
- ½ teaspoon baking soda
- 4 ounces white mushrooms, trimmed and halved if small or quartered if large
- 1 tablespoon olive oil
- 1 onion, chopped fine
- 3 garlic cloves, minced
- 1 tablespoon tomato paste
- 2 teaspoons minced fresh oregano or 1 teaspoon dried
- ⅛ teaspoon red pepper flakes
- 1 (28-ounce) can tomato puree
- 1 (14.5-ounce) can diced tomatoes, drained
- ¼ cup grated Parmesan cheese, plus extra for serving
- 12 ounces gluten-free penne

1. Toss beef with water, 1 teaspoon salt, ¼ teaspoon pepper, and baking soda in bowl until thoroughly combined. Let sit for 20 minutes.

2. Meanwhile, pulse mushrooms in food processor until finely chopped, about 8 pulses, scraping down bowl as needed. Heat oil in large saucepan over medium-high heat until just smoking. Add processed mushrooms and onion and cook until vegetables are softened and well browned, 8 to 10 minutes.

3. Stir in garlic, tomato paste, oregano, and pepper flakes and cook until fragrant, about 30 seconds. Stir in tomato puree, diced tomatoes, ½ teaspoon salt, and ½ teaspoon pepper and bring to gentle simmer. Stir in meat mixture and cook, breaking meat into small pieces with wooden spoon, until cooked through and sauce has thickened, about 30 minutes. Stir in Parmesan and season with salt and pepper to taste.

4. Meanwhile, bring 4 quarts water to boil in large pot. Add pasta and 1 tablespoon salt and cook, stirring often, until al dente. Reserve ½ cup cooking water, then drain pasta and return it to pot. Add sauce to pasta and toss to combine. Add reserved cooking water as needed to adjust consistency. Serve, passing Parmesan separately.

SMART SHOPPING **Tomato Puree**

Tomato puree is cooked and strained to remove the tomato seeds, making it smoother and thicker than other canned tomato products. In the test kitchen we have found that tomato puree works well when we want a thick sauce. With its thick consistency and strong tomato flavor, Muir Glen Tomato Puree is our favorite.

Soba Noodles with Pork and Vegetables

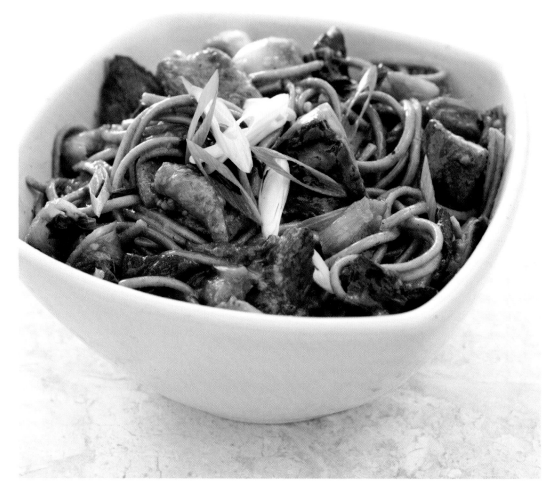

G-F TESTING LAB

SOBA NOODLES   Many brands of soba noodles also contain wheat; make sure to read the ingredient label and buy noodles made with only buckwheat flour. See page 24 for more details. Do not substitute other types of noodles for the soba noodles. Note that because of the salty ingredients, we don't salt the cooking water for the noodles in this recipe.

✓ WHY THIS RECIPE WORKS

Soba noodles have a strong flavor that demands an equally flavorful combination of sauce and add-ins. Meaty country-style pork ribs are a great starting point. Baby bok choy lent appealing crunch, while earthy shiitake mushrooms gave the dish savory depth. For our sauce, we started with gluten-free tamari. Ordinarily, we would reach for oyster sauce for a hit of briny sweetness, but we discovered oyster sauce contains gluten. After some tinkering, we found a combination of brown sugar and fish sauce provided a similar flavor without the gluten. Sesame oil added nutty richness, chili-garlic sauce brought the right amount of heat, and sake contributed clean complexity. We prefer this dish made with sake, but an equal amount of vermouth can be substituted. One large head of bok choy (stems and leaves separated and sliced ½ inch wide) can be substituted for the baby bok choy; add the stems with the mushrooms, and the leaves with the cooked pork.

Soba Noodles with Pork, Shiitakes, and Bok Choy

SERVES 4

- ¼ cup gluten-free tamari or soy sauce (see page 121)
- 3 tablespoons packed brown sugar
- 2 tablespoons fish sauce
- 4 teaspoons sake (Japanese rice wine)
- 1 tablespoon Asian chili-garlic sauce
- 1 tablespoon toasted sesame oil
- 1 pound boneless country-style pork ribs, trimmed and sliced crosswise into ⅛-inch-thick strips
- 6 garlic cloves, minced
- 1 tablespoon grated fresh ginger
- 4 teaspoons vegetable oil
- 6 heads baby bok choy (4 ounces each), sliced crosswise ½ inch wide
- 10 ounces shiitake mushrooms, stemmed and quartered
- 8 ounces gluten-free dried soba noodles
- 2 scallions, sliced thin on bias

1. Whisk tamari, sugar, fish sauce, sake, chili-garlic sauce, and sesame oil together in medium bowl. Measure 3 tablespoons of mixture into separate bowl and stir in pork; cover and refrigerate for at least 15 minutes or up to 1 hour. In separate bowl, combine garlic, ginger, and 1 teaspoon vegetable oil.

2. Heat 1 teaspoon vegetable oil in 12-inch nonstick skillet over high heat until just smoking. Add half of pork in single layer and cook without stirring for 1 minute. Stir and continue to cook until browned, about 2 minutes; transfer to clean bowl. Repeat with 1 teaspoon vegetable oil and remaining pork; transfer to bowl.

3. Wipe now-empty skillet clean with paper towels, add remaining 1 teaspoon vegetable oil, and heat over high heat until just smoking. Add bok choy and mushrooms and cook, stirring often, until vegetables are browned, 5 to 7 minutes. Clear center of skillet, add garlic-ginger mixture, and mash into pan until fragrant, about 30 seconds; stir into vegetables. Stir in cooked pork with any accumulated juice. Stir in tamari mixture and simmer until sauce has thickened, about 1 minute. Remove from heat and cover to keep warm.

4. Meanwhile, bring 4 quarts water to boil in large pot. Add noodles and cook, stirring often, until tender. Reserve ½ cup cooking water, then drain noodles and return them to pot. Add pork mixture and toss to combine. Add reserved cooking water as needed to adjust consistency. Sprinkle individual portions with scallions and serve.

SMART SHOPPING

Boneless Country-Style Pork Ribs

These meaty boneless ribs have enough marbling to stay moist and flavorful during long simmering times, making them a good choice for braising, but they also cook relatively quickly, especially when cut into smaller pieces. Look for ribs that have striations of fat throughout the meat, and avoid those that look very lean.

Soba Noodles with Roasted Eggplant

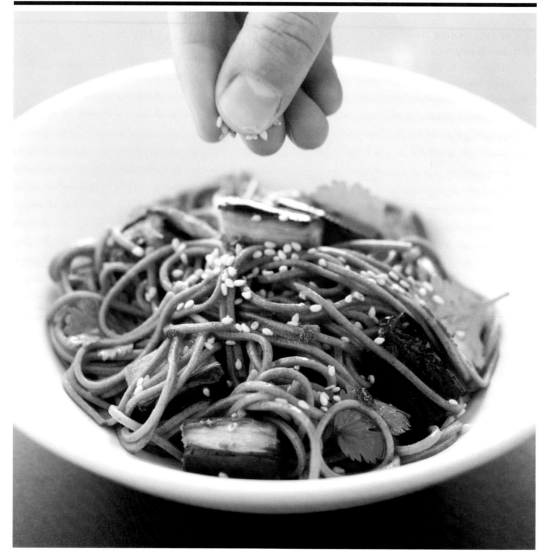

G-F TESTING LAB

SOBA NOODLES   Many brands of soba noodles also contain wheat; make sure to read the ingredient label and buy noodles made with only buckwheat flour. See page 24 for more details. Do not substitute other types of noodles for the soba noodles. Note that because of the salty ingredients, we don't salt the cooking water for the noodles in this recipe.

With its creamy texture and mild flavor, eggplant is a perfect foil to nutty buckwheat soba noodles. Roasting proved an easy, hands-off way to cook the eggplant, and tossing it with wheat-free tamari and vegetable oil beforehand helped to season it. For the sauce, we turned once again to tamari for savory richness. An oyster sauce substitute—a combination of fish sauce and brown sugar—that we'd just developed for another soba noodle recipe lent just the right briny sweetness. Asian chili-garlic sauce and toasted sesame oil provided a nice balance of sweet and spicy flavors, while a bit of sake contributed a clean flavor that gave the sauce complexity. Finishing with cilantro and sesame seeds kept the recipe simple while adding freshness, complementary nutty flavor, and visual appeal. We prefer this dish made with sake, but an equal amount of vermouth can be substituted.

Soba Noodles with Roasted Eggplant and Sesame

SERVES 4

¼	**cup vegetable oil**
2	**pounds eggplant, cut into 1-inch pieces**
¼	**cup gluten-free tamari or soy sauce**
3	**tablespoons packed brown sugar**
2	**tablespoons toasted sesame oil**
4	**teaspoons sake (Japanese rice wine)**
1	**tablespoon Asian chili-garlic sauce**
1	**tablespoon fish sauce**
8	**ounces gluten-free dried soba noodles**
¾	**cup fresh cilantro leaves**
2	**teaspoons sesame seeds, toasted**

1. Adjust oven rack to middle position and heat oven to 450 degrees. Line large rimmed baking sheet with aluminum foil and brush with 1 tablespoon vegetable oil. Toss eggplant with remaining 3 tablespoons vegetable oil and 1 tablespoon tamari in large bowl, then spread onto prepared baking sheet. Roast until well browned and tender, 25 to 30 minutes, stirring halfway through roasting.

2. In small saucepan, whisk remaining 3 tablespoons tamari, sugar, sesame oil, sake, chili-garlic sauce, and fish sauce together. Cook over medium heat until sugar has dissolved, about 1 minute; cover and set aside.

3. Meanwhile, bring 4 quarts water to boil in large pot. Add noodles and cook, stirring often, until tender. Reserve ½ cup cooking water, then drain noodles and return them to pot. Add sauce and roasted eggplant and toss to combine. Add reserved cooking water as needed to adjust consistency. Sprinkle individual portions with cilantro and sesame seeds and serve.

SMART SHOPPING

Gluten-Free Tamari and Soy Sauce

Tamari is sold alongside soy sauce on the supermarket shelf, but the two are not the same. While soy sauce is a blend of fermented wheat and soybeans, tamari traditionally is made from fermented soybeans and contains no wheat. However, some brands today do contain a little wheat, so it's still important to read the label. It has a more pungent flavor than soy sauce, but we've found it usually works well as a soy sauce substitute. We have also noticed gluten-free soy sauce recently at the supermarket. This product is made with soybeans and rice rather than wheat and is another wheat-free option.

SMART SHOPPING **Asian Hot Chili Sauces**

Used both in cooking and as a condiment, these sauces come in a variety of styles. Sriracha contains garlic and is made from chiles that are ground into a smooth paste. Chili-garlic sauce also contains garlic and is similar to Sriracha, but the chiles are coarsely ground. Sambal oelek is made purely from ground chiles. Without the addition of garlic or other spices, it provides heat but not the same complexity of flavor. Once opened, these sauces will keep for several months in the refrigerator.

Drunken Noodles with Chicken

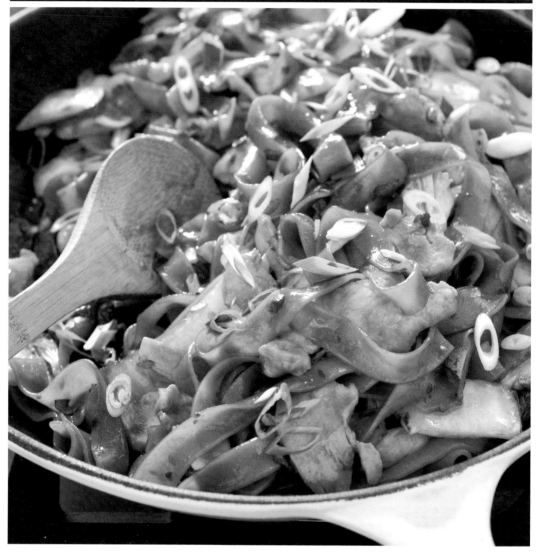

G-F TESTING LAB

RICE NOODLES We prefer ⅜-inch-wide noodles here, but ¼-inch-wide rice noodles can be substituted (however, do not substitute other types of noodles for the rice noodles). Even if the package directions suggest boiling rice noodles, we strongly recommend that you soak them in hot tap water. The soaking time will be longer but there's no risk of overcooking these delicate noodles; while the noodles soak, you can prep the other ingredients. See page 24 for more details about buying and soaking rice noodles. If using ¼-inch-wide noodles, reduce soaking time in step 1 to 20 minutes.

✅ WHY THIS RECIPE WORKS

Called drunken noodles because it is a supposed hangover cure, this dish features wide rice noodles in a spicy, potent sauce and lots of basil. We soaked wide rice noodles in hot water until they were just pliable so that we could finish cooking them in the sauce and infuse them with flavor. Chicken and napa cabbage, which we quickly stir-fried one after the other, made it a filling entrée. We found that tossing the chicken with tamari and letting it sit before cooking boosted its flavor and helped to keep it moist. After setting the meat and vegetables aside, we added the noodles to the skillet, along with a mixture of tamari, lime juice, dark brown sugar, and chili-garlic sauce. Waiting to add the basil until the last minute ensured its color stayed fresh.

Drunken Noodles with Chicken

SERVES 4

- 12 ounces (⅜-inch-wide) dried flat rice noodles
- 12 ounces boneless, skinless chicken breasts, trimmed and sliced into ¼-inch-thick strips
- 1 tablespoon plus ¼ cup gluten-free tamari or soy sauce (see page 121)
- ¾ cup packed dark brown sugar
- ⅓ cup lime juice (3 limes), plus lime wedges for serving
- ¼ cup water
- ¼ cup Asian chili-garlic sauce
- ¼ cup vegetable oil
- ½ head napa cabbage, cored and cut into 1-inch pieces (6 cups)
- 1½ cups coarsely chopped fresh Thai basil, Italian (sweet) basil, or cilantro
- 4 scallions, sliced thin on bias

1. Cover noodles with very hot tap water in large bowl and stir to separate. Let noodles soak until softened, pliable, and limp but not fully tender, 35 to 40 minutes; drain.

2. Meanwhile, toss chicken with 1 tablespoon tamari in bowl, cover, and refrigerate for at least 10 minutes or up to 1 hour. In separate bowl, whisk together remaining ¼ cup tamari, sugar, lime juice, water, and chili-garlic sauce; set aside.

3. Heat 2 teaspoons oil in 12-inch nonstick skillet over high heat until just smoking. Add chicken in single layer and cook without stirring for 1 minute. Stir and continue to cook until nearly cooked through, about 2 minutes; transfer to clean bowl.

4. Add 1 teaspoon oil to now-empty skillet and heat over high heat until just smoking. Add cabbage and cook, stirring often, until spotty brown, 3 to 5 minutes; transfer to bowl with chicken.

5. Wipe now-empty skillet clean with paper towels, add remaining 3 tablespoons oil, and heat over medium-high heat until shimmering. Add drained rice noodles and tamari mixture and cook, tossing gently, until sauce has thickened and noodles are well coated and tender, 5 to 10 minutes. Stir in chicken-cabbage mixture and basil and cook until chicken is warmed through, about 1 minute. Sprinkle with scallions and serve with lime wedges.

TEST KITCHEN TIP
Slicing Chicken for Stir-Fries

To make it easier to cut, freeze the chicken for 15 minutes.

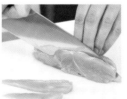 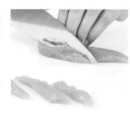

1. Slice breasts across grain into ¼-inch-wide strips that are 1½ to 2 inches long. Cut center in half so they are same length as end pieces.

2. Cut tenderloins on diagonal to produce pieces of meat about same size as strips of breast meat.

Singapore Noodles with Shrimp

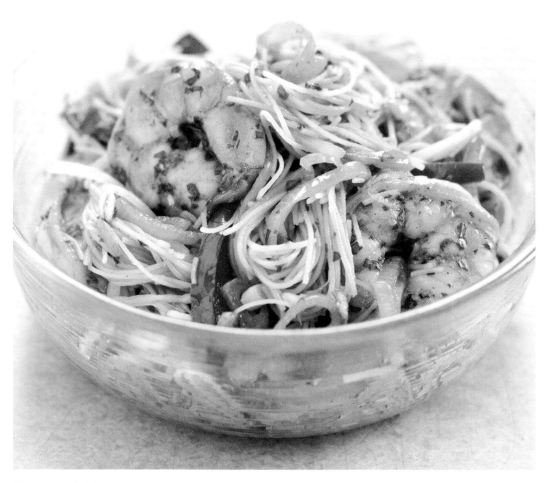

G-F TESTING LAB

RICE NOODLES   Do not substitute other types of noodles for the rice vermicelli here. Even if the package directions suggest boiling rice noodles, we strongly recommend that you soak them in hot tap water. The soaking time will be longer but there's no risk of overcooking these delicate noodles; while the noodles soak, you can prep the other ingredients. See page 24 for more details about buying and soaking rice noodles.

☑ WHY THIS RECIPE WORKS

Also known as curry noodles, this dish is Asian comfort food at its best: a big bowl of tender rice vermicelli swathed in a fragrant, curry-laced sauce. Boiling the noodles was a nonstarter—we knew they would only turn sticky and gummy. Instead, it's best to soak them in hot water until just barely tender, then finish cooking them through at the end with the sauce. As for the curry powder, 1 tablespoon provided the right hit of flavor but didn't go overboard. To make the recipe substantial, we added shrimp, and tossing them with a bit of the curry and some sugar ensured that they had great flavor and browned nicely. Once we had browned the shrimp, we set them aside and built our sauce, then returned the noodles and shrimp to the pot, along with a full cup of liquid (chicken broth provided the right savory balance) and finished cooking. Shallots and bell pepper added sweetness and texture. Finally, with minced cilantro for clean, citrusy notes and bean sprouts for crunch, this colorful dish proved both visually appealing and flavorful.

Singapore Noodles with Shrimp
SERVES 4

8 ounces dried rice vermicelli
1 pound extra-large shrimp (21 to 25 per pound), peeled, deveined, and tails removed
1 tablespoon curry powder
⅛ teaspoon sugar
2 tablespoons vegetable oil
6 shallots, sliced thin
2 red bell peppers, stemmed, seeded, and cut into ¼-inch-wide strips
2 garlic cloves, minced
1 cup chicken broth
⅓ cup gluten-free tamari or soy sauce (see page 121)
1 tablespoon mirin
1 teaspoon Sriracha sauce
4 ounces (2 cups) bean sprouts
½ cup minced fresh cilantro

1. Cover noodles with very hot tap water in large bowl and stir to separate. Let noodles soak until softened, pliable, and limp but not fully tender, about 20 minutes; drain.

2. Meanwhile, pat shrimp dry with paper towels and toss with ½ teaspoon curry powder and sugar in bowl. Heat 1 tablespoon oil in Dutch oven over high heat until just smoking. Add shrimp in single layer and cook, without stirring, until beginning to brown, about 1 minute. Stir shrimp and continue to cook until spotty brown and just pink around edges, about 30 seconds; transfer to clean bowl.

3. Add remaining 1 tablespoon oil to now-empty pot and heat over medium heat until shimmering. Add shallots, bell peppers, and remaining 2½ teaspoons curry powder and cook until vegetables are softened, 3 to 5 minutes. Stir in garlic and cook until fragrant, about 30 seconds.

4. Stir in drained noodles, shrimp with any accumulated juice, broth, tamari, mirin, and Sriracha and cook, tossing gently, until noodles are well coated, 2 to 3 minutes. Stir in bean sprouts and cilantro. Serve.

TEST KITCHEN TIP **Deveining Shrimp**

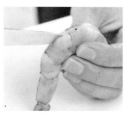 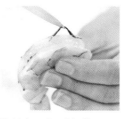

1. Hold shrimp firmly in one hand, then use paring knife to cut down back side of shrimp, about ⅛- to ¼-inch deep, to expose vein.

2. Using tip of knife, gently remove vein. Wipe knife against paper towel to remove vein and discard.

Pad Thai with Shrimp

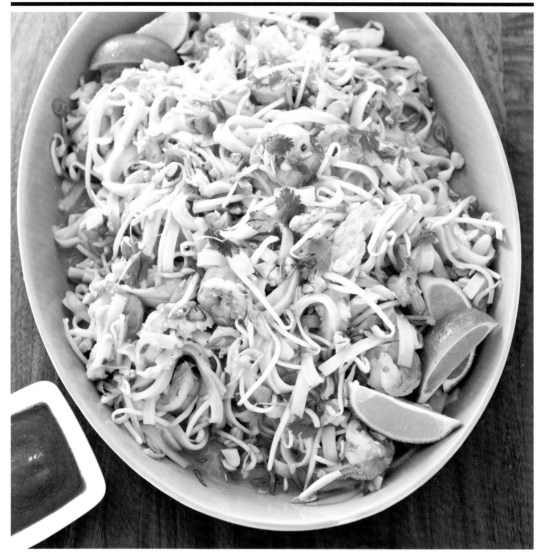

RICE NOODLES Do not substitute other types of noodles for the rice noodles. Even if the package directions suggest boiling rice noodles, we strongly recommend that you soak them in hot tap water. The soaking time will be longer but there's no risk of overcooking these delicate noodles; while the noodles soak, you can prep the other ingredients. See page 24 for more details about buying and soaking rice noodles.

✔ WHY THIS RECIPE WORKS

With its sweet-and-sour, salty-spicy sauce, plump, sweet shrimp, and tender rice noodles, pad thai is Thailand's best-known noodle dish and it's naturally gluten-free. Making pad thai at home can be a chore thanks to a lengthy ingredient list with hard-to-find items. We found we could achieve just the right balance of flavors while keeping it simple by using a combination of fish sauce, lime juice, rice vinegar, and brown sugar for the sauce. With this flavorful base, we found we didn't even need to season the shrimp; we merely sautéed them in the pan until barely pink at the edges, then stirred them in later to finish cooking. To get the texture of the rice noodles just right, we first soaked them in hot water so they'd start to soften, then stir-fried them in the pan. Scrambled eggs, chopped peanuts, bean sprouts, and thinly sliced scallions completed our easy, authentic-tasting pad thai.

Pad Thai with Shrimp
SERVES 4

- 8 ounces (¼-inch-wide) dried flat rice noodles
- ⅓ cup water
- ¼ cup lime juice (2 limes)
- 3 tablespoons fish sauce
- 3 tablespoons packed brown sugar
- 1 tablespoon rice vinegar
- ¼ cup vegetable oil
- 12 ounces medium shrimp (41 to 50 per pound), peeled, deveined, and tails removed
- 3 garlic cloves, minced
- 2 large eggs, lightly beaten
- ¼ teaspoon salt
- 6 tablespoons chopped unsalted roasted peanuts
- 6 ounces (3 cups) bean sprouts
- 5 scallions, sliced thin on bias
  Lime wedges
  Fresh cilantro leaves
  Sriracha sauce

1. Cover noodles with very hot tap water in large bowl and stir to separate. Let noodles soak until softened, pliable, and limp but not fully tender, about 20 minutes; drain. In separate bowl, whisk water, lime juice, fish sauce, sugar, rice vinegar, and 2 tablespoons oil together.

2. Pat shrimp dry with paper towels. Heat 1 tablespoon oil in 12-inch nonstick skillet over high heat until just smoking. Add shrimp in single layer and cook, without stirring, until beginning to brown, about 1 minute. Stir shrimp and continue to cook until spotty brown and just pink around edges, about 30 seconds; transfer to bowl.

3. Add remaining 1 tablespoon oil and garlic to now-empty skillet and cook over medium heat until fragrant, about 30 seconds. Stir in eggs and salt and cook, stirring vigorously, until eggs are scrambled, about 20 seconds.

4. Add drained noodles and fish sauce mixture. Increase heat to high and cook, tossing gently, until noodles are evenly coated. Add cooked shrimp, ¼ cup peanuts, bean sprouts, and three-quarters of scallions. Continue to cook, tossing constantly, until noodles are tender, about 2 minutes. (If necessary, add 2 tablespoons water to skillet and continue to cook until noodles are tender.)

5. Transfer noodles to serving platter and sprinkle with remaining peanuts and remaining scallions. Serve, passing lime wedges, cilantro, and Sriracha sauce separately.

SMART SHOPPING Fish Sauce

Fish sauce is a salty, amber-colored liquid made from fermented fish. Naturally gluten-free, fish sauce lends dishes a salty complexity that is impossible to replicate with other ingredients. Color correlates with flavor in fish sauce; the lighter the sauce, the lighter the flavor. Fish sauce will keep indefinitely without refrigeration.

Spicy Basil Noodles with Crispy Tofu

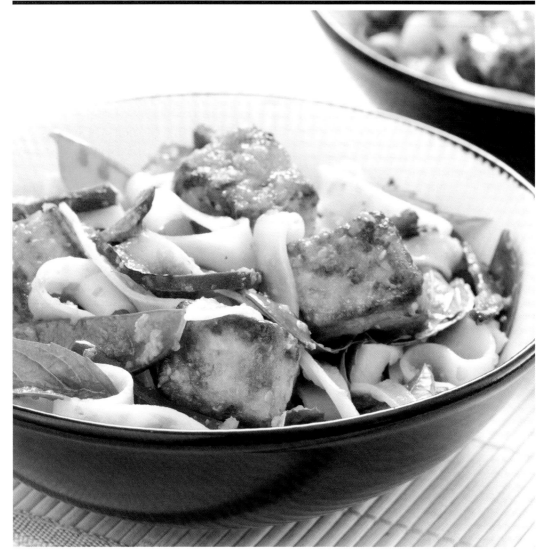

G-F TESTING LAB

RICE NOODLES   We prefer ⅜-inch-wide noodles here, but ¼-inch-wide rice noodles will work fine (however, do not substitute other types of noodles for the rice noodles). Even if the package directions suggest boiling rice noodles, we strongly recommend that you soak them in hot tap water. The soaking time will be longer but there's no risk of overcooking these delicate noodles; while the noodles soak, you can prep the other ingredients. See page 24 for more details about buying and soaking rice noodles. If using ¼-inch-wide noodles, reduce soaking time in step 1 to 20 minutes.

✓ WHY THIS RECIPE WORKS

This brightly flavored Thai dish combines rice noodles with plenty of basil and a spicy, aromatic sauce. For the right amount of subtle heat, we made a paste of chiles, garlic, and shallots in the food processor. Briefly cooking this paste deepened its flavor and mellowed the harshness of the raw aromatics. Fish sauce, brown sugar, lime juice, and chicken broth added sweet and savory notes. We found a full 2 cups of basil was required to provide the dish's trademark fresh flavor and color. Pan-fried tofu offered both creamy and crispy textures that paired well with the noodles, and giving it a properly crisped exterior required a two-step approach. First, we let the tofu drain on paper towels for 20 minutes and blotted it dry. Next, we tossed it in cornstarch, which encouraged browning and gave it the right crisp coating. Extra-firm tofu is the best choice here, but firm tofu will work. This dish is quite spicy; use the lesser amount of chiles if you want a less spicy dish. For more heat, add the chile seeds.

Spicy Basil Noodles with Crispy Tofu, Snap Peas, and Bell Pepper

SERVES 4

12	ounces (⅜-inch-wide) dried flat rice noodles
14	ounces extra-firm tofu, cut into 1-inch cubes
6–8	Thai, serrano, or jalapeño chiles, stemmed and seeded
6	garlic cloves, peeled
4	shallots, peeled
2	cups chicken broth
¼	cup fish sauce
¼	cup packed brown sugar
3	tablespoons lime juice (2 limes)
½	cup cornstarch
	Salt and pepper
7	tablespoons vegetable oil
6	ounces snap peas, strings removed
1	red bell pepper, stemmed, seeded, cut into ¼-inch-wide strips, and halved crosswise
2	cups fresh Thai basil or Italian (sweet) basil leaves

1. Cover noodles with very hot tap water in large bowl and stir to separate. Let noodles soak until softened, pliable, and limp but not fully tender, 35 to 40 minutes; drain. Spread tofu over paper towel–lined baking sheet, let drain for 20 minutes, then gently press dry with paper towels.

2. Pulse chiles, garlic, and shallots in food processor into smooth paste, about 30 pulses, scraping down bowl as needed. Whisk broth, fish sauce, sugar, and lime juice together in bowl.

3. Adjust oven rack to upper-middle position and heat oven to 200 degrees. Spread cornstarch into shallow dish or pie plate. Season tofu with salt and pepper, then dredge in cornstarch and transfer to plate. Heat 3 tablespoons oil in 12-inch nonstick skillet over medium-high heat until just smoking. Add tofu and cook, turning as needed, until all sides are crisp and browned, about 8 minutes; transfer to paper towel–lined plate and keep warm in oven.

4. Wipe now-empty skillet clean with paper towels, add 1 tablespoon oil, and heat over high heat until just smoking. Add snap peas and bell pepper and cook, stirring often, until vegetables are crisp-tender and beginning to brown, 3 to 5 minutes; transfer to bowl.

5. Add remaining 3 tablespoons oil to now-empty skillet and heat over medium-high heat until shimmering. Add processed chile mixture and cook until moisture evaporates and color deepens, 3 to 5 minutes. Add drained noodles and broth mixture and cook, tossing gently, until sauce has thickened and noodles are well coated and tender, 5 to 10 minutes.

6. Stir in cooked vegetables and basil and cook until basil wilts slightly, about 1 minute. (If necessary, add up to ¼ cup hot tap water, 1 tablespoon at a time, to adjust consistency.) Top individual portions with crispy tofu and serve.

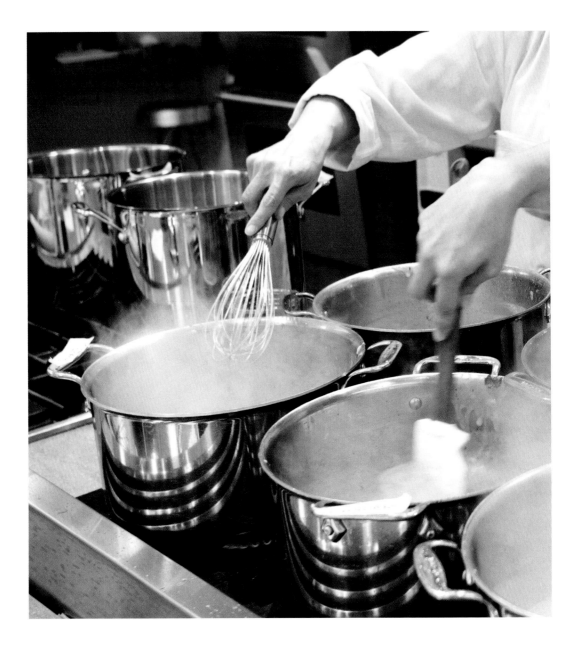

COMFORT FOODS

Lasagna with Hearty Tomato-Meat Sauce

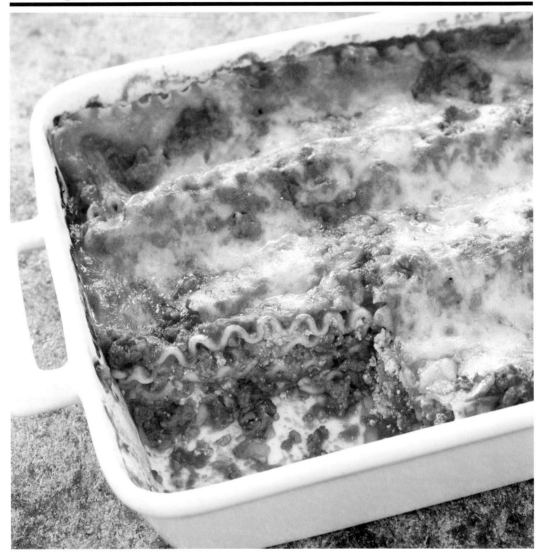

G-F TESTING LAB

LASAGNA NOODLES	We had good luck using Tinkyada lasagna noodles (see page 24 for more details), which require boiling, but be careful not to overcook the noodles or they can fall apart when handled.

✔ WHY THIS RECIPE WORKS

When it comes to making a gluten-free version of a classic meat-sauce lasagna, we quickly discovered that it's all about the noodles. As with wheat noodles, you have two options—no-boil and boil-before-use—when selecting among the various gluten-free options. No-boil noodles, a standard in the test kitchen when it comes to making traditional lasagna, failed us in the gluten-free universe. These noodles varied drastically from brand to brand. They came out unevenly cooked, gummy, starchy, or brittle, or they completely disintegrated. Old-fashioned boil-before-use noodles produced more consistent results, with tender noodles that held up in the oven. Still, our preferred noodles were more delicate than the traditional ones, so we made sure to boil them only until just tender, and we opted for a sauce with a smooth consistency to avoid chunks that might weigh down and break apart the noodles in the assembled casserole. Prepared along with a classic ricotta filling, this lasagna impressed everyone in the test kitchen. If you can't find meatloaf mix, you can substitute 8 ounces each of 85 percent lean ground beef and ground pork. You can use whole-milk or part-skim mozzarella and ricotta in this recipe.

Lasagna with Hearty Tomato-Meat Sauce
SERVES 6 TO 8

NOODLES AND SAUCE

12 gluten-free lasagna noodles (10 ounces)
    Salt and pepper
4 teaspoons olive oil
1 (28-ounce) can diced tomatoes, drained
1 onion, chopped fine
6 garlic cloves, minced
1 pound meatloaf mix
¼ cup heavy cream
1 (28-ounce) can tomato puree

FILLING

16 ounces (2 cups) whole-milk ricotta cheese
2½ ounces Parmesan cheese, grated (1¼ cups)
½ cup chopped fresh basil
1 large egg, lightly beaten
½ teaspoon salt
½ teaspoon pepper
1 pound mozzarella cheese, shredded (4 cups)

1. FOR THE NOODLES AND SAUCE: Adjust oven rack to middle position and heat oven to 375 degrees. Bring 4 quarts water to boil in large pot. Add lasagna noodles and 1 tablespoon salt and cook, stirring frequently, until just tender. Drain noodles, return to pot, and toss with 1 teaspoon olive oil. Spread oiled noodles out on baking sheet; set aside.

2. Pulse diced tomatoes in food processor until almost smooth, about 5 pulses. Heat remaining 1 tablespoon oil in Dutch oven over medium heat until shimmering. Add onion and cook, stirring occasionally, until softened, about 5 minutes. Add garlic and cook until fragrant, about 30 seconds.

3. Stir in meatloaf mix, ½ teaspoon salt, and ½ teaspoon pepper, increase heat to medium-high, and cook, breaking up any large pieces with wooden spoon, until no longer pink, about 4 minutes. Add cream, bring to simmer, and cook, stirring occasionally, until liquid evaporates and only rendered fat remains, about 4 minutes. Stir in processed diced tomatoes and tomato puree, and bring to simmer. Reduce heat to low and simmer until sauce has thickened and is reduced to about 6 cups, 15 to 20 minutes. (Sauce can be cooled, covered, and refrigerated for up to 2 days; reheat before assembling lasagna.)

4. FOR THE FILLING: Meanwhile, combine ricotta, 1 cup Parmesan, basil, egg, salt, and pepper in bowl.

5. Spread ½ cup meat sauce evenly over bottom of 13 by 9-inch baking dish (avoiding larger pieces of meat). Arrange 3 noodles in single layer on top of sauce. Spread each noodle evenly with 3 tablespoons ricotta mixture and sprinkle entire layer with 1 cup mozzarella. Spoon 1½ cups meat sauce over top. Repeat layering of noodles, ricotta, mozzarella, and sauce two more times. For final layer, arrange remaining 3 noodles on top and cover completely with remaining 1 cup sauce. Sprinkle with remaining 1 cup mozzarella, then sprinkle with remaining ¼ cup Parmesan.

6. Cover dish tightly with aluminum foil sprayed with vegetable oil spray. Bake for 20 minutes. Remove foil and continue to bake until cheese is spotty brown and edges are just bubbling, 20 to 25 minutes longer. Let lasagna cool for 15 minutes before serving.

SMART SHOPPING **Diced Tomatoes**

Diced tomatoes are best for rustic tomato sauces with a chunky texture, such as our Spaghetti and Meatballs (page 112), Penne with Weeknight Meat Sauce (page 116), and Spaghetti with Puttanesca Sauce (page 110). Diced tomatoes may also be processed with their juice in a food processor and used in place of crushed tomatoes when called for in a recipe. They are available packed both in juice and in puree; we favor diced tomatoes packed in juice because they have a fresher flavor. Overall, our preferred brand is Hunt's Diced Tomatoes, which tasters liked most for its fresh flavor and good balance of sweet and tart notes.

TEST KITCHEN TIP **Assembling Lasagna**

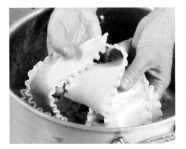

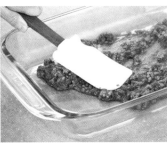

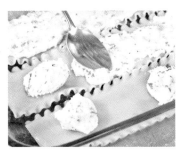

1. Boil lasagna noodles until just tender, drain, and toss with olive oil. When cool enough to handle, lay noodles out flat on baking sheet.

2. Avoiding larger pieces of meat, spread ½ cup meat sauce evenly over bottom of 13 by 9-inch baking dish. Arrange 3 noodles in single layer on top of sauce.

3. Dollop each noodle with 3 tablespoons ricotta mixture, then spread evenly using back of spoon. Sprinkle entire layer with 1 cup mozzarella.

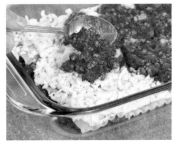

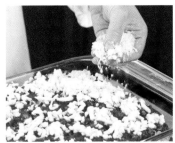

4. Spoon 1½ cups meat sauce over top of mozzarella layer. Repeat layering of noodles, ricotta, mozzarella, and sauce 2 more times.

5. For final layer, arrange last 3 noodles on top and cover with remaining sauce. Sprinkle with remaining mozzarella, then sprinkle with remaining Parmesan.

Spinach and Tomato Lasagna

✔ WHY THIS RECIPE WORKS

To make the greens the star, we stirred some chopped spinach into a basic tomato sauce. Frozen spinach worked just as well as fresh and was easier since it didn't require washing. Next came the classic ricotta layer. Here was another opportunity to add spinach by adding it to the ricotta and eggs mixture. We spread our spinach-packed ricotta between layers of noodles and tomato sauce and moved our casserole to the oven. Even though the spinach was already chopped, with so much of it in the lasagna, the texture was noticeably uneven. To avoid clumps of spinach, we used the food processor to chop it into small pieces. The ricotta layer also seemed a little thick and dry. Reserving some of the liquid from draining the spinach, then adding it to the ricotta mixture, boosted the spinach flavor of the whole lasagna and also helped make the ricotta mixture easier to spread. Since we had the food processor out for the spinach, we tried processing the ricotta with the eggs and spinach liquid before stirring in the spinach. This extra step was worth it; the ricotta mixture became appealingly smooth and creamy. You can thaw the spinach overnight in the refrigerator instead of microwaving it. But do warm the spinach liquid to help smooth the ricotta.

Spinach and Tomato Lasagna
SERVES 6 TO 8

20	ounces frozen chopped spinach
12	gluten-free lasagna noodles (10 ounces)
	Salt and pepper
2	tablespoons olive oil
1	onion, chopped fine
5	garlic cloves, minced
⅛	teaspoon red pepper flakes
2	(28-ounce) cans crushed tomatoes
6	tablespoons chopped fresh basil
16	ounces (2 cups) whole-milk ricotta cheese
3	ounces Parmesan cheese, grated (1½ cups)
2	large eggs
12	ounces mozzarella cheese, shredded (3 cups)

1. Adjust oven rack to middle position and heat oven to 375 degrees. Microwave spinach in large bowl, covered, until thawed, 10 to 15 minutes, stirring halfway through. Squeeze spinach dry, reserving ¼ cup liquid. Pulse spinach in food processor until ground, 8 to 10 pulses, scraping down bowl every few pulses. Wipe out large bowl with paper towels. Transfer spinach to now-empty bowl; set aside.

2. Bring 4 quarts water to boil in large pot. Add lasagna noodles and 1 tablespoon salt and cook, stirring frequently, until just tender. Drain noodles, return to pot, and toss with 1 teaspoon olive oil. Spread oiled noodles out on baking sheet; set aside.

3. Meanwhile, heat remaining 5 teaspoons oil in large saucepan over medium heat until shimmering. Add onion and cook until softened, about 5 minutes. Stir in garlic and pepper flakes and cook until fragrant, about 30 seconds. Add ½ cup processed spinach, tomatoes, 1 teaspoon salt, and ½ teaspoon pepper and cook until slightly thickened, about 10 minutes. Off heat, stir in 3 tablespoons basil.

4. Process reserved spinach liquid and ricotta in food processor until smooth, about 30 seconds. Add remaining 3 tablespoons basil, Parmesan, eggs, 1 teaspoon salt, and ½ teaspoon pepper and process until combined. Stir ricotta mixture into remaining spinach.

5. Spread 1¼ cups tomato sauce evenly over bottom of 13 by 9-inch baking dish. Arrange 3 noodles in single layer on top of sauce. Spread 1 cup ricotta mixture evenly over noodles and sprinkle entire layer with ⅔ cup mozzarella. Spoon 1¼ cups tomato sauce over top. Repeat layering of noodles, ricotta mixture, mozzarella, and tomato sauce two more times. For final layer, arrange remaining 3 noodles on top and cover completely with remaining tomato sauce. Sprinkle with remaining 1 cup mozzarella.

6. Cover dish tightly with aluminum foil sprayed with vegetable oil spray. Place on rimmed baking sheet, and bake until bubbling around edges, about 40 minutes. Remove foil and continue to bake until cheese is melted, about 10 minutes longer. Let lasagna cool for 15 minutes before serving.

Eggplant Parmesan

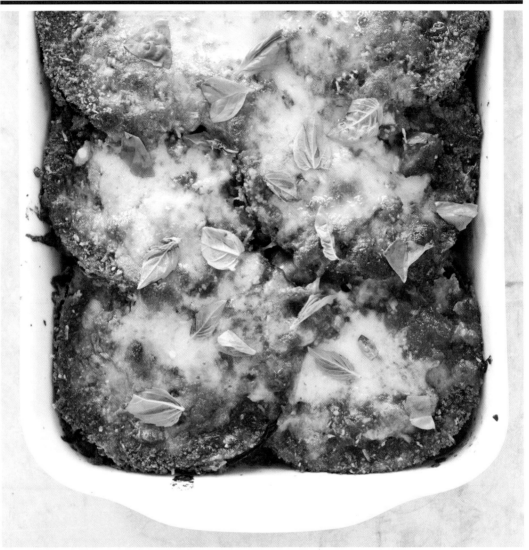

G-F TESTING LAB

BREAD   You can use store-bought bread or our Classic Sandwich Bread (page 170) to make the bread crumbs. Our favorite store-bought brand is Udi's Gluten Free White Sandwich Bread (see page 22 for complete tasting). Weights of gluten-free sandwich bread vary from brand to brand; if you are not using Udi's, we recommend going by weight rather than number of slices. Bread may clump together during toasting; make sure to break it apart into fine crumbs before breading.

WHY THIS RECIPE WORKS

In past experience with classic recipes, dipping the eggplant slices in flour, then egg, then bread crumbs had always delivered an even, crisp coating that stayed in place. We found replacing the flour with cornstarch worked equally well for a gluten-free version. The coating clung well, and the starch also helped with crispness. The biggest challenge was the bread-crumb coating itself. After trying several options, we settled on making our own fresh crumbs in the food processor. But unlike traditional homemade bread crumbs, those made with store-bought gluten-free bread didn't coat the eggplant slices evenly. The solution involved both toasting the crumbs and adding some extra ingredients (see page 139 for more details). Traditionally, cooking the coated eggplant before assembling this casserole is key to keeping the coating crisp and in place. The same proved true with our gluten-free version. Baking the breaded slices in the oven was appealingly hands-off, but the eggplant turned out tasting stale. Pan frying won out, with eggplant surrounded by a perfectly light and crunchy golden exterior. Layered with a simple basil-tomato sauce, Parmesan, and mozzarella and baked, our eggplant remained crisp, tender, and flavorful—better results than with most traditional versions. Be sure to avoid saucing the outer edges of the eggplant slices in step 5 so that they remain crisp once baked. You can use whole-milk or part-skim mozzarella in this recipe.

Eggplant Parmesan
SERVES 6 TO 8

EGGPLANT

- 10 slices (about 10 ounces) gluten-free sandwich bread, torn into quarters
- 2 ounces Parmesan cheese, grated (1 cup)
- 1 cup cornstarch
  Salt and pepper
- 4 large eggs
- 1½ pounds eggplant, sliced into ¼-inch-thick rounds
- ½ cup vegetable oil, plus extra as needed

TOMATO SAUCE

- 3 (14.5-ounce) cans diced tomatoes
- 2 tablespoons extra-virgin olive oil
- 4 garlic cloves, minced
- ¼ teaspoon red pepper flakes
- ½ cup chopped fresh basil, plus 10 torn leaves for garnish
  Salt and pepper
- 8 ounces mozzarella, shredded (2 cups)
- 1 ounce Parmesan cheese, grated (½ cup)

1. FOR THE EGGPLANT: Adjust oven rack to lower-middle position and heat oven to 425 degrees. Process bread in food processor until evenly ground, about 30 seconds (you should have about 4 cups). Spread crumbs in even layer on rimmed baking sheet and bake, stirring occasionally, until golden brown, 7 to 10 minutes. Transfer crumbs to shallow dish, breaking up any large clumps into fine crumbs. (Do not turn off oven.) Stir in Parmesan, 1 tablespoon cornstarch, ½ teaspoon salt, and ¼ teaspoon pepper. Beat eggs in second shallow dish. Combine remaining cornstarch and ½ teaspoon pepper in large zipper-lock bag.

2. Set wire rack in rimmed baking sheet. Working with half of eggplant slices at a time, place eggplant in bag of cornstarch, seal bag, and shake bag to coat eggplant. Using tongs, remove eggplant pieces from bag, shaking off excess cornstarch, dip in eggs, then coat with bread crumbs, pressing gently to adhere. Place breaded eggplant slices on prepared wire rack.

3. Heat oil in 12-inch nonstick skillet over medium-high heat until shimmering. Cook eggplant in batches until well browned on both sides, about 4 minutes, flipping halfway through cooking; add extra oil to pan as needed. Transfer cooked eggplant to clean wire rack set in rimmed baking sheet.

4. FOR THE TOMATO SAUCE: Process 2 cans diced tomatoes and their juice in food processor until almost smooth, about 5 seconds. Heat oil, garlic, and pepper flakes in large saucepan over medium-high heat, stirring occasionally, until fragrant and garlic is light golden, about 2 minutes. Stir in processed tomatoes and remaining can of diced tomatoes and their juice and bring to boil. Reduce heat to medium-low and simmer, stirring occasionally, until sauce has thickened and reduced to 4 cups, about 15 minutes. Stir in chopped basil and season with salt and pepper to taste.

5. Spread 1 cup tomato sauce evenly over bottom of 13 by 9-inch baking dish. Layer in half of fried eggplant slices, overlapping slices to fit.

Spoon 1 cup sauce over eggplant and sprinkle with 1 cup mozzarella. Layer in remaining eggplant and spoon 1 cup sauce over eggplant, leaving majority of eggplant exposed, then sprinkle with remaining 1 cup mozzarella and Parmesan. Bake until bubbling and cheese is browned, 13 to 15 minutes. Let cool for 10 minutes, then scatter torn basil leaves over top and serve, passing remaining 1 cup tomato sauce separately.

TEST KITCHEN TIP **Achieving a Crisp Eggplant Coating**

Cornstarch works well in lieu of the all-purpose flour used in a traditional coating. Homemade bread crumbs made from store-bought or homemade gluten-free sandwich bread are the best breading, but because these crumbs are fluffy and sticky, you need to toast them before coating the eggplant. Adding Parmesan directly to the coating boosts flavor, while more cornstarch further boosts browning and crispness.

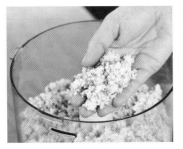

1. Process bread in food processor until evenly ground, about 30 seconds. (Crumbs will be sticky.)

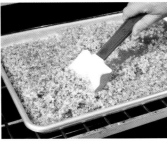

2. Spread processed bread crumbs on rimmed baking sheet and bake, stirring occasionally, until crumbs are evenly golden brown.

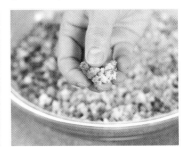

3. Transfer crumbs to shallow dish, breaking up any large clumps into fine crumbs, then stir in Parmesan and cornstarch.

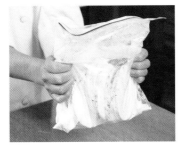

4. Place half of eggplant slices in bag of cornstarch, seal bag, and shake bag to coat eggplant evenly.

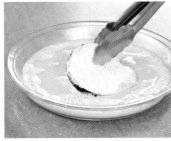

5. Using tongs, thoroughly coat eggplant with beaten eggs, allowing excess to drip off.

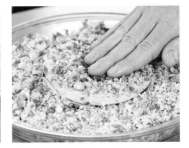

6. Dredge eggplant in bread crumbs, pressing gently to adhere and making sure all sides are evenly coated.

Coating Eggplant Parmesan

THE PROBLEM You might think that making a gluten-free version of Eggplant Parmesan would be easy since, after all, it just requires finding an alternative way to bread the eggplant. But we found this task was more complex than expected: Not only did we face unexpected hurdles in nailing down the best gluten-free coating, but we also had to find the best technique for actually coating the eggplant—and for cooking the eggplant slices once coated.

THE STORE-BOUGHT NITTY-GRITTY Store-bought gluten-free bread crumbs are certainly convenient and easy to work with. However, their texture is very hard and fine, like cornmeal. After breading the eggplant with these crumbs, we tried both baking and frying the coated eggplant. Neither worked well; both versions tasted dry, bland, and gritty.

PASS ON THE PANKO With their delicate, ultra-crisp texture, these Japanese-style bread crumbs work well in a number of traditional coating applications. We were hopeful when we found several gluten-free brands at the supermarket, but none of them impressed us. They all had an overly tough texture right out of the box and turned rock-hard once the eggplant was breaded and cooked (once again, both baking and frying delivered equally poor results).

PLAIN? NO GAIN Just to make sure we weren't missing an easy solution, we tested roasting the eggplant plain, then layering it into the dish with the cheese and tomato sauce—no coating, crumbs or otherwise. The result was a pretty tasty eggplant casserole, but everyone in the test kitchen agreed that without the coating it just wasn't eggplant Parmesan.

BREAD FLUFF We learned right away that gluten-free sandwich bread, with its high starch content and lack of structure, simply didn't act like regular bread when ground into crumbs in the food processor—it broke down into fluffy, sticky pieces that clumped together in one solid mess. They were difficult to work with.

THE SOLUTION THAT STUCK We then tried spreading the sticky homemade bread crumbs onto a baking sheet and toasting them in the oven in the hope that they would dry out. This worked perfectly. Since some crumbs still clumped, we found that adding some cornstarch filled in the gaps and also boosted browning and crispness, while mixing in some grated Parmesan helped boost the flavor of the coating. A standard breading procedure (dipping in flour, then egg, then bread crumbs) worked well when we substituted cornstarch for the flour. We also tried substituting tapioca starch, rice flour, and potato starch in place of the flour, but only the cornstarch helped the crumbs stay crisp and formed a uniform coating that stayed in place around the eggplant. Finally, we tested both baking and frying. The coating on the baked version tasted stale and dry. The fried eggplant, with a light, crunchy texture and authentic flavor, won hands down.

Easy Stovetop Macaroni and Cheese

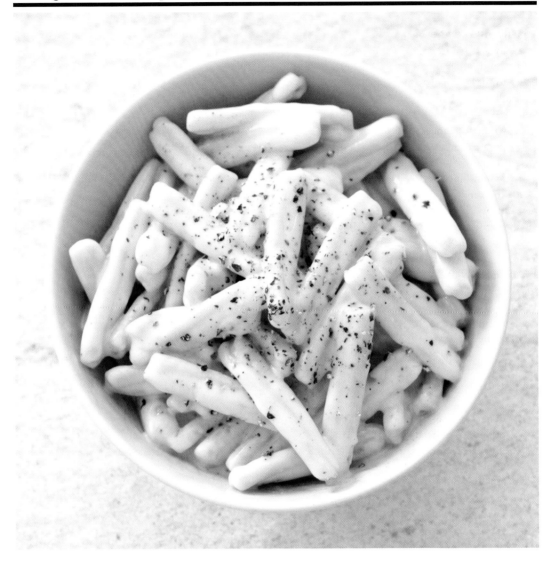

G-F TESTING LAB

PASTA   Our favorite brand is Jovial Gluten Free Brown Rice Pasta (see pages 25–26 for complete tasting). This brand does not make a traditional macaroni shape, but it does offer caserecce, which is shaped like a very narrow, twisted, and rolled tube. Cooking times for gluten-free pasta vary from brand to brand. Make sure to taste the pasta often, as it can overcook quickly.

Our favorite version of mac and cheese is rich, cheesy, and indulgent—but it relies on a béchamel sauce for its base. This sauce, which calls for whisking milk into a butter-flour roux, ensures smooth, thick results in the final mac and cheese. For equally creamy results without the flour, we found that a can of evaporated milk plus a couple of eggs were the key to success. The evaporated milk added just the right richness and creaminess, while the eggs worked as the thickener. (We also tried half-and-half, but it lost out because it curdled.) We cooked the pasta, then returned it to the pot and added our eggs and evaporated milk with the cheese, plus a little dry mustard and cayenne for a flavor boost. Ready for the table in about 20 minutes, our gluten-free mac and cheese was not only super-cheesy and creamy but also fast and easy. You can substitute Monterey Jack or Colby cheese if desired, but the flavor will be less pronounced.

Easy Stovetop Macaroni and Cheese
SERVES 4

    12 **ounces gluten-free caserecce (see page 140) or elbow macaroni**
        Salt and pepper
     2 **large eggs**
     1 **(12-ounce) can evaporated milk**
     ½ **teaspoon dry mustard, dissolved in 1 teaspoon water**
     4 **tablespoons unsalted butter**
    12 **ounces sharp cheddar cheese, shredded (3 cups)**
        Pinch cayenne pepper

1. Bring 4 quarts water to boil in large pot. Stir in pasta and 1 tablespoon salt and cook, stirring often, until pasta is al dente. Meanwhile, whisk eggs, half of evaporated milk, mustard mixture, and ¼ teaspoon salt together in bowl.

2. Drain pasta and return it to pot. Add butter and cook over low heat, stirring constantly, until melted. Stir in egg mixture, half of cheese, and cayenne. Cook, gradually stirring in remaining milk and cheese, until mixture is hot and creamy, about 5 minutes.

3. Let mixture sit off heat until sauce has thickened slightly, 2 to 5 minutes. Season with salt and pepper to taste. Serve.

SMART SHOPPING

Evaporated Milk vs. Condensed Milk

Evaporated and condensed milk both begin the same way: by heating milk in a vacuum so that 60 percent or more of the water evaporates. The resulting thick liquid is then either given a high-temperature treatment to sterilize it, making evaporated milk, or sweetened to preserve it, making condensed milk. Both evaporated and condensed milk have about twice the concentration of fat and protein as regular whole milk. However, condensed milk is about 45 percent sugar and is used for baking—not for savory casseroles or macaroni and cheese—so make sure to pick up the right product when shopping.

Baked Macaroni and Cheese

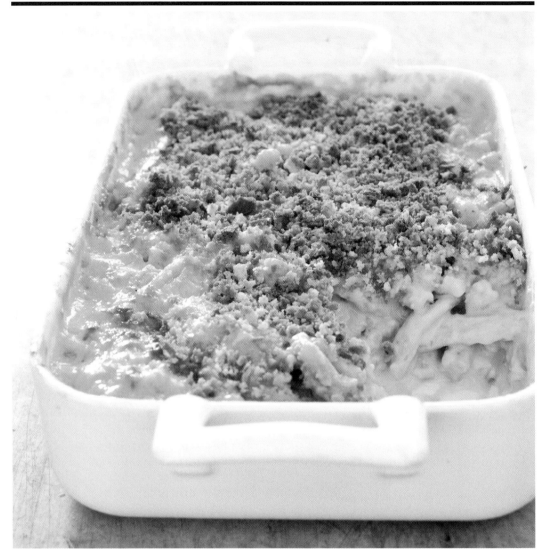

G-F TESTING LAB

PASTA	Our favorite brand is Jovial Gluten Free Brown Rice Pasta (see pages 25–26 for complete tasting). This brand does not make a traditional macaroni shape, but it does offer caserecce, which is shaped like a very narrow, twisted, and rolled tube. Cooking times for gluten-free pasta vary from brand to brand.
BREAD	You can use store-bought bread or our Classic Sandwich Bread (page 170) to make the bread crumbs. Our favorite store-bought brand is Udi's Gluten Free White Sandwich Bread (see page 22 for complete tasting). Weights of gluten-free sandwich bread vary from brand to brand; if you are not using Udi's, we recommend going by weight rather than number of slices. Bread may clump together during toasting; make sure to break it apart into fine crumbs before sprinkling over the pasta.

Baked macaroni and cheese is the king of all casseroles. At its finest, it emerges from the oven with a crisp crumb topping and creamy, cheesy pasta below. Our favorite traditional baked mac and cheese relies on béchamel sauce for its base. This sauce, which calls for whisking milk into a butter-flour roux, ensures smooth, creamy results in the final dish. For equally creamy results without the flour, we relied on cornstarch (first mixed with milk to prevent clumping), which thickened our sauce to the perfect consistency. (We kept our sauce mixture loose so that it could withstand the heat of the oven without drying out.) For the cheese, we found that a mix of Colby cheese (for meltability) and cheddar cheese (for rich flavor) delivered an appealing casserole that baked up smooth and creamy. Adding a little dry mustard and cayenne helped to boost the cheesy flavor even more. Now, all we needed was the perfect bread-crumb topping. The simple fix was pulsing gluten-free bread and melted butter in the food processor and then toasting the coated crumbs in the oven. Once baked on top of our casserole, the crumbs provided the ideal crisp counterpoint to our tender pasta and creamy cheese sauce. You can substitute Monterey Jack for the Colby cheese if desired, but the flavor will be less pronounced. Make sure to taste the pasta often, as it can overcook quickly.

Baked Macaroni and Cheese
SERVES 4

3	slices (about 3 ounces) gluten-free sandwich bread, torn into quarters
2	tablespoons unsalted butter, melted, plus 4 tablespoons unsalted butter
12	ounces gluten-free caserecce (see page 142) or elbow macaroni
	Salt and pepper
2½	cups whole milk
2	tablespoons cornstarch
1	garlic clove, minced
½	teaspoon dry mustard
⅛	teaspoon cayenne pepper
1	cup chicken broth
12	ounces Colby cheese, shredded (3 cups)
6	ounces extra-sharp cheddar cheese, shredded (1½ cups)

1. Adjust oven rack to middle position and heat oven to 400 degrees. Pulse bread and melted butter in food processor until coarsely ground, about 12 pulses. Spread crumbs in even layer on rimmed baking sheet and bake, stirring occasionally, until lightly browned, 6 to 8 minutes. Let cool on wire rack. (Do not turn off oven.) Once crumbs have cooled slightly, break up any large clumps into fine crumbs.

2. Meanwhile, bring 4 quarts water to boil in large pot. Stir in pasta and 1 tablespoon salt and cook, stirring often, until pasta is al dente. Drain pasta and leave in colander.

3. Whisk ½ cup milk and cornstarch together in small bowl. Add remaining 4 tablespoons butter to now-empty pot and return to medium heat until melted. Stir in garlic, mustard, and cayenne and cook until fragrant, about 30 seconds. Whisk in remaining 2 cups milk and chicken broth and bring to simmer. Whisk in cornstarch mixture, return to simmer, and continue cooking, whisking often, until large bubbles form on surface and mixture is slightly thickened, 8 to 10 minutes. Off heat, gradually whisk in Colby and cheddar until completely melted. Season with salt and pepper to taste.

4. Stir drained pasta into cheese sauce, breaking up any clumps, until well combined. Pour pasta mixture into 8-inch square baking dish (or other 2-quart casserole dish) and sprinkle with bread crumbs. Bake until golden brown and bubbling around edges, about 15 minutes. Let cool for 10 minutes before serving.

All-American Meatloaf

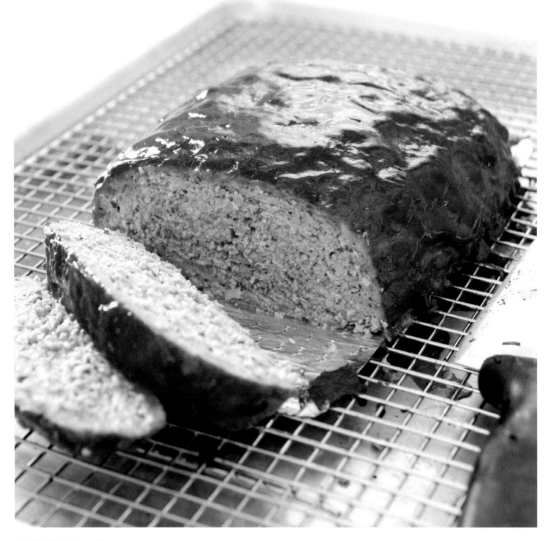

G-F TESTING LAB

POTATO FLAKES   Make sure to buy potato flakes, not potato granules, which have a slightly metallic taste.

✔ WHY THIS RECIPE WORKS

For a tender, moist meatloaf, we've learned that the key is adding a panade—a paste of bread (or similar ingredient, such as crackers) and milk—to the meat mixture. We wanted to make an equally tender gluten-free version, but substituting store-bought gluten-free sandwich bread was a no-go. The bread never broke down into a proper paste, and it delivered a tough, chewy meatloaf. From there we tried more adventurous ingredients: ground oats (an addition found in many older recipes), corn tortillas, potato flakes, and gelatin. All produced a loaf that was nicely bound, but the potato flakes were the winner in the end. They had the right neutral flavor and blended seamlessly into the mixture, and their starchy makeup worked just like bread, absorbing liquid and keeping the loaf tender. A combination of beef and pork provided better flavor and texture than traditional store-bought meatloaf mix. Since ground beef will cook up tough if overworked, we mixed all the ingredients with the ground pork first, then worked in the ground beef.

All-American Meatloaf
SERVES 6

- ½ cup ketchup
- ¼ cup packed light brown sugar
- 4 teaspoons cider vinegar
- 1 tablespoon vegetable oil
- 2 onions, chopped fine
- 4 garlic cloves, minced
- 1 teaspoon minced fresh thyme or ½ teaspoon dried
- 2 large eggs
- ½ cup milk
- 2 teaspoons Dijon mustard
- 2 teaspoons Worcestershire sauce
- 1 teaspoon salt
- ½ teaspoon pepper
- ⅓ cup potato flakes
- ⅓ cup minced fresh parsley
- 1 pound ground pork
- 1 pound 85 percent lean ground beef

1. Adjust oven rack to upper-middle position and heat oven to 350 degrees. Fold heavy-duty aluminum foil to form 9 by 5-inch rectangle. Center foil on wire rack set in rimmed baking sheet. Poke holes in foil with skewer (about ½ inch apart). Spray foil with vegetable oil spray.

2. Stir ketchup, sugar, and vinegar together in bowl and set aside. Heat oil in 12-inch nonstick skillet over medium-high heat until shimmering. Add onions and cook until softened, about 5 minutes. Stir in garlic and thyme and cook until fragrant, about 30 seconds. Transfer to large bowl and let cool for 5 minutes.

3. Whisk in eggs, milk, mustard, Worcestershire, salt, and pepper. Stir in potato flakes and parsley. Add pork and knead with hands until thoroughly combined. Add beef and continue to knead until uniform.

4. Transfer meat mixture to foil rectangle and shape into 9 by 5-inch loaf. Brush half of ketchup mixture over meatloaf. Bake meatloaf for 40 minutes.

5. Brush meatloaf with remaining ketchup mixture and continue to bake until center of loaf registers 160 degrees, 30 to 35 minutes. Let meatloaf cool for 15 minutes before slicing. Serve.

TEST KITCHEN TIP
Avoiding Greasy Meatloaf

We cook our meatloaf free-form on a wire rack to let the rendered fat drip away. The foil, which should be coated with vegetable oil spray, ensures that the meatloaf doesn't stick.

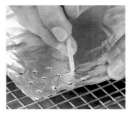

Set rack inside rimmed baking sheet and top with 9 by 5-inch rectangle of aluminum foil. Using skewer, poke holes in foil about ½ inch apart to allow fat to drain away.

Keeping Meatloaf Tender

THE PROBLEM Unlike a hamburger, meatloaf is cooked until well done, which means that avoiding dry, tough meat can be particularly tricky. In the test kitchen, we've known for a long time that incorporating a panade—a paste made from bread (or similar ingredient, such as crackers) and milk—is a simple technique for delivering an ultra-tender, moist meatloaf. How does a panade work? The starches in the bread absorb liquid from the milk to form a gel that coats and lubricates the protein molecules in the meat, preventing the molecules from linking together and shrinking into a tough matrix. The result: a thoroughly cooked meatloaf that is also tender and juicy. So how could we accomplish the same thing without using traditional bread?

NOT A SIMPLE SWAP Swapping an equal amount of our winning gluten-free sandwich bread for regular sandwich bread in the panade seemed like an obvious solution. Too bad it didn't work. While regular sandwich bread turns into a starchy paste when mixed with milk, the gluten-free bread didn't. Instead, it broke down into small, spongy pieces, and the finished meatloaf tasted tough and chewy. Why? The higher level of starch in gluten-free bread forms more-crystalline starch as the bread cools and rests. This crystalline starch is very heat-resistant, even in moist foods, so gluten-free bread will never fully break down, including in a panade and baked meatloaf.

AN OLD-FASHIONED ATTEMPT Many recipes in older cookbooks call for adding oats to meatloaf. Imagining they could function much like bread by absorbing moisture, we started by grinding oats (we tested both old-fashioned and quick-cooking) in the food processor, then softening them in milk before combining them with the meat. But this also didn't pass muster. Tasters didn't care for the noticeable oat flavor in the loaf, and there were bits of oat that never really softened, leaving stale-tasting bits throughout.

AN IDEA THAT DIDN'T GEL In the past we've had good luck using gelatin in conjunction with a panade in meatballs and meatloaf to deliver a tender, juicy result. We wondered if we could get gelatin alone to deliver the outcome we were after. We let a little bit hydrate with the milk and eggs before combining the mixture with the meat. Unfortunately, this didn't solve our problem. The resulting meatloaf was really juicy—but the meat had a rubbery texture. Why? Since gelatin is soluble in water, it doesn't do much to separate the meat proteins and keep them from binding together to form a tough, rubbery network when the meat is cooked. While the gelatin kept the meat juicy, it didn't deliver at all on the tender front.

A CORNY TEST Adding corn tortillas that we'd processed to fine crumbs actually worked very well. This meatloaf was very tender and moist, but the problem was that the corn flavor tasted out of place here.

FLAKES TAKE FIRST Sold as an easy way to make mashed potatoes at the last minute, potato flakes are a convenience product we don't often use in the test kitchen. Yet they turned out to be the solution we needed. The starch in potato flakes, which are made from dehydrated spuds, functioned just like the starch in wheat-based bread, absorbing moisture and dissolving seamlessly into the meat mixture. And unlike potato flour, dehydrated potato flakes are less likely to clump when combined with liquid. They created a gel when combined with the milk and coated the protein molecules in the meat. The result? A tender, juicy meatloaf without the need for bread.

Fried Chicken

WHY THIS RECIPE WORKS

There's a lot of debate about the best way to make fried chicken, but it's pretty much a given that flour is going to be in the recipe. Typically, the chicken is dredged in flour, then a buttermilk-egg batter, then another coating of flour. The flour plays two basic roles. The starch in flour delivers a coating that will be brown and crisp, while the protein in flour allows the coating to cling to the chicken and stay in place. Could we develop a recipe that delivered moist chicken coated with a crisp, mahogany crust—without traditional flour helping us out? Once the chicken was brined (we knew from experience this would ensure juicy meat), we ran a battery of gluten-free coating tests to see if any could match all-purpose flour. We tried cornstarch, rice flour, potato flour, potato starch, cornmeal, and corn flour. Cornstarch produced the crispiest crust, and although it has less binding powder than flour (because it contains a lot less protein), this coating still clung nicely to the chicken. However, the coating was thin and lacked flavor. Mixing the cornstarch with cornmeal delivered a more substantial and more flavorful crust that fried up perfectly. Following a classic three-step breading process, we gave the chicken a very light coating of cornstarch, then dipped it in a buttermilk-egg mixture, then dredged it in a final coating of seasoned cornstarch and cornmeal. We found that adding both baking soda and baking powder to the buttermilk produced just enough carbon dioxide to lighten the coating. Letting the dredged chicken sit for 30 minutes before frying evenly hydrated the coating and prevented any dry spots. This fried chicken fried up as juicy, crisp, and brown as the traditional standby. A whole 4-pound chicken, cut into 10 pieces (4 breast pieces, 2 drumsticks, 2 thighs, 2 wings), can be used instead of the chicken parts. Skinless chicken pieces are also an acceptable substitute, but the meat will come out slightly drier. If using kosher chicken, do not brine in step 1.

Fried Chicken
SERVES 4

	Salt
¼	cup sugar
3½	pounds bone-in chicken pieces (split breasts cut in half, drumsticks, and/or thighs), trimmed
1	cup cornstarch
1	large egg
1	teaspoon baking powder (see page 20)
½	teaspoon baking soda
1	cup buttermilk
1	cup cornmeal (see page 149)
1½	teaspoons garlic powder
1½	teaspoons paprika
¼	teaspoon cayenne pepper
3–4	quarts peanut or vegetable oil

1. Whisk 1 quart cold water, ¼ cup salt, and sugar together in large bowl until sugar and salt dissolve. Add chicken, cover, and refrigerate for 1 hour. Remove chicken from brine and pat dry with paper towels. Set wire rack in rimmed baking sheet and line plate with triple layer of paper towels.

2. Place ½ cup cornstarch in large zipper-lock bag. Beat egg, baking powder, and baking soda together in medium bowl; stir in buttermilk (mixture will bubble and foam). Whisk remaining ½ cup cornstarch, cornmeal, garlic powder, paprika, cayenne, and 1 teaspoon salt together in shallow dish.

3. Working with half of chicken at a time, place chicken in bag of cornstarch, seal bag, and shake bag to coat chicken. Using tongs, remove chicken pieces from bag, shaking off excess cornstarch, dip in buttermilk mixture, then coat with cornmeal mixture, pressing gently to adhere. Place dredged chicken on prepared wire rack, skin side up. Cover loosely with plastic wrap and let sit 30 minutes.

4. Meanwhile, add oil to large Dutch oven until it measures about 2 inches deep, and heat over

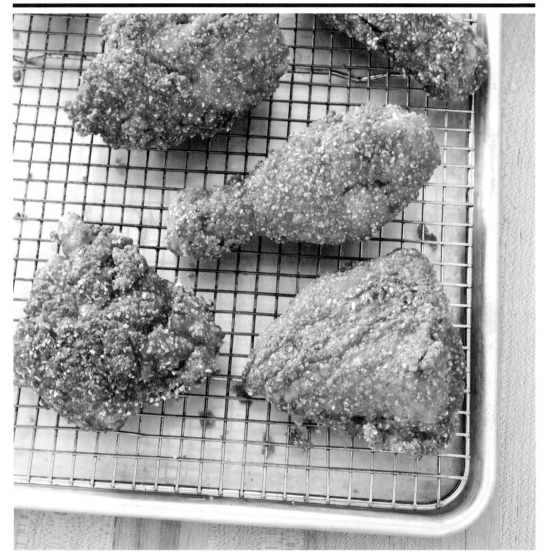

G-F TESTING LAB

CORNMEAL　　The test kitchen's favorite cornmeal for most applications, including this recipe, is finely ground Whole-Grain Arrowhead Mills Cornmeal. This brand has been processed in a gluten-free facility, but not all brands are. Make sure to read the label. See page 149 for more details on buying cornmeal.

medium-high heat to 350 degrees. Adjust oven rack to middle position and heat oven to 200 degrees. Carefully place half of chicken in pot, skin side down, cover, and fry, stirring occasionally to prevent pieces from sticking together, until deep golden brown, 7 to 11 minutes. Adjust burner, if necessary, to maintain oil temperature between 300 and 325 degrees. (After 4 minutes, check chicken pieces for even browning and rearrange if some pieces are browning faster than others.) Turn chicken pieces over and continue to cook until breast pieces register 160 degrees and drumsticks and/or thighs register 175 degrees, 6 to 8 minutes. (Smaller pieces may cook faster than larger pieces. Remove pieces from pot as they reach correct temperature.) Drain chicken briefly on paper towel–lined plate, then transfer to clean wire rack set in rimmed baking sheet and keep warm in oven.

5. Return oil to 350 degrees and repeat with remaining chicken. Serve.

SMART SHOPPING **Cornmeal**

Different recipes require different grinds and types of cornmeal. Here's what you need to know.

GRIND SIZES: While some brands label their cornmeal as fine-, medium-, or coarse-ground, many may not. And what is one brand's fine grind is another brand's medium or even coarse. We consider grains that are about the size of couscous to be coarse-ground. "Regular" cornmeal (like Quaker or Arrowhead Mills) is finely ground.

WHOLE GRAIN VS. DEGERMINATED: Whole grain cornmeal has the hull and germ of each kernel still intact. Because of that, we have found it adds a full corn flavor to baked goods, but it will never completely break down in liquid. Degerminated corn kernels have had their hard hull and germ removed and cook more evenly in polenta.

STONE-GROUND: While companies like Quaker use smooth steel rollers to produce very fine, uniform cornmeal, stone grinding produces grains of varying sizes that create a more varied texture. Keep in mind that stone-ground cornmeal can be ground fine, medium, or coarse.

INSTANT AND QUICK-COOKING: These varieties have superfine grains that are parcooked in order to reduce the cooking time They cook up gluey and lack corn flavor, so we don't use them.

TEST KITCHEN TIP **Frying Chicken**

Frying can be intimidating, but it's really simple if you follow a few basic directions. The key to success is maintaining the proper temperature for the frying oil. If it's too hot, the exterior of the food will burn before the interior cooks through, but if it's too cool the coating will never crisp up and will instead be greasy. Make sure to use a candy or instant-read thermometer to ensure your oil is at the right temperature.

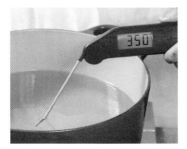
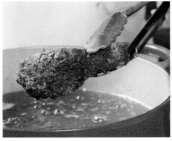
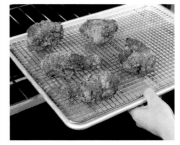

1. Add oil to Dutch oven until it measures 2 inches deep. Heat oil over medium-high heat until it registers 350 degrees (this will take about 10 to 15 minutes).

2. Carefully place half of chicken pieces in hot oil and fry until deep golden brown and breasts register 160 degrees and drumsticks and/or thighs register 175 degrees.

3. Drain chicken briefly on paper towel–lined plate, then transfer to clean wire rack set in rimmed baking sheet and place in 200-degree oven while frying remaining chicken.

Crispy Pan-Fried Pork Chops

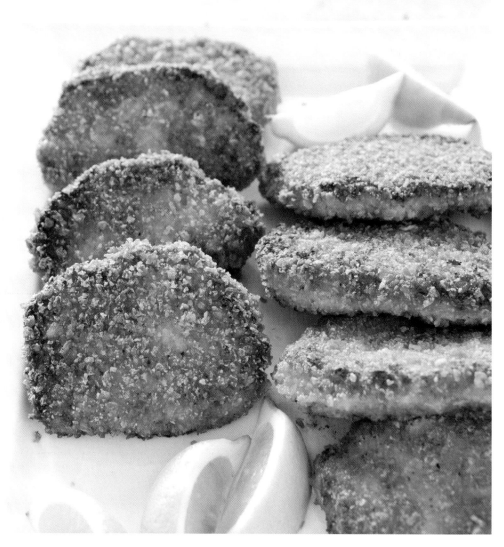

G-F TESTING LAB

CORNFLAKES   Not all brands of cornflakes are gluten-free and not all brands are processed in a gluten-free facility; make sure to read the label.

✔ WHY THIS RECIPE WORKS

Boneless pork chops are lean and mild, a trait that often translates to bland and boring. A crunchy cornflake coating can be just the thing to give this approachable cut a boost. For a light, crisp exterior, we dipped the chops in cornstarch to absorb moisture. Buttermilk helped the cornflakes adhere, while minced garlic and mustard lent needed flavor. Two more tricks guaranteed our coating stayed in place. First, we scored the chops in a crosshatch pattern to enable the cornstarch to cling securely to the chops. And second, we let the breaded chops rest to give the cornstarch time to absorb moisture and form a thick coating that would turn crisp once cooked. We prefer natural to enhanced pork (pork that has been injected with a salt solution to increase moistness). Don't let the cooked chops drain on the paper towels for longer than 30 seconds, or the heat will steam the crust and make it soggy. Omit the sugar if using cornflakes that are already sweetened.

Crispy Pan-Fried Pork Chops
SERVES 4

- ⅓ cup cornstarch
- 1 cup buttermilk
- 1 tablespoon Dijon mustard
- 2 teaspoons sugar (optional)
- 1 garlic clove, minced
- 3½ cups cornflakes
- Salt and pepper
- 8 (3- to 4-ounce) boneless pork chops, ½ to ¾ inch thick, trimmed
- ⅔ cup vegetable oil
- Lemon wedges

1. Place cornstarch in large zipper-lock bag. In shallow dish, whisk buttermilk, mustard, sugar (if using), and garlic until combined. Process cornflakes, ¼ teaspoon salt, and ½ teaspoon pepper in food processor until cornflakes are finely ground, about 10 seconds. Transfer cornflake mixture to second shallow dish.

2. Adjust oven rack to middle position and heat oven to 200 degrees. Set wire rack in rimmed baking sheet. With sharp knife, cut 1⁄16-inch-deep slits on both sides of chops, spaced ½ inch apart, in crosshatch pattern. Season chops with salt and pepper.

3. Working with half of chops at a time, place chops in bag of cornstarch, seal bag, and shake bag to coat chops. Using tongs, remove chops from bag, shaking off excess cornstarch, coat in buttermilk mixture, then coat with cornflake mixture, pressing gently to adhere. Place breaded chops on prepared wire rack. Let coated chops sit for 10 minutes.

4. Heat ⅓ cup oil in 12-inch nonstick skillet over medium-high heat until shimmering. Place 4 chops in skillet and cook until golden brown and crispy, 2 to 5 minutes. Carefully flip chops and continue to cook until second side is golden brown and crispy, and center of chop registers 145 degrees, 2 to 5 minutes longer. Transfer chops to paper towel–lined plate and let drain 30 seconds on each side. Transfer to clean wire rack set in rimmed baking sheet and keep warm in oven. Discard oil in skillet and wipe clean with paper towels. Repeat process with remaining ⅓ cup oil and remaining pork chops. Serve with lemon wedges.

TEST KITCHEN TIP **Building a Sturdy Coating**

Making shallow cuts in the chops releases juices and sticky meat proteins that dampen the cornstarch and help the coating adhere.

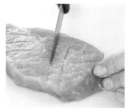

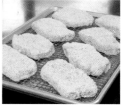

1. With sharp knife, cut 1⁄16-inch-deep slits on both sides of chops, spaced ½ inch apart, in crosshatch pattern.

2. Let breaded chops sit for 10 minutes to enable cornstarch to absorb moisture and form an adhesive paste.

Crispy Chicken Fingers

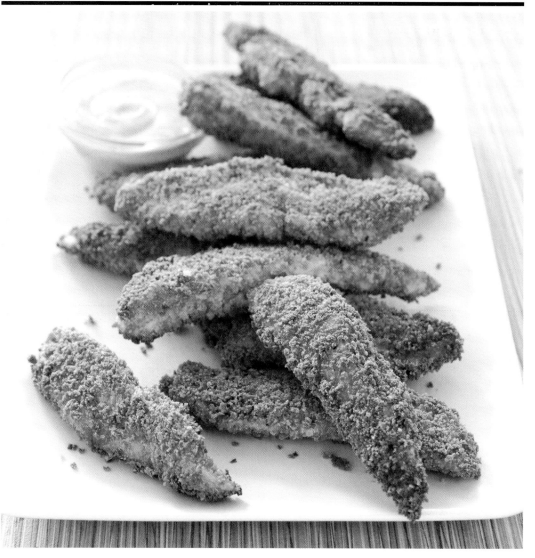

G-F TESTING LAB

BREAD   You can use store-bought bread or our Classic Sandwich Bread (page 170) to make the bread crumbs. Our favorite store-bought brand is Udi's Gluten Free White Sandwich Bread (see page 22 for complete tasting). Weights of gluten-free sandwich bread vary from brand to brand; if you are not using Udi's, we recommend going by weight rather than number of slices. Bread may clump together during toasting; make sure to break it apart into fine crumbs before breading.

✓ WHY THIS RECIPE WORKS

Fast and appealing to both kids and adults, breaded chicken fingers are a weeknight staple in many households. For a gluten-free coating that cooked up crisp, flavorful, and perfectly browned, we took a few tricks from our Eggplant Parmesan recipe (page 136). We started by processing store-bought gluten-free sandwich bread in the food processor (we knew store-bought crumbs would cook up dry and taste stale). And because these crumbs break down into fluffy, sticky clumps, we then toasted them to dry them out and give us fine, dry crumbs that coated the chicken more evenly. Still, there were some bare spots. Adding some cornstarch to the crumbs ensured an evenly browned coating. The same breading method—dipping in cornstarch, then egg, then the bread crumbs—that we'd used for our Eggplant Parmesan worked equally well here (although we skipped adding cheese to the crumbs for a simpler coating). As for the cooking method, pan-fried won out over oven-baked, delivering chicken fingers with a crisper exterior surrounding perfectly moist, flavorful chicken.

Crispy Chicken Fingers
SERVES 4

- **6 slices (about 6 ounces) gluten-free sandwich bread, torn into quarters**
- **½ cup cornstarch**
- **Salt and pepper**
- **2 large eggs**
- **1½ pounds boneless, skinless chicken breasts, trimmed and cut lengthwise on slight diagonal into ¾-inch-wide strips**
- **¾ cup vegetable oil**

1. Adjust oven rack to lower-middle position and heat oven to 425 degrees. Process bread in food processor until evenly ground, about 30 seconds. Spread crumbs in even layer on rimmed baking sheet and bake, stirring occasionally, until golden brown, 7 to 10 minutes. Reduce oven temperature to 200 degrees.

2. Transfer crumbs to shallow dish, breaking up any large clumps into fine crumbs. Stir in 1 tablespoon cornstarch, ½ teaspoon salt, and ¼ teaspoon pepper. Beat eggs in second shallow dish. Place remaining cornstarch in large zipper-lock bag.

3. Set wire rack in rimmed baking sheet. Pat chicken dry with paper towels and season with salt and pepper. Working with half of chicken at a time, place chicken in bag of cornstarch, seal bag, and shake bag to coat chicken. Using tongs, remove chicken pieces from bag, shaking off excess cornstarch, dip in eggs, then coat with bread-crumb mixture, pressing gently to adhere. Place breaded chicken on prepared wire rack.

4. Heat oil in 12-inch nonstick skillet over medium-high heat until just smoking. Add half of chicken and cook until golden brown on all sides, 4 to 6 minutes, flipping halfway through cooking. Drain chicken briefly on paper towels, then transfer to paper towel–lined plate and keep warm in oven. Repeat with remaining breaded chicken. Serve.

TEST KITCHEN TIP **Cutting Chicken Fingers**

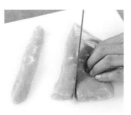

After trimming each chicken breast, slice it lengthwise on slight diagonal into long, ¾-inch-wide strips.

Shepherd's Pie

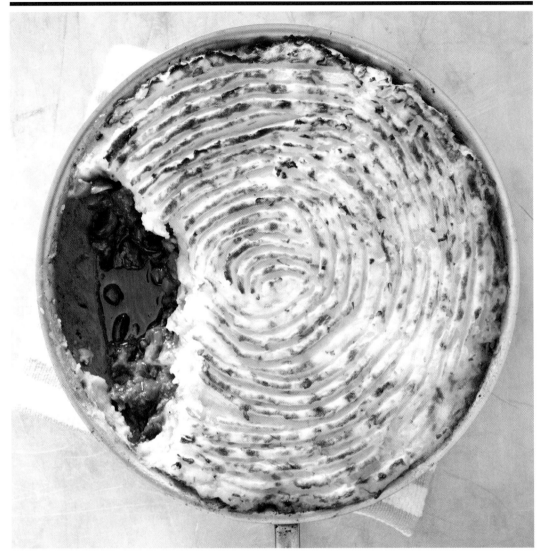

G-F TESTING LAB

CORNSTARCH   Cornstarch takes the place of the flour in the traditional recipe. See page 20 for details on this ingredient.

✔ WHY THIS RECIPE WORKS

We wanted a streamlined, modern take on this dish—with a flavorful gravy that coated the meat without relying on flour. Making the recipe from start to finish in a skillet kept it streamlined, and swapping in ground beef for the usual chunks of meat saved us from a lengthy braising time. To keep the meat tender, we knew from experience it would help to toss it with baking soda and water, then let it rest briefly (a trick we also used with our Penne with Weeknight Meat Sauce, page 116). In lieu of flour for thickening power, we turned to cornstarch. Combining it with a little water to make a slurry kept it from clumping and ensured that it dispersed evenly in the gravy. Don't use ground beef that's fattier than 93 percent or the dish will be greasy. You will need a 10-inch broiler-safe skillet for this recipe.

Shepherd's Pie
SERVES 4 TO 6

- 1½ pounds 93 percent lean ground beef
- 3 tablespoons water
- Salt and pepper
- ½ teaspoon baking soda
- 2½ pounds russet potatoes, peeled and cut into 1-inch chunks
- 4 tablespoons unsalted butter, melted
- ½ cup milk
- 1 large egg yolk
- 8 scallions, green parts only, sliced thin
- 2 teaspoons vegetable oil
- 1 onion, chopped
- 4 ounces white mushrooms, trimmed and chopped
- 1 tablespoon tomato paste
- 2 garlic cloves, minced
- 2 tablespoons Madeira or ruby port
- 1¼ cups beef broth
- 2 teaspoons Worcestershire sauce
- 2 sprigs fresh thyme
- 1 bay leaf
- 2 carrots, peeled and chopped
- 4 teaspoons cornstarch

1. Toss beef with 2 tablespoons water, 1 teaspoon salt, ¼ teaspoon pepper, and baking soda in bowl until thoroughly combined. Set aside for 20 minutes.

2. Meanwhile, place potatoes in medium saucepan; add water to just cover and 1 tablespoon salt. Bring to boil over high heat. Reduce heat to medium-low and simmer until potatoes are soft, 8 to 10 minutes. Drain potatoes and return to saucepan. Return saucepan to low heat and cook, shaking pot occasionally, until moisture has evaporated, about 1 minute. Remove pan from heat and mash potatoes well. Stir in melted butter. Whisk together milk and egg yolk, then stir into potatoes. Stir in scallions and season with salt and pepper. Cover and set aside.

3. Heat oil in broiler-safe 10-inch skillet over medium heat until shimmering. Add onion, mushrooms, ½ teaspoon salt, and ¼ teaspoon pepper and cook, stirring occasionally, until vegetables are just starting to soften, 4 to 6 minutes. Stir in tomato paste and garlic and cook until bottom of skillet is dark brown, about 2 minutes. Add Madeira and cook, scraping up any browned bits, until evaporated, about 1 minute. Add broth, Worcestershire, thyme, bay leaf, and carrots and bring to boil, scraping up any browned bits. Reduce heat to medium-low, add beef in 2-inch chunks, and bring to gentle simmer. Cover and cook until beef is cooked through, 10 to 12 minutes, breaking up meat chunks with 2 forks halfway through cooking. Stir cornstarch and remaining 1 tablespoon water together, then stir mixture into filling and continue to simmer until slightly thickened, about 1 minute. Discard thyme and bay leaf. Season with salt and pepper to taste.

4. Adjust oven rack 5 inches from broiler element and heat broiler. Place mashed potatoes in large zipper-lock bag and snip off a corner to create 1-inch opening. Pipe potatoes in even layer over filling. Smooth potatoes with back of spoon, then use tines of fork to make ridges over surface. Place skillet on rimmed baking sheet and broil until potatoes are golden brown and crusty and filling is bubbly, 10 to 15 minutes. Let cool for 10 minutes before serving.

Chicken Pot Pie

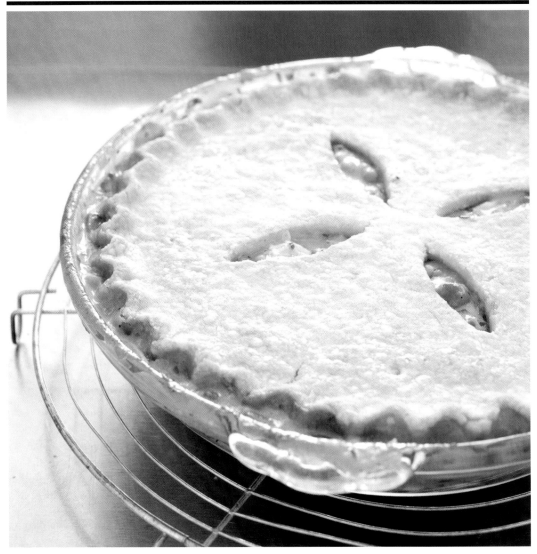

G-F TESTING LAB

FLOUR SUBSTITUTION	King Arthur Gluten-Free Multi-Purpose Flour 1½ ounces = ¼ **cup**	Bob's Red Mill GF All-Purpose Baking Flour 1½ ounces = **5 tablespoons**

King Arthur makes the filling a tad starchier and Bob's Red Mill makes the filling a bit darker in color, but both options work well. King Arthur makes the crust a bit more delicate and crumbly, and it doesn't brown quite as well as our flour blend in this recipe. Bob's Red Mill makes the crust slightly drier and less tender.

✔ WHY THIS RECIPE WORKS

With its flaky pastry topping and flour-thickened gravy, chicken pot pie might be the most quintessential comfort food—so it's all the more disappointing that it's typically off-limits for anyone avoiding gluten. We knew we'd be using our own gluten-free pie dough for the topping, so we moved on to tackle finding a roux replacement that would deliver an equally velvety, rich sauce. We tested every gluten-free thickener we could think of: arrowroot, tapioca starch, potato starch, potato flour, white rice flour, gelatin, and even xanthan gum. The latter two turned the sauce gloppy and unappetizing, while most of the starches produced fillings that were slimy and oddly translucent. Finally, we turned to our own flour blend. While perhaps not as straightforward as using a single starch or flour, it amounted to minimal extra work since we needed it for the pastry topping anyway. We found that just 1½ ounces provided sufficient thickening power, and because it contains a combination of flours and starches, it didn't turn the gravy slimy, like starches alone, or gritty, like flour alone. The rest of the filling came together very easily. We followed the classic method for building the sauce, lightly browning aromatic vegetables in butter before adding tomato paste for color and flavor. We then stirred in the flour blend, making sure to cook it briefly before whisking in the chicken broth. We poached whole chicken breasts (or thighs, if you like more flavorful dark meat) in the sauce. When the chicken was cooked through, it was cooled, shredded, and stirred back into the sauce along with peas and cream. Once our classic filling was prepared, we unrolled the dough over the hot filling and popped it in the oven. But instead of baking up nice and flaky, the dough turned out gummy because of all the liquid. So instead we first parbaked the rolled-out dough until it was golden, then slid it over the filling. All the assembled pie needed was about 10 minutes in the oven to finish cooking through and unify the flaky crust and hearty, comforting filling. If you don't have a rimless baking sheet to use for baking the crust, use an inverted rimmed baking sheet.

Chicken Pot Pie
SERVES 4 TO 6

- 1 recipe Single-Crust Pie Dough (page 247)
- 4 tablespoons unsalted butter
- 1 onion, chopped fine
- 2 carrots, peeled and sliced ¼ inch thick
- 1 celery rib, sliced ¼ inch thick
  Salt and pepper
- 1 teaspoon tomato paste
- 1 teaspoon minced fresh thyme
- 1½ ounces (⅓ cup) ATK Gluten-Free Flour Blend (page 13)
- 2 cups chicken broth
- 1½ pounds boneless, skinless chicken breasts and/or thighs, trimmed
- ½ cup frozen green peas
- ¼ cup heavy cream
- 3 tablespoons minced fresh parsley
- 1 tablespoon dry sherry

1. Roll pie dough between 2 sheets of parchment paper into 10-inch circle. Remove top parchment sheet. Fold in outer ½-inch rim of dough (creating 9½-inch circle). Using index finger of one hand and thumb and index finger of other hand, crimp folded edge of dough to make attractive fluted rim. Using paring knife, cut 4 oval-shaped vents, each about 2 inches long and ½ inch wide, in center of dough. Transfer dough, still on parchment, to baking sheet and chill in freezer until firm, about 15 minutes.

2. Adjust oven racks to upper-middle and lower-middle positions and heat oven to 400 degrees. Bake shaped dough on upper-middle rack until golden brown and crisp, 18 to 20 minutes. Transfer crust, still on sheet, to wire rack and let cool slightly. (Do not turn off oven.)

3. Meanwhile, melt butter in Dutch oven over medium-high heat. Add onion, carrots, celery, ¼ teaspoon salt, and ¼ teaspoon pepper and cook until tender and lightly browned, about 8 minutes. Stir in tomato paste and thyme and cook until browned, about 2 minutes. Stir in flour blend and cook until golden, about 1 minute.

4. Slowly whisk in chicken broth until no lumps remain. Add chicken, cover, and bring to simmer. Reduce heat to medium-low and continue to simmer, covered, stirring occasionally, until chicken registers 160 degrees for breasts and 175 degrees for thighs, and sauce has thickened, 15 to 18 minutes. Remove pot from heat. Transfer chicken to large bowl and let cool slightly. Using two forks, shred into bite-size pieces.

5. Stir peas, heavy cream, parsley, and sherry into thickened sauce, then stir in shredded chicken with any accumulated juices. Season with salt and pepper to taste. Pour mixture into 9½-inch deep-dish pie plate and place parbaked pie crust on top of filling. Bake on lower-middle rack until crust is deep golden brown and filling is bubbly, about 10 minutes. Let pot pie cool for 5 to 10 minutes before serving.

TEST KITCHEN TIP **Preparing Pot Pie Crust**

Because the pastry crust will turn gummy if baked start to finish over the hot pie filling, we roll it out to fit our pie and first parbake it alone, then slide it on top of the filling. It needs to bake only about 10 minutes longer before it's done.

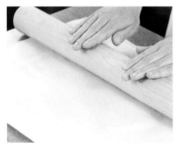

1. Roll dough between 2 sheets of parchment into 10-inch circle. Remove top parchment.

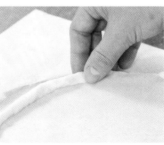

2. Fold in outer ½-inch rim of dough, creating 9½-inch circle.

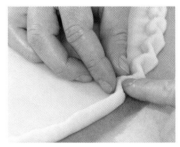

3. Using index finger of one hand and thumb and index finger of other hand, crimp folded edge of dough to make fluted rim.

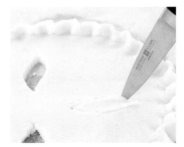

4. Cut 4 oval-shaped vents, each about 2 inches long and ½ inch wide, in dough. Transfer dough, still on parchment, to baking sheet and freeze until firm.

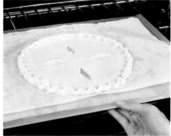

5. Bake crust, still on baking sheet, on upper-middle rack until golden brown, 18 to 20 minutes.

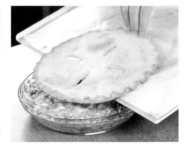

6. Carefully slide parbaked pie crust on top of warm filling.

Cheese Quiche

✔ WHY THIS RECIPE WORKS

Since most quiche fillings are naturally gluten-free, the challenge of a good gluten-free quiche recipe lies squarely in the crust. We had just developed our recipe for a flaky gluten-free pie dough, so we thought baking a custardy cheese quiche filling in a parbaked crust would be a quick and easy win. To our surprise, the golden-brown parbaked crust turned unappealingly soggy after we'd filled it and returned it to the oven to cook the custard through. To preserve its light, flaky texture, we realized we needed to create a moisture barrier between the crust and the filling. Sprinkling cheese over the bottom of the crust during the last few minutes of parbaking allowed the cheese to melt into an even layer that provided the perfect defense it needed. Dry Parmesan worked best here since it didn't turn rubbery. For the filling, we opted to use cheddar since it melted seamlessly into the custard. To ensure every bit of cheese made it into the final quiche, we added the cheddar to the pie shell before the custard since sometimes not all of the custard mixture fit into the pie shell. Even after the shell had been filled and had baked for 45 minutes, this crust was still perfectly crisp. And no one would have guessed it was gluten-free. Be sure to add the custard to the pie shell while the shell is still warm so that the quiche will bake evenly; if the crust has cooled, simply rewarm it in the oven for about 5 minutes before adding the custard. The center of the quiche will be soft and will jiggle slightly when it comes out of the oven, but the filling will continue to set (and sink somewhat) as it cools. See page 248 for details on fitting pie dough into a pie plate. This basic recipe is easy to adapt and we offer four simple variations on page 161.

Cheese Quiche
SERVES 6 TO 8

- 1 recipe Single-Crust Pie Dough (page 247)
- 1 ounce Parmesan cheese, grated (½ cup)
- 5 large eggs
- 2 cups half-and-half
- 1 tablespoon minced fresh chives
- ¼ teaspoon salt
- ¼ teaspoon pepper
- 4 ounces cheddar cheese, shredded (1 cup)

1. Adjust oven rack to lower-middle position and heat oven to 375 degrees. Roll dough into 12-inch circle between 2 large sheets of plastic wrap. Remove top plastic, gently invert dough over 9-inch pie plate, and ease dough into plate. Remove remaining plastic, and trim dough ½ inch beyond lip of pie plate. Tuck overhanging dough under itself to be flush with edge of pie plate. Crimp dough evenly around edge using your fingers. Cover dough loosely in plastic and freeze until chilled and firm, about 15 minutes.

2. Remove plastic and bake until crust is light golden brown in center, about 20 minutes. Remove crust from oven, sprinkle bottom of crust evenly with Parmesan, and continue to bake until cheese has melted, about 5 minutes. Transfer pie plate to wire rack. Reduce oven temperature to 350 degrees. (Crust must still be warm when filling is added.)

3. While crust bakes, whisk eggs, half-and-half, chives, salt, and pepper together in large liquid measuring cup. Place warm pie shell on rimmed baking sheet, sprinkle cheddar into bottom of pie shell, and place in oven. Carefully pour egg mixture into shell until it reaches about ¼ inch from top edge of crust (you may have extra egg mixture).

4. Bake quiche until top is lightly browned, center is set but soft, and knife inserted about 1 inch from edge comes out clean, 35 to 45 minutes. Let quiche cool for at least 1 hour or up to 3 hours before serving.

VARIATIONS

Quiche Lorraine

Substitute 1 cup shredded Gruyère for cheddar. Fry 4 slices finely chopped bacon in 10-inch skillet over medium heat until crisp, about 8 minutes. Transfer bacon to paper towel–lined plate and pour off all but

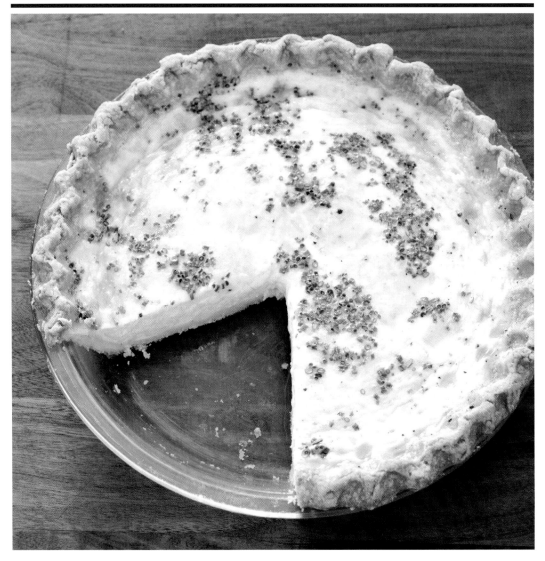

G-F TESTING LAB

FLOUR SUBSTITUTION	King Arthur makes the crust a bit more delicate and crumbly, and it doesn't brown quite as well as our flour blend in this recipe. Bob's Red Mill makes the crust slightly drier and less tender.

2 teaspoons bacon fat left in skillet. Add 1 small finely chopped onion to skillet and cook over medium heat until lightly browned, about 5 minutes. Cool slightly, and stir into egg mixture along with bacon.

Leek and Goat Cheese Quiche

Substitute 1 cup crumbled goat cheese for cheddar. Melt 2 tablespoons unsalted butter in 10-inch skillet over medium-high heat. Add 2 finely chopped leeks, white and light green parts only, and cook until softened, about 6 minutes. Cool slightly, and stir into egg mixture.

Asparagus and Gruyère Quiche

Substitute 1 cup shredded Gruyère for cheddar and stir 1 bunch asparagus, trimmed and sliced on bias into ¼-inch-thick pieces, into egg mixture.

Spinach and Feta Quiche

Omit chives and substitute 1 cup crumbled feta for cheddar. Stir 1 (10-ounce) package frozen chopped spinach, thawed and squeezed dry, into egg mixture.

TEST KITCHEN TIP **Making Perfect Quiche**

For a crisp crust and perfectly cooked filling, we not only parbake our gluten-free crust, but also sprinkle Parmesan partway through the parbaking time to create a moisture barrier against the filling. Pouring the custard into the pie shell after it's on the oven rack is easier than trying to transfer the shell with its very liquid-y filling to the oven. Cheddar makes a good choice for the cheese in the filling because it melts well into the custard. To ensure maximum cheesy flavor, we add the cheddar before the custard because there likely wouldn't be enough room for all of it if the custard filling were poured in first. We pull the quiche from the oven before it is completely set since it will finish cooking as it cools.

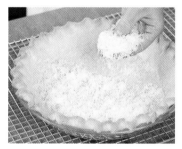 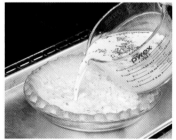 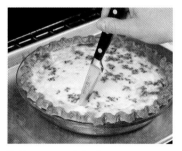

1. Sprinkle Parmesan over bottom of parbaked crust and bake until just melted and set, about 5 minutes. Reduce oven temperature as directed.

2. Place warm pie shell on rimmed baking sheet, sprinkle cheddar into pie shell, and place in oven. Carefully pour egg mixture into shell until it reaches about ¼ inch from top edge of crust (you may have extra egg mixture).

3. Remove quiche from oven when top is browned and knife inserted about 1 inch from edge comes out clean. Center of quiche should jiggle slightly (it will continue to cook as it cools).

Tamale Pie

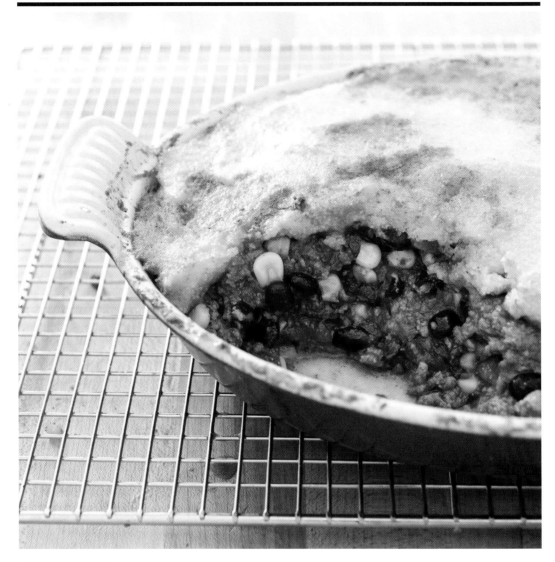

CORNMEAL Coarse-ground degerminated cornmeal such as yellow grits (with grains the size of couscous) works best in this recipe. Avoid instant and quick-cooking products, as well as whole-grain, stone-ground, and regular cornmeal. Not all brands of cornmeal are processed in a gluten-free facility; make sure to read the label. See page 149 for more details on buying cornmeal.

✓ WHY THIS RECIPE WORKS

With its spicy mixture of meat and vegetables—and cornbread topping that soaks up all the flavors—a good tamale pie is hard to beat. But most tamale pies rely on a cornbread layer that includes flour. We tried making a tamale pie using our own recipe for gluten-free cornbread (see page 190), spreading the batter over the prepared filling and baking the pie like a traditional recipe, but without all-purpose flour in the mix to provide structure, it disintegrated into the filling. Clearly our cornbread, while fine baked in a skillet and great served alongside a bowl of chili, didn't have the necessary structure to bake through on top of a liquid-y tamale pie filling. Looking for an alternative with a similarly rustic corn flavor, we landed on polenta. We prepared the filling in a skillet and the polenta in a separate pot, then spread the polenta over the filling and baked it all together for about 30 minutes. For the tamale pie filling itself, we turned to a flavorful, simple combination of ground beef and black beans. A cup of Monterey Jack melted into the mixture and helped thicken it to just the right texture. Ground pork or turkey can be substituted for the beef.

Tamale Pie
SERVES 6

- 3 tablespoons vegetable oil
- 1 pound 90 percent lean ground beef
- 1 onion, chopped fine
- 1 jalapeño chile, stemmed, seeded, and minced
  Salt and pepper
- 1½ tablespoons chili powder
- 2 garlic cloves, minced
- 1½ teaspoons minced fresh oregano or ¾ teaspoon dried

- 1 (15-ounce) can black beans, rinsed
- 1 (14.5-ounce) can diced tomatoes
- 1 cup fresh or frozen corn (thawed if frozen)
- 4 ounces Monterey Jack cheese, shredded (1 cup)
- 2½ cups water
- ¾ cup coarse-ground cornmeal

1. Adjust oven rack to lower-middle position and heat oven to 375 degrees. Heat 1 tablespoon oil in 12-inch skillet over medium-high heat until just smoking. Add ground beef and cook, breaking up large clumps, until just beginning to brown, about 4 minutes.

2. Stir in onion, jalapeño, and ¼ teaspoon salt and cook until softened, about 5 minutes. Stir in chili powder, garlic, and oregano and cook until fragrant, about 30 seconds. Stir in beans, tomatoes and their juice, and corn and simmer until almost all liquid has evaporated, about 3 minutes. Off heat, stir cheese into beef mixture and season with salt and pepper to taste. Transfer mixture to 9½-inch deep-dish pie plate or 3-quart baking dish.

3. Bring water to boil in large saucepan over high heat. Add ¼ teaspoon salt, then slowly pour in cornmeal while whisking vigorously to prevent clumping. Reduce heat to medium and cook, whisking constantly, until cornmeal thickens, about 3 minutes. Stir in remaining 2 tablespoons oil.

4. Spread cornmeal mixture over top of beef mixture and seal against edge of dish. Cover with aluminum foil that has been sprayed with vegetable oil spray, and bake until crust is set and pie is heated through, about 30 minutes. Let cool for 5 to 10 minutes before serving.

Golden Cornbread and Sausage Stuffing

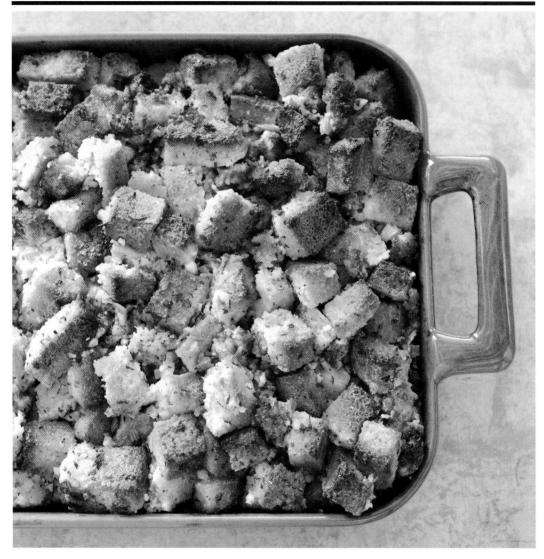

G-F TESTING LAB

CORNMEAL   The test kitchen's favorite cornmeal for baking is finely ground Whole-Grain Arrowhead Mills Cornmeal. This brand has been processed in a gluten-free facility, but not all brands are. Make sure to read the label. See page 149 for more details on buying cornmeal.

✅ WHY THIS RECIPE WORKS

We set out to make a gluten-free cornbread stuffing that would have everyone asking for more. Using our own gluten-free cornbread recipe seemed like a reasonable starting point, but it turned to mush in a stuffing recipe. The first key was adding tapioca flour, which helps the cornbread absorb moisture without disintegrating. The second key was adding cornstarch to the broth mixture, as the cornbread soaked up the liquid like a sponge. The cornbread absorbed just enough of the cornstarch-thickened, gravylike liquid to turn into a cohesive, scoopable casserole without getting mushy. Many cornbread stuffing recipes require first baking cornbread, then drying it out so that it will hold up. To keep our recipe simple, we baked the cornbread in a thin layer in a large baking sheet, purposely overbaking it so the cornbread is dried and ready to absorb the broth.

Golden Cornbread and Sausage Stuffing
SERVES 8 TO 10

CORNBREAD
- 10 **ounces (2 cups) cornmeal**
- 4 **ounces (1 cup) tapioca flour**
- 1 **tablespoon baking powder (see page 20)**
- ¾ **teaspoon baking soda**
- ¼ **teaspoon salt**
- 4 **large eggs**
- 1 **cup whole milk**
- 3 **tablespoons unsalted butter, melted**

STUFFING
- 6 **tablespoons unsalted butter**
- 1 **pound bulk pork sausage**
- 2 **onions, chopped fine**
- 2 **celery ribs, chopped fine**
- 2 **tablespoons minced fresh thyme**
- 2 **tablespoons minced fresh sage**
- 2 **garlic cloves, minced**
- 3 **cups chicken broth**
- 1 **cup half-and-half**
- 1 **teaspoon pepper**
- 2 **tablespoons cornstarch**

1. FOR THE CORNBREAD: Adjust oven rack to middle position and heat oven to 350 degrees. Line rimmed baking sheet with parchment paper and spray with vegetable oil spray. Whisk cornmeal, tapioca flour, baking powder, baking soda, and salt together in large bowl. In separate bowl, whisk together eggs and milk, then whisk into flour mixture until combined. Stir in melted butter.

2. Spread batter evenly into prepared pan. Bake until top is deep golden brown and edges have pulled away from sides of pan, about 20 minutes, rotating sheet halfway through baking. Let cool 10 minutes, then flip out onto wire rack and let cool to room temperature. Cut cornbread into ½-inch pieces. Increase oven temperature to 400 degrees.

3. FOR THE STUFFING: Spray 13 by 9-inch baking dish with vegetable oil spray. Melt butter in large saucepan over medium-high heat. Add sausage and cook, breaking meat into small pieces, until sausage loses its raw color, about 5 minutes. Transfer sausage to very large bowl, leaving fat in pan.

4. Add onions and celery to fat in saucepan and cook over medium-high heat until softened, about 8 minutes. Stir in thyme, sage, and garlic and cook until fragrant, about 30 seconds. Whisk in 2½ cups broth, half-and-half, and pepper, and bring to simmer. Whisk together remaining ½ cup broth and cornstarch in bowl, and slowly whisk into simmering mixture. Simmer until slightly thickened, about 10 minutes.

5. Add cornbread to bowl with sausage (but don't mix it in). Pour broth mixture over cornbread and stir gently to combine, being careful not to break cornbread into smaller pieces. Cover with plastic wrap and let sit, stirring occasionally, until all liquid is absorbed, about 15 minutes. Transfer mixture to prepared baking dish. Bake until top is golden brown, about 40 minutes. Let stuffing cool 10 minutes before serving. (Stuffing can be cooled and refrigerated for up to 1 day. Reheat, covered with foil, in 400-degree oven.)

Wild Rice Dressing

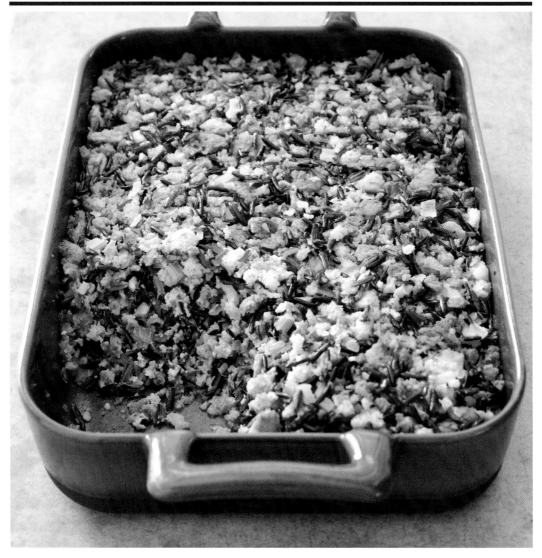

G-F TESTING LAB

BREAD   You can use store-bought bread or our Classic Sandwich Bread (page 170) to make the bread crumbs. Our favorite store-bought brand is Udi's Gluten Free White Sandwich Bread (see page 22 for complete tasting). Weights of gluten-free sandwich bread vary from brand to brand; if you are not using Udi's, we recommend going by weight rather than number of slices. Bread may clump together during toasting; make sure to break it apart into fine crumbs.

✓ WHY THIS RECIPE WORKS

After developing a classic Southern-style cornbread stuffing, we set out to make a wild rice stuffing that could straddle the line between rustic and elegant on the Thanksgiving table. We knew the rice would be combined with plenty of flavorful ingredients, so even though it meant a slightly diluted flavor, we settled on cooking it like pasta—in plenty of liquid—since that would guarantee even cooking and the fewest blown-out grains. A combination of chicken broth and water gave the rice the right amount of meaty flavor. To bind the grains, we wanted to use a custard for richness plus just enough gluten-free sandwich bread to hold it all together. For the custard, we tried a combination of cream and eggs, but this was too rich by itself so we added some liquid reserved from cooking the rice to lighten it up and reinforce the rice's flavor. We made gluten-free bread crumbs in the food processor from store-bought bread, then toasted the crumbs to ensure they dried out and didn't clump when we combined them with the rice. Drizzling the casserole with butter and covering it with foil before baking ensured the rice grains on top didn't dry out and infused the bread with a complementary nutty richness. Depending on the brand, wild rice absorbs varying quantities of liquid. If you have less than 1½ cups of leftover cooking liquid, make up the difference with additional chicken broth. To make this recipe vegetarian, you can substitute vegetable broth for the chicken broth.

Wild Rice Dressing
SERVES 10 TO 12

- 2 cups chicken broth
- 2 cups water
- 1 bay leaf
- 2 cups wild rice
- 10 slices (about 10 ounces) gluten-free sandwich bread, torn into pieces
- 8 tablespoons unsalted butter
- 2 onions, chopped fine
- 3 celery ribs, chopped fine
- 4 garlic cloves, minced
- 1 tablespoon minced fresh sage or 1½ teaspoons dried
- 1 tablespoon minced fresh thyme or 1½ teaspoons dried
- 1½ cups heavy cream
- 2 large eggs
- ¾ teaspoon salt
- ½ teaspoon pepper

1. Bring broth, water, and bay leaf to boil in medium saucepan over medium-high heat. Stir in rice, reduce heat to low, cover, and simmer until rice is tender, 35 to 45 minutes. Strain contents of pan through fine-mesh strainer into large liquid measuring cup. Transfer rice to bowl; discard bay leaf. Reserve 1½ cups cooking liquid.

2. Adjust oven rack to lower-middle position and heat oven to 325 degrees. Pulse 5 slices bread in food processor until only pea-size pieces remain and transfer to rimmed baking sheet. Repeat with remaining 5 slices bread and transfer to sheet. Bake bread crumbs until deep golden brown, about 15 to 17 minutes, stirring occasionally and rotating sheet halfway through baking. Let bread crumbs cool completely, about 10 minutes. (Do not turn off oven.)

3. Melt 4 tablespoons butter in 12-inch skillet over medium heat. Add onions and celery and cook until softened and golden, 8 to 10 minutes. Add garlic, sage, and thyme and cook until fragrant, about 30 seconds. Stir in reserved cooking liquid, remove from heat, and cool 5 minutes.

4. Whisk cream, eggs, salt, and pepper together in large bowl. Slowly whisk in onion mixture. Stir in rice and toasted bread crumbs until well combined, then transfer to 13 by 9-inch baking dish. Melt remaining 4 tablespoons butter in now-empty skillet and drizzle evenly over dressing. Cover dish with aluminum foil and bake until set, 45 to 55 minutes. Remove foil and let cool 15 minutes. Serve. (The dressing can be cooled and refrigerated for up to 1 day. Reheat, covered with foil, in 325-degree oven.)

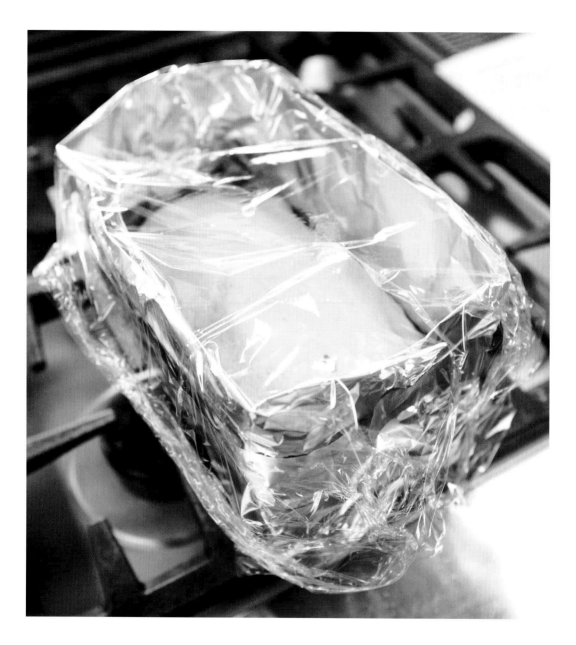

YEAST BREADS, SAVORY LOAVES, AND PIZZA

Classic Sandwich Bread

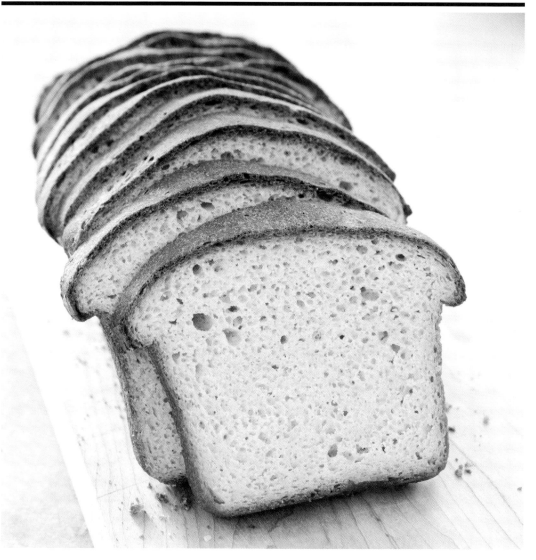

G-F TESTING LAB

FLOUR SUBSTITUTION	King Arthur Gluten-Free Multi-Purpose Flour 14 ounces = **2⅓ cups plus ¼ cup**	Bob's Red Mill GF All-Purpose Baking Flour 14 ounces = **2½ cups plus ⅓ cup**
	Note that bread made with King Arthur will have a slightly tighter crumb, and bread made with Bob's Red Mill will be denser and will have a distinct bean flavor.	
OAT FLOUR	If you do not have oat flour, you can process 4 ounces old-fashioned rolled oats in a food processor or spice grinder until finely ground, about 1 minute. Do not use quick oats; they have a dusty texture that doesn't work in this recipe.	
PSYLLIUM HUSK	Do not omit the powdered psyllium husk; it is crucial to the structure of the bread. For more information, see page 16.	

✓ WHY THIS RECIPE WORKS

Most gluten-free sandwich bread recipes turn out squat bricks with a cardboard texture. We wanted a reliable recipe that produced a light-textured sandwich loaf—something large enough to actually slice for sandwiches. We began with our classic sandwich bread mixing method in a stand mixer fitted with a dough hook but found that the bread significantly improved when we replaced the dough hook with the paddle. The starches in the gluten-free flour blend need to be hydrated, and mixing with a paddle for 6 minutes was the best way to get the job done. (At first the dough will seem very soupy, but as the starches hydrate it will become thicker and start to look like cookie dough.) To build a tall loaf with a nice crumb, we needed more protein and turned to oat flour for help. While many other recipes in this book rely on xanthan gum to provide structure, we preferred psyllium husk in this recipe (as well as in all other bread recipes) because it resulted in a more delicate crumb. Psyllium helped build a stronger protein network that trapped gas and steam—which was key to producing a tall loaf. We also liked its earthy flavor, which seemed out of place in cookies but was perfect in bread. Adding baking powder as well as the usual yeast was also key to getting a good rise. Milk is the classic choice for sandwich bread, but we achieved a better rise with water—and a lot of it. An egg and some milk powder added more protein and structure, and the milk powder was also key for flavor and browning. The high water content was essential to produce steam and enable the loaf to rise, but we found it necessary to prolong the baking time to drive off moisture once the loaf was set. (Shorter baking times yielded a gummy crumb.) To help the dough rise, we fashioned a collar out of foil and attached it to the top of the loaf pan, much as you might do when making a soufflé. Do not substitute soy milk powder for the milk powder in this recipe, as it will negatively impact the flavor and structure of the bread. Note that this recipe calls for an 8½ by 4½-inch loaf pan; if using a 9 by 5-inch loaf pan, the dough will not rise as high and the bread will not be quite as tall.

Classic Sandwich Bread
MAKES 1 LOAF

2	cups warm water (110 degrees)
2	large eggs
2	tablespoons unsalted butter, melted and cooled
14	ounces (3 cups plus 2 tablespoons) ATK Gluten-Free Flour Blend (page 13)
4	ounces (1⅓ cups) gluten-free oat flour
1½	ounces (½ cup) nonfat dry milk powder
3	tablespoons powdered psyllium husk
2	tablespoons sugar
2¼	teaspoons instant or rapid rise yeast
2	teaspoons baking powder (see page 20)
1½	teaspoons salt

1. Spray 8½ by 4½-inch loaf pan with vegetable oil spray. Whisk water, eggs, and melted butter together in bowl. Using stand mixer fitted with paddle, mix flour blend, oat flour, milk powder, psyllium, sugar, yeast, baking powder, and salt together on low speed until combined. Slowly add water mixture and let dough come together, about 1 minute, scraping down bowl as needed. Increase speed to medium and beat until sticky and uniform, about 6 minutes. (Dough will resemble cookie dough.)

2. Using rubber spatula, scrape dough into prepared loaf pan and press it gently into corners with wet hands; smooth top of dough and spray with water. Tightly wrap double layer of aluminum foil around pan so that top edge of foil rests at least 1 inch above rim of pan; secure foil collar with staples. Cover loosely with plastic wrap and let rise at room temperature until dough has risen by 50 percent (½ inch above rim of pan), about 1 hour.

3. Adjust oven rack to middle position and heat oven to 350 degrees. Remove plastic and spray loaf with water. Bake until top is golden, crust is firm, and loaf sounds hollow when tapped, about 1½ hours, rotating pan halfway through baking.

4. Transfer pan to wire rack and let bread cool for 10 minutes. Remove loaf from pan and let cool completely on rack, about 2 hours. Serve. (Once cooled, bread can be wrapped in double layer of plastic wrap and stored at room temperature for up to 3 days. See freezing instructions below.)

VARIATION

Oatmeal-Honey Sandwich Bread

We prefer our flour blend, but you can substitute 12 ounces of another blend. We strongly recommend weighing the flour; if you opt to measure by volume, you will need 1⅔ cups plus ½ cup King Arthur Gluten-Free Multi-Purpose Flour or 2¼ cups plus 2 tablespoons Bob's Red Mill GF All-Purpose Baking Flour. Note that bread made with King Arthur will be slightly spongy, and bread made with Bob's Red Mill will be denser and slightly wet and will have a distinct bean flavor.

Reduce water to 1¾ cups. Reduce ATK Gluten-Free Flour Blend to 12 ounces (2⅔ cups) and increase oat flour to 6 ounces (2 cups). Substitute 3 tablespoons honey for sugar. Sprinkle top of loaf with 2 tablespoons old-fashioned rolled oats after spraying with water in step 3. Increase baking time to 2 hours.

TEST KITCHEN TIP **Working with Gluten-Free Sandwich Bread Dough**

Most experienced bakers know that bread dough is properly kneaded when it transitions from sticky to smooth. This change doesn't occur when making gluten-free bread dough. The mixing process is important for hydrating the flour and combining the ingredients, but when the dough is properly mixed it will still be quite sticky and it will look like thick cookie dough. As a result, the dough goes right from the mixing bowl to the loaf pan in this recipe. Don't attempt hand kneading on the counter.

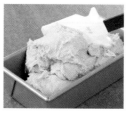

Using rubber spatula, scrape dough into greased 8½ by 4½-inch loaf pan. Using wet hands, press dough gently into corners of pan; smooth top of dough and spray with water.

TEST KITCHEN TIP

Cooling and Storing Gluten-Free Bread

Like its traditional counterparts, gluten-free bread needs to cool completely before being sliced, or the interior of the loaf will be gummy. Gluten-free breads have a shorter shelf life than bread made with wheat flour. As baked bread cools, its starches begin to crystallize, trapping water inside the hardened crystal structures. This process of "retrogradation" (more commonly known as staling) explains why bread becomes firm and appears to dry out as it sits on the counter. Gluten-free flour blends have a higher starch content than wheat flour has, so this effect is amplified in gluten-free breads.

We have found that most gluten-free breads will keep for a few days if wrapped tightly in a double layer of plastic wrap. After the first day, the bread is best toasted. As with traditional breads, refrigerating any gluten-free bread will speed up the staling process, so keep them on the counter.

TEST KITCHEN TIP

Freezing Gluten-Free Bread

We have found that freezing fully cooled loaves is a good option for most gluten-free breads. For sandwich breads, we like to slice the bread before freezing so that we can pull individual slices from the freezer as needed. This applies to Classic Sandwich Bread, Oatmeal-Honey Sandwich Bread, Multigrain Sandwich Bread, and Cinnamon-Raisin Bread. For Hearty Country Flax Bread and Olive-Rosemary Bread, freeze leftover bread in a single piece, defrost it at room temperature, and then reheat the bread in a 400-degree oven for about 10 minutes to recrisp the crust. (You can also slice these two breads before freezing and then take out pieces one at a time for toasting.) Don't keep any gluten-free bread in the freezer for longer than one month.

Classic Sandwich Bread

A good gluten-free sandwich bread is hard to come by. Among supermarket options, our tasters felt that most were inedible. (See page 22 for more detail.) Whether store-bought or homemade, most gluten-free loaves are short and dense, but with some clever engineering we were able to create a tall loaf that could actually be used for sandwiches.

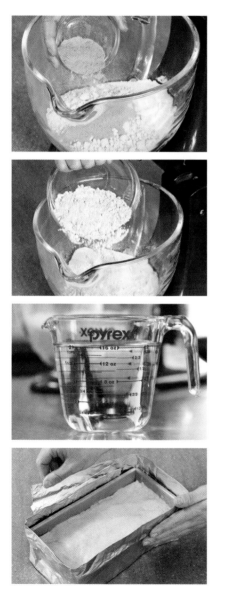

1. ADD PSYLLIUM: The gluten proteins in wheat flour build structure in traditional sandwich breads. After testing various options, we concluded that powdered psyllium husk was the best substitute. It acts like a binding agent and strengthens the proteins in gluten-free flours so they can hold gas and steam during baking without weighing the bread down or producing a gummy texture. (See page 21 for more detail about psyllium.)

2. ADD MILK POWDER AND OAT FLOUR: Most sandwich breads are made with milk, but we found that most gluten-free loaves, including this one, rose better with water. To make up for the lost flavor, we turned to milk powder. It added a rich dairy flavor and ensured a brown crust. Bread flour is a common choice for sandwich bread because its high protein content contributes to a better rise and lighter crumb. To increase the protein content in our recipe we tested a variety of whole-grain gluten-free flours before landing on oat flour, which got the job done without imparting an out-of-place flavor.

3. ADD EXTRA WATER AND BAKE IT LONGER: While the hydration level of a typical sandwich bread is around 68 percent (meaning that there are 68 grams of water for every 100 grams of flour), our gluten-free loaves turned out small and dense when we used this hydration level. Adding more water (enough to boost the hydration level to 89 percent) produced more steam and helped create a loaf with good rise. Because the dough is so wet, we found it necessary to extend the baking time and drive off some of the excess moisture once the loaf had risen and set and the steam had done its job.

4. USE A FOIL COLLAR: Because there is less protein in gluten-free bread dough than in traditional bread dough, gluten-free bread has a hard time rising straight up in the oven. In many tests, loaves rose well but then spilled over the sides of the pan, causing a real mess. Many recipes solve this problem by making smaller loaves. Instead, we engineered a taller pan by attaching a foil collar, just as you might do when making a soufflé in a ceramic soufflé dish. The collar, which should extend at least 1 inch above the rim of the pan, ensures that the loaf will rise up rather than out.

Multigrain Sandwich Bread

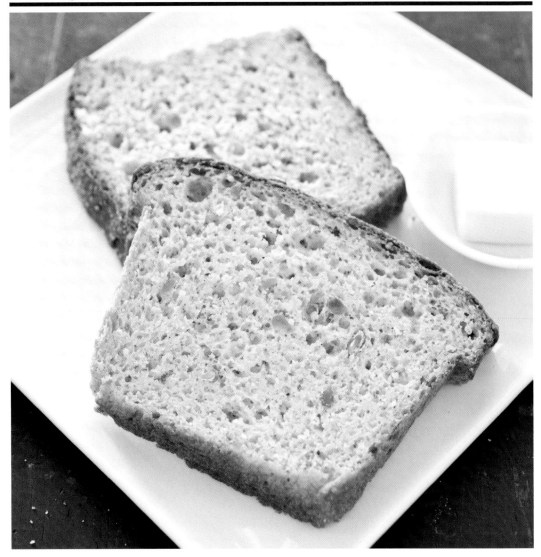

G-F TESTING LAB

FLOUR SUBSTITUTION	King Arthur Gluten-Free Multi-Purpose Flour 11½ ounces = **1¾ cups plus ⅓ cup**	Bob's Red Mill GF All-Purpose Baking Flour 11½ ounces = **2⅓ cups**
	Note that bread made with King Arthur will have a slightly denser crumb, and bread made with Bob's Red Mill will be a bit drier and will have a distinct bean flavor.	
HOT CEREAL MIX	Bob's Red Mill Gluten-Free Mighty Tasty Hot Cereal contains four grains: brown rice, corn, sweet white sorghum, and buckwheat. Note that other brands of hot cereal mixes may not work the same in this recipe because they all absorb water differently.	
PSYLLIUM HUSK	Do not omit the powdered psyllium husk; it is crucial to the structure of the bread. For more information, see page 16.	

✔ WHY THIS RECIPE WORKS

We were looking for bread tender enough for sandwiches, without sacrificing a hearty multigrain flavor. We started with our sandwich bread recipe, which calls for 14 ounces of flour blend and 4 ounces of oat flour. The obvious first step was to replace the oat flour with several grains. We tested a variety of whole-grain flours, alone and in combinations. The more flours we added, the more we liked this bread, but shopping for small amounts of multiple flours was a hassle. To simplify this recipe, we turned to hot cereal mixes, which contain multiple whole grains in one package. The shopping was now easy, but the whole grains were making the loaf quite dense. Extra yeast and baking powder solved this problem. We also had to change the amount of water, as the cereal mix did not absorb the water as easily as the oat flour did in our classic recipe. Now the only thing missing from our bread was the welcome crunch of seeds. Sunflower seeds were able to distinguish themselves in the loaf and added a nutty richness. Two final tweaks gave this bread even more character: using honey instead of granulated sugar, and swapping out the butter for vegetable oil to keep the loaf from overbrowning. (We also reduced the oven temperature from 350 degrees to 325 degrees for the same reason.) Do not substitute soy milk powder for the milk powder in this recipe, as it will negatively impact the flavor and structure of the bread. If you don't eat dairy, you're better off omitting the milk powder, although the structure of the bread will suffer a bit. Note that this recipe calls for an 8½ by 4½-inch loaf pan; if using a 9 by 5-inch loaf pan, the dough will not rise as high and the bread will not be quite as tall.

Multigrain Sandwich Bread
MAKES 1 LOAF

- 1½ cups warm water (110 degrees)
- 2 large eggs
- 2 tablespoons vegetable oil
- 2 tablespoons honey

- 11½ ounces (2⅓ cups plus ¼ cup) ATK Gluten-Free Flour Blend (page 13)
- 4 ounces (¾ cup) Bob's Red Mill Gluten-Free Mighty Tasty Hot Cereal
- 1½ ounces (½ cup) nonfat dry milk powder
- 3 tablespoons powdered psyllium husk
- 1 tablespoon instant or rapid-rise yeast
- 1 tablespoon baking powder (see page 20)
- 1½ teaspoons salt
- 2 tablespoons unsalted sunflower seeds

1. Spray 8½ by 4½-inch loaf pan with vegetable oil spray. Whisk water, eggs, oil, and honey together in bowl. Using stand mixer fitted with paddle, mix flour blend, hot cereal mix, milk powder, psyllium, yeast, baking powder, and salt together on low speed until combined. Slowly add water mixture and let dough come together, about 1 minute, scraping down bowl as needed. Increase speed to medium and beat until sticky and uniform, about 6 minutes. Reduce speed to low, add sunflower seeds, and mix until incorporated. (Dough will resemble cookie dough.)

2. Using rubber spatula, scrape dough into prepared loaf pan and press it gently into corners with wet hands; smooth top of dough and spray with water. Tightly wrap double layer of aluminum foil around pan so that top edge of foil rests at least 1 inch above rim of pan; secure foil collar with staples. Cover loosely with plastic wrap and let rise at room temperature until dough has risen by 50 percent (½ inch above rim of pan), about 1 hour.

3. Adjust oven rack to middle position and heat oven to 325 degrees. Remove plastic and spray loaf with water. Bake until top is golden, crust is firm, and loaf sounds hollow when tapped, about 1½ hours, rotating pan halfway through baking.

4. Transfer to wire rack and let bread cool in pan for 10 minutes. Remove loaf from pan and let cool completely on rack, about 2 hours. Serve. (Once cooled, bread can be wrapped in double layer of plastic wrap and stored at room temperature for up to 3 days. See freezing instructions on page 172.)

Cinnamon-Raisin Bread

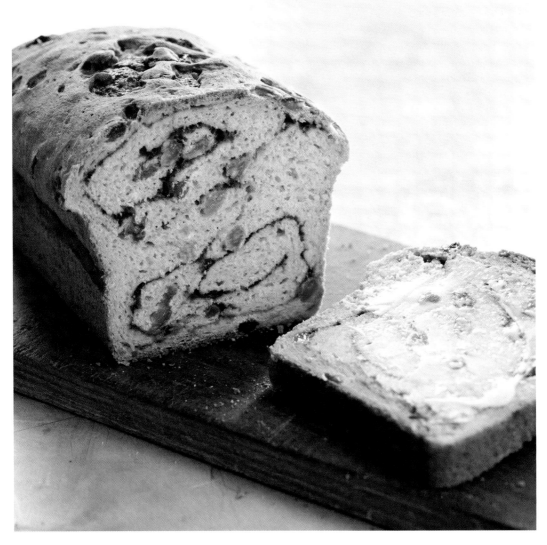

G-F TESTING LAB

FLOUR SUBSTITUTION	King Arthur Gluten-Free Multi-Purpose Flour 14 ounces = **2⅓ cups plus ¼ cup**	Bob's Red Mill All-Purpose GF Baking Flour 14 ounces = **2½ cups plus ⅓ cup**
	Note that bread made with King Arthur will be slightly spongy, and bread made with Bob's Red Mill will be denser and slightly wet and will have a distinct bean flavor.	
OAT FLOUR	If you do not have oat flour, you can process 4 ounces old-fashioned rolled oats in a food processor or spice grinder until finely ground, about 1 minute. Do not use quick oats; they have a dusty texture that doesn't work in this recipe.	
PSYLLIUM HUSK	Do not omit the powdered psyllium husk; it is crucial to the structure of the bread. For more information, see page 16.	

✓ WHY THIS RECIPE WORKS

Cinnamon-raisin bread is always appealing (at least in theory), but it often falls flat. It is either dry, with a scant amount of filling, or overly sweet and gooey—more like cinnamon buns than bread. We wanted to develop a fluffy, sweet loaf with a soft crumb, plenty of raisins, and a generous cinnamon swirl. That said, we didn't want something so sticky that slices couldn't go into the toaster without setting off the smoke alarm. Using our sandwich bread as the base for this recipe, we started by adding an extra tablespoon of sugar, which made the bread plenty sweet. We discovered that the raisins were best added to the finished dough (so they didn't get blown apart during the kneading process). We then switched our focus to the cinnamon filling. Most traditional recipes mix together brown or granulated sugar, cinnamon, and salt and simply spread this mixture over the dough and roll it up tight. But every time we tried this method, our loaves were marred by gaping holes. After way too many failures, we realized that the layer of cinnamon sugar was too thin and ran out during baking. Switching to confectioners' sugar and increasing the amount of cinnamon produced a filling that stayed in place. When powdery confectioners' sugar absorbed water from the dough, it formed a sticky paste. This paste was then thickened by the cornstarch in the sugar and by the cinnamon. Unfortunately the confectioners' sugar did not completely melt. We needed more moisture than could be supplied by the dough. Lightly spraying the filling with water once it was in place guaranteed that the powdery sugar became a paste, with no dry bits. Our loaf was close to perfect, but to guarantee that our filling could be tasted with every bite, we divided the dough in half, spread the filling over each piece, then stacked the two pieces in a loaf pan. We finally had the bread we were wanting—slightly sweet and evenly streaked with cinnamon sugar, and with no holes. Do not substitute soy milk powder for the milk powder in this recipe, as it will negatively impact the flavor and structure of the bread. Note that this recipe calls for an 8½ by 4½-inch loaf pan; if using a 9 by 5-inch loaf pan, the dough will not rise as high and the bread will not be quite as tall.

Cinnamon-Raisin Bread

MAKES 1 LOAF

FILLING

- 2 ounces (½ cup) confectioners' sugar
- 4 teaspoons ground cinnamon
- ½ teaspoon salt

DOUGH

- 2 cups warm water (110 degrees)
- 2 large eggs
- 2 tablespoons unsalted butter, melted and cooled
- 14 ounces (3 cups plus 2 tablespoons) ATK Gluten-Free Flour Blend (page 13)
- 4 ounces (1⅓ cups) gluten-free oat flour
- 1½ ounces (½ cup) nonfat dry milk powder
- 3 tablespoons powdered psyllium husk
- 3 tablespoons granulated sugar
- 2¼ teaspoons instant or rapid-rise yeast
- 2 teaspoons baking powder (see page 20)
- 1½ teaspoons salt
- 1 cup (5 ounces) golden raisins

1. FOR THE FILLING: Combine all ingredients in bowl.

2. FOR THE DOUGH: Spray 8½ by 4½-inch loaf pan with vegetable oil spray. Whisk water, eggs, and melted butter together in bowl. Using stand mixer fitted with paddle, mix flour blend, oat flour, milk powder, psyllium, granulated sugar, yeast, baking powder, and salt together on low speed until just combined. Slowly add water mixture and let dough come together, about 1 minute, scraping down bowl as needed. Increase speed to medium and beat until sticky and uniform, about 6 minutes. (Dough will be very sticky.) Reduce speed to low, add raisins, and mix until incorporated, 30 to 60 seconds.

3. Spray large sheet of parchment paper with vegetable oil spray. With wet hands, transfer half of dough to prepared parchment. Clean and wet hands again. Pat dough into rough 11 by 8-inch rectangle. Sprinkle half of filling mixture evenly over dough, leaving ½-inch border on all sides; spray filling lightly with water. With short side facing you, use parchment to roll dough into tight cylinder. Pinch seam closed and place seam side up in prepared pan. Repeat with second piece of dough and remaining filling; place in pan, seam side down, on top of first piece of dough. Smooth top of dough and spray with water. Tightly wrap double layer of aluminum foil around pan so that top edge of foil rests at least 1 inch above rim of pan; secure foil collar with staples. Cover loosely with plastic wrap and let rise at room temperature until dough has risen by 50 percent (½ inch above rim of pan), about 1 hour.

4. Adjust oven rack to middle position and heat oven to 350 degrees. Remove plastic and spray loaf with water. Bake until top is golden, crust is firm, and loaf sounds hollow when tapped, about 1½ hours, rotating pan halfway through baking.

5. Transfer to wire rack and let bread cool in pan for 10 minutes. Remove loaf from pan and let cool completely on rack, about 2 hours. Serve. (Once cooled, bread can be wrapped in double layer of plastic wrap and stored at room temperature for up to 3 days. See freezing instructions on page 172.)

TEST KITCHEN TIP **Shaping Cinnamon-Raisin Bread**

Dividing the dough in half and spreading the filling over each piece ensures even distribution of the cinnamon sugar filling in the baked loaf. Make sure to spray the filling (once in place) with water. (A plant mister is perfect for this task.) The water turns the filling into a paste that stays in place as the loaf rises and bakes.

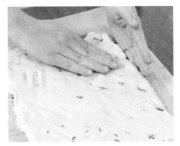
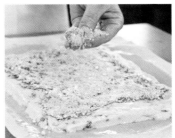
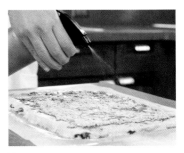

1. With wet hands, transfer half of dough to greased parchment. Clean and wet hands. Pat dough into rough 11 by 8-inch rectangle.

2. Sprinkle half of filling mixture evenly over dough, leaving ½-inch border on all sides.

3. Spray filling lightly with water. Filling should be speckled with water over entire surface.

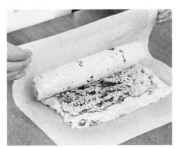
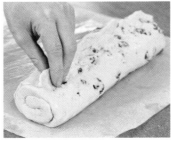
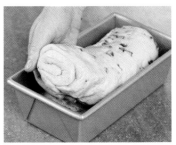

4. With short side facing you, use parchment to help roll dough into tight cylinder by rolling it gently away from you.

5. Turn loaf seam side up, pinch closed, and place seam side up in prepared pan.

6. Repeat with second piece of dough and remaining filling. Place this piece of dough seam side down on top of first piece. Smooth top and spray with water.

Hearty Country Flax Bread

✓ WHY THIS RECIPE WORKS

A good rustic bread has a chewy but soft interior crumb and a hearty crust. Classic recipes contain as few as four ingredients—flour, water, yeast, and salt. Protein content is especially important when making any rustic bread because these loaves are baked free-form, rather than in a loaf pan. All that protein gives the dough enough structure to rise up (rather than just out). We knew our gluten-free flour blend would need help. As with sandwich breads, we found that psyllium worked better than either xanthan or guar gum at strengthening the protein network, but it was far from sufficient. We needed to supplement our flour blend with higher-protein flour and tested flours made from teff, quinoa, millet, and flax. We had good results with most of these flours, but our tasters preferred the earthy but still mellow flavor of ground flaxseeds. With the addition of flax, we found that the dough did not absorb water as easily so we cut back on the liquid. As with our sandwich breads, we found that a little sugar helped the yeast do its job and that the milk powder improved flavor and browning. While our loaf was tasting better, it was still spreading way too much in the oven and seemed to lack structure. Adding eggs (something standard in sandwich bread but quite unusual in rustic breads) boosted the protein content and helped with structure. Adding baking soda (another unusual addition) helped create a more delicate crumb. (The flaxseeds are slightly acidic, so baking soda worked better than baking powder in this recipe.) The ingredient list was in good shape, but the loaf was still spreading too much during proofing and baking. Up to this point, we had been letting the loaf rise on a piece of parchment and then transferring the loaf (still on the parchment) to a preheated baking stone, just as we would when making conventional rustic bread. We solved our spread problems by transferring the shaped dough to a small skillet for rising and baking. The sides of the pan prevented excess spread and ensured that the loaf emerged from the oven with good height and a light crumb. Placing the skillet onto a preheated baking stone in the oven produced a really crisp bottom crust.

We had one last problem to tackle—the dough was sometimes splitting during baking. We found that cutting the top of the loaf with a sharp bread knife allowed the crust to expand and prevented the bread from splitting in the oven. Also spraying the loaf with water right before it went into the oven delayed the formation of a crust during the longer baking time, allowing the bread to fully expand without tearing or splitting. Using more yeast than usual (a full tablespoon) helped with the rise, as did starting the loaf in a hot oven (set to 400 degrees) and then turning down the heat so the loaf could cook through. Do not substitute soy milk powder for the milk powder in this recipe, as it will negatively impact the flavor and structure of the bread. If you don't eat dairy, you're better off omitting the milk powder although the structure of the bread will suffer a bit.

Hearty Country Flax Bread
MAKES 1 LOAF

1¾	cups warm water (110 degrees)
2	large eggs
14	ounces (3 cups plus 2 tablespoons) ATK Gluten-Free Flour Blend (page 13)
3	ounces (¾ cup) ground flaxseeds
1½	ounces (½ cup) nonfat dry milk powder
3	tablespoons powdered psyllium husk
2	tablespoons sugar
1	tablespoon instant or rapid-rise yeast
1½	teaspoons salt
¾	teaspoon baking soda

1. Whisk water and eggs together in bowl. Using stand mixer fitted with paddle, mix flour blend, ground flaxseeds, milk powder, psyllium, sugar, yeast, salt, and baking soda together on low speed until combined. Slowly add water mixture and let dough come together, about 1 minute, scraping down bowl as needed. Increase speed to medium and beat until sticky and uniform, about 6 minutes. (Dough will resemble cookie dough.)

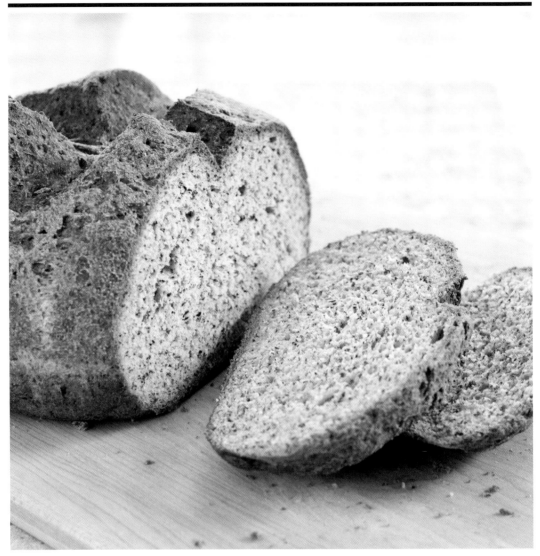

G-F TESTING LAB

FLOUR SUBSTITUTION	King Arthur Gluten-Free Multi-Purpose Flour 14 ounces = **2⅓ cups plus ¼ cup**	Bob's Red Mill GF All-Purpose Baking Flour 14 ounces = **2½ cups plus ⅓ cup**
	Note that bread made with King Arthur will be slightly gummy, and bread made with Bob's Red Mill will be denser and a bit drier and will have an extremely earthy flavor.	
PSYLLIUM HUSK	Do not omit the powdered psyllium husk; it is crucial to the structure of the bread. For more information, see page 16.	

2. Spray 18 by 12-inch sheet of parchment paper with vegetable oil spray. Using rubber spatula, transfer dough to prepared parchment and shape into 6½-inch ball with wet hands. Place dough (still on parchment) inside ovensafe 8-inch skillet. Using sharp serrated knife or single-edge razor blade, make two ½-inch-deep, 4-inch-long slashes in X shape across top of dough. Spray dough with water. Cover loosely with plastic wrap and let rise at room temperature until dough has risen by 50 percent, about 2 hours.

3. One hour before baking, adjust oven rack to lowest position, place baking stone on rack, and heat oven to 400 degrees. Remove plastic and spray loaf with water. Reduce oven temperature to 350 degrees and place skillet on baking stone. Bake until top of bread is well browned, crust is firm, and loaf sounds hollow when tapped, about 1½ hours, rotating skillet halfway through baking.

4. Carefully remove loaf from skillet, transfer to wire rack (discard parchment), and let bread cool completely, about 2 hours. Serve. (Once cooled, bread can be wrapped in double layer of plastic wrap and stored at room temperature for up to 3 days. See freezing instructions on page 172.)

SMART SHOPPING **Flaxseeds**

Flaxseeds are similar in size to sesame seeds and have a sweet, wheaty flavor. They are naturally gluten-free and are sold both whole and ground in most supermarkets. Flaxseeds are one of the highest sources known for the omega-3 fatty acid called alpha-linolenic acid (ALA), which is found only in certain plant foods and oils and must be supplied by our diet for good health. Whole seeds have a longer shelf life, but we preferred ground flaxseeds in our bread because we wanted to use them as a flour rather than as a stir-in. As an added bonus, grinding flaxseeds improves the release of nutrients. If you can't find ground flaxseeds, you can grind whole seeds in a spice grinder or food processor. Like other nuts and seeds, store flaxseeds in the freezer.

TEST KITCHEN TIP **Shaping Hearty Country Flax Bread**

Letting our rustic loaf rise and bake in an ovensafe 8-inch skillet helped prevent spread, ensuring our bread had a better, taller rise. A small cast-iron skillet or conventional skillet with a metal handle is ideal for this recipe. If you prefer, use a single-edge razor blade rather than a serrated knife in step 3. Once the dough has been slashed and sprayed with water, cover it loosely with plastic wrap and let it rise as directed.

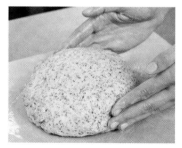

1. Using rubber spatula, transfer dough to greased parchment and shape into 6½-inch ball with wet hands.

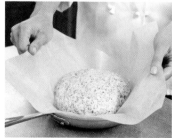

2. Place dough (still on parchment) inside ovensafe 8-inch skillet.

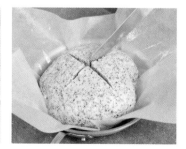

3. Using serrated knife, make two ½-inch-deep, 4-inch-long slashes in X shape across top of dough. Spray dough with water, cover with plastic, and let rise.

Olive-Rosemary Bread

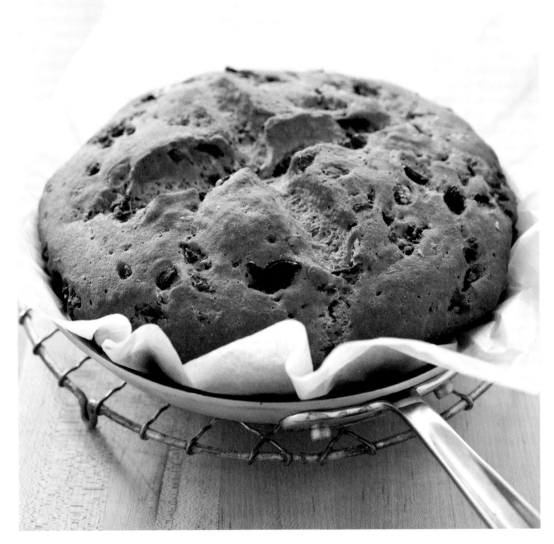

G-F TESTING LAB

FLOUR SUBSTITUTION	King Arthur Gluten-Free Multi-Purpose Flour 12 ounces = **1⅔ cups plus ½ cup**	Bob's Red Mill GF All-Purpose Baking Flour 12 ounces = **2¼ cups plus 2 tablespoons**
	Note that bread made with Bob's Red Mill will have a strong earthy, beany flavor that clashes somewhat with the rosemary in this recipe.	
OAT FLOUR	If you do not have oat flour, you can process 4 ounces old-fashioned rolled oats in a food processor or spice grinder until finely ground, about 1 minute. Do not use quick oats; they have a dusty texture that doesn't work in this recipe.	
PSYLLIUM HUSK	Do not omit the powdered psyllium husk; it is crucial to the structure of the bread. For more information, see page 16.	

✓ WHY THIS RECIPE WORKS

We used our Hearty Country Flax Bread (page 179) as a starting point for this recipe. While we liked the earthy flavor of ground flax in the country bread, it clashed with the olives and rosemary. We had better results when we replaced the ground flax with milder-tasting oat flour. While the flavors were right, the crumb was very dense and the crust was overly thick. Adding another egg and a few tablespoons of olive oil made the crumb softer, while brushing the loaf with an additional tablespoon of oil just before baking helped to soften the crust. Finally, two teaspoons of lemon juice softened the crumb even further, providing a great contrast to the hearty (but no longer tough) crust. The hydration level in this dough is pretty high, and we found that it needed a longer, slower baking process than the basic country bread. We had the best results baking the loaf in a relatively cool 325-degree oven for 2 hours (yes, this is correct). As with the country bread, this loaf will spread out rather than rise up unless it is proofed and baked in an ovenproof skillet. However, due to the long baking time, we found that placing the skillet on a heated baking stone caused the crust to become too dark and hard. When the dough has risen, simply brush it with oil and place the skillet with the risen dough right into the oven. Do not substitute soy milk powder for the milk powder in this recipe, as it will negatively impact the flavor and structure of the bread. If you don't eat dairy, you're better off omitting the milk powder, although the structure of the bread will suffer a bit. For tips on shaping this bread, see the steps on page 181.

Olive-Rosemary Bread
MAKE 1 LOAF

- 1½   cups warm water (110 degrees)
- 3   large eggs
- 3   tablespoons olive oil
- 2   teaspoons lemon juice
- 12   ounces (2⅔ cups) ATK Gluten-Free Flour Blend (page 13)
- 4   ounces (1⅓ cups) gluten-free oat flour

- 1½   ounces (½ cup) nonfat dry milk powder
- 3   tablespoons powdered psyllium husk
- 2   tablespoons sugar
- 1   tablespoon instant or rapid-rise yeast
- 1   teaspoon salt
- ¾   teaspoon baking soda
- 1   cup pitted kalamata olives, rinsed and chopped
- 2   tablespoons chopped fresh rosemary

1. Whisk water, eggs, 2 tablespoons oil, and lemon juice together in bowl. Using stand mixer fitted with paddle, mix flour blend, oat flour, milk powder, psyllium, sugar, yeast, salt, and baking soda together on low speed until combined. Slowly add water mixture and let dough come together, about 1 minute, scraping down bowl as needed. Increase speed to medium and beat until sticky and uniform, about 6 minutes. (Dough will resemble cookie dough.) Stir in olives and rosemary with rubber spatula.

2. Spray 18 by 12-inch sheet of parchment paper with vegetable oil spray. Using rubber spatula, transfer dough to prepared parchment and shape into 6½-inch ball with wet hands. Place dough (still on parchment) inside ovensafe 8-inch skillet. Using sharp serrated knife or single-edge razor blade, make two ½-inch-deep, 4-inch-long slashes in X shape across top of dough. Spray dough with water. Cover loosely with plastic wrap and let rise at room temperature until dough has risen by 50 percent, about 1½ hours.

3. Adjust oven rack to lowest position and heat oven to 325 degrees. Remove plastic and brush with remaining 1 tablespoon olive oil. Bake until top of bread is dark golden brown, crust is firm, and loaf sounds hollow when tapped, about 2 hours, rotating skillet halfway through baking.

4. Carefully remove loaf from skillet, transfer to wire rack (discard parchment), and let bread cool completely, about 2 hours. Serve. (Once cooled, bread can be wrapped in double layer of plastic wrap and stored at room temperature for up to 3 days. See freezing instructions on page 172.)

Dinner Rolls

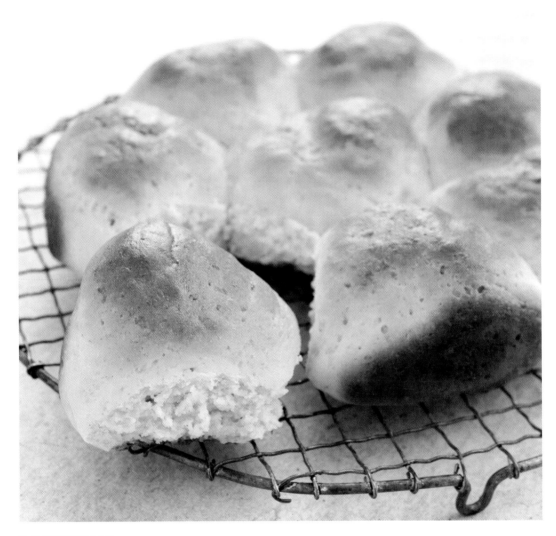

G-F TESTING LAB

FLOUR SUBSTITUTION	King Arthur Gluten-Free Multi-Purpose Flour 15 ounces = **2¾ cups**	Bob's Red Mill GF All-Purpose Baking Flour 15 ounces = **3 cups**
	Note that rolls made with King Arthur will be slightly pasty, and rolls made with Bob's Red Mill will have a strong bean flavor and a darker color. The dough made with Bob's Red Mill will be a bit looser and harder to shape, but the rolls will rise just fine and bake up nicely.	
PSYLLIUM HUSK	Do not omit the powdered psyllium husk; it is crucial to the structure of the rolls. For more information, see page 16.	

WHY THIS RECIPE WORKS

Store-bought gluten-free dinner rolls are tough and bland, and many homemade recipes aren't much better. We wanted rich, tender, pull-apart dinner rolls, so we started with our favorite test kitchen recipe and substituted our gluten-free flour blend plus some psyllium to boost structure. This approach produced rolls with great buttery flavor, but tasters complained that the rolls were greasy. Cutting back on the amount of butter and adding a small amount of nonfat milk powder lent a rich flavor without any added greasiness. The bigger problem was the texture of the crumb—it was dense and a bit tough. The dough needed more liquid. We tested both milk and water, and tasters agreed that the water worked best given all the butter, milk powder, and eggs in the dough. This helped, but our rolls needed something more. Up to this point we had been relying solely on yeast, and we wondered if adding a chemical leavener would create a more open crumb and further tenderize our rolls. We tested various combinations and found that 2 teaspoons of baking powder plus the standard packet of yeast produced rolls with the desired airy crumb. We had one more trick up our sleeve. In other kitchen tests, we discovered the tenderizing effect of lemon juice in our pie dough, so we made one last batch of rolls with some lemon juice in the mix. These rolls were perfect—pillowy soft with a light crumb and rich buttery flavor. The rolls are best eaten the day they are made.

Dinner Rolls
MAKES 8 ROLLS

- 1⅓ cups warm water (110 degrees), plus 1 teaspoon water
- 2 teaspoons lemon juice
- 2 large eggs, plus 1 large yolk
- 15 ounces (3⅓ cups) ATK Gluten-Free Flour Blend (page 13)
- 1½ ounces (½ cup) nonfat dry milk powder
- 2 tablespoons powdered psyllium husk
- 2 tablespoons sugar
- 2¼ teaspoons instant or rapid-rise yeast
- 2 teaspoons baking powder (see page 20)
  Salt
- 6 tablespoons unsalted butter, cut into 6 pieces and softened

1. Spray 9-inch round cake pan with vegetable oil spray. Whisk 1⅓ cups warm water, lemon juice, and 1 egg plus yolk together in bowl. Using stand mixer fitted with paddle, mix flour blend, milk powder, psyllium, sugar, yeast, baking powder, and 1½ teaspoons salt together on low speed until combined. Slowly add water mixture and let dough come together, about 1 minute, scraping down bowl as needed. Add butter, increase speed to medium, and beat until sticky and uniform, about 6 minutes.

2. Working with generous ⅓ cup dough at a time, shape into rough rounds using wet hands, and arrange rolls in prepared pan (1 in center and 7 spaced evenly around edges). Cover loosely with plastic wrap and let rise at room temperature until doubled in size (rolls should press against each other), about 1 hour. (Risen rolls can be refrigerated for up to 4 hours.)

3. Adjust oven rack to middle position and heat oven to 375 degrees. Lightly beat remaining 1 egg, 1 teaspoon water, and pinch salt in bowl until combined. Remove plastic and brush rolls with egg wash. Bake until tops are golden brown, 35 to 40 minutes, rotating pan halfway through baking.

4. Let rolls cool in pan on wire rack for 10 minutes, then invert onto rack; reinvert rolls and let cool for 10 to 15 minutes. Break rolls apart and serve warm.

TEST KITCHEN TIP **Shaping Dinner Rolls**

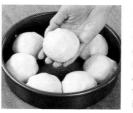

Baking rolls in cake pan helps them to rise up rather than out. Divide dough into 8 pieces, shape into rounds, and arrange in greased pan with 1 piece of dough in center.

English Muffins

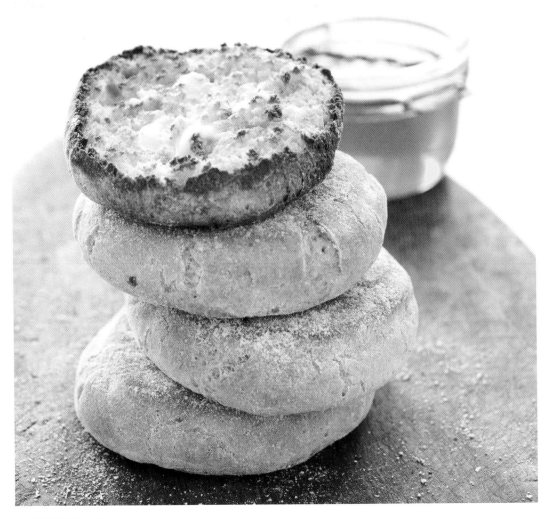

G-F TESTING LAB

FLOUR SUBSTITUTION	King Arthur Gluten-Free Multi-Purpose Flour 14 ounces = **2⅓ cups plus ¼ cup**	Bob's Red Mill GF All-Purpose Baking Flour 14 ounces = **2½ cups plus ⅓ cup**
	Note that English muffins made with King Arthur will be slightly starchy, and English muffins made with Bob's Red Mill will be darker and will have a distinct bean flavor.	
OAT FLOUR	If you do not have oat flour, you can process 4 ounces old-fashioned rolled oats in a food processor or spice grinder until finely ground, about 1 minute. Do not use quick oats; they have a dusty texture that doesn't work in this recipe.	
PSYLLIUM HUSK	Do not omit the powdered psyllium husk; it is crucial to the structure of the muffins. For more information, see page 16.	

WHY THIS RECIPE WORKS

Our Classic Sandwich Bread proved to be a good starting point for this recipe—the dough has the necessary flavor and richness—and the classic technique worked well. We portioned the dough into rough balls and let them rise on two rimmed baking sheets until nearly doubled in size. The dough was rather sticky, and we had trouble dusting them with cornmeal (which helps create the distinctive crunch on the exterior of any good English muffin). We found it easier to sprinkle the rimmed baking sheet with cornmeal and then sprinkle more cornmeal over the top of the risen dough rounds. In order to create their distinctive shape and crumb, it's necessary to flatten the dough rounds both before and during griddling. While some classic recipes cook the muffins entirely on the stovetop, we thought the crusts became much too hard. One minute of griddling per side was sufficient. We then transferred the muffins to a baking sheet and finished by baking them in the oven to ensure they were cooked through but not overly browned. Do not substitute soy milk powder for the milk powder in this recipe, as it will negatively impact the flavor and structure of the English muffins.

English Muffins
MAKES 10 MUFFINS

3¾	ounces (¾ cup) cornmeal
2	cups warm water (110 degrees)
2	large eggs
2	tablespoons unsalted butter, melted and cooled
14	ounces (3 cups plus 2 tablespoons) ATK Gluten-Free Flour Blend (page 13)
4	ounces (1⅓ cups) gluten-free oat flour
1½	ounces (½ cup) nonfat dry milk powder
3	tablespoons powdered psyllium husk
2	tablespoons sugar
2¼	teaspoons instant or rapid-rise yeast
2	teaspoons baking powder (see page 20)
1½	teaspoons salt
3	teaspoons vegetable oil

1. Sprinkle ½ cup cornmeal evenly over 2 rimmed baking sheets. Whisk water, eggs, and melted butter together in bowl. Using stand mixer fitted with paddle, mix flour blend, oat flour, milk powder, psyllium, sugar, yeast, baking powder, and salt together on low speed until combined. Slowly add water mixture and let dough come together, about 1 minute, scraping down bowl as needed. Increase speed to medium and beat until sticky and uniform, about 6 minutes. (Dough will resemble cookie dough.)

2. Working with ⅓ cup dough at a time, shape into rough balls using wet hands, and space at least 1½ inches apart on prepared sheets (5 per sheet). Cover loosely with lightly greased plastic wrap and let rise at room temperature until doubled in size, about 1 hour.

3. Adjust oven rack to lower-middle position and heat oven to 350 degrees. Remove plastic and, using greased metal spatula, press dough balls into ¾-inch-thick rounds (about 3½ inches in diameter). Dust tops of muffins with remaining ¼ cup cornmeal.

4. Heat 1 teaspoon oil in 12-inch skillet over medium heat until shimmering, about 2 minutes. Wipe out skillet with paper towel, leaving thin film of oil on bottom and sides of pan. Carefully lay 4 muffins in pan and cook until bottoms are just set, about 1 minute, occasionally pressing down on muffins with spatula to prevent doming.

5. Flip muffins and continue to cook until set on second side, about 1 minute longer. Transfer muffins to clean baking sheet lined with parchment. Repeat with remaining 2 teaspoons oil and remaining muffins in 2 more batches, wiping skillet clean before each batch and transferring muffins to same baking sheet.

6. Bake until golden brown and firm, 30 to 35 minutes, rotating sheet halfway through baking. Transfer muffins to wire rack and let cool for at least 20 minutes before splitting with fork and toasting. Serve. (Once cooled, unsplit English muffins can be stored in zipper-lock bag for up to 2 days. See page 209 for freezing instructions.)

Cheddar Cheese Bread

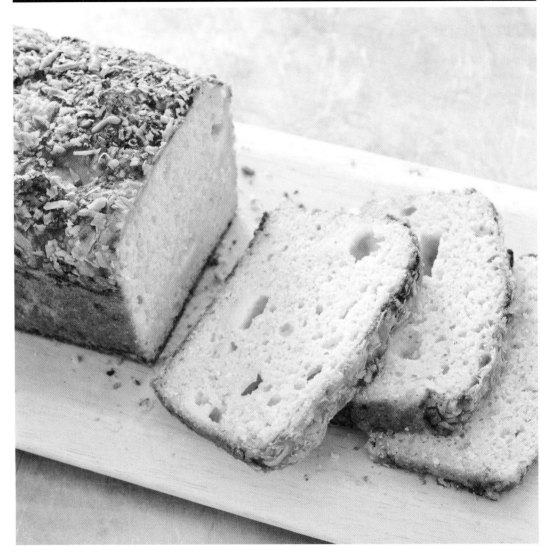

G-F TESTING LAB

FLOUR SUBSTITUTION	King Arthur Gluten-Free Multi-Purpose Flour 12½ ounces = **2¼ cups**	Bob's Red Mill GF All-Purpose Baking Flour 12½ ounces = **2½ cups**

Note that bread made with King Arthur will be somewhat pasty, and bread made with Bob's Red Mill will be wetter and will have a distinct bean flavor.

✓ WHY THIS RECIPE WORKS

Studded with pockets of cheese and featuring a crunchy cheese crust, cheddar cheese bread is a comforting loaf that is just as good fresh from the oven as it is transformed into the ultimate grilled cheese. These loaves are typically dense, so we knew we were going to rely heavily on leaveners. Baking powder alone wasn't enough to give this springy dough the right lift, but the addition of a small amount of baking soda did the trick. Tangy sour cream along with cayenne and ground black pepper complemented the sharp cheddar perfectly. Grating the Parmesan on the large holes of a box grater and sprinkling it over the top of the loaf and in the bottom of the pan added a nice texture; do not grate it fine or use pregrated Parmesan. A mild, soft Asiago cheese, crumbled into ¼- to ½-inch pieces, is a nice substitute for the cheddar. The texture of the bread improves as it cools, so resist the urge to slice the loaf while it is piping hot.

Cheddar Cheese Bread

MAKES 1 LOAF

3	ounces Parmesan cheese, grated on large holes of box grater (1 cup)
12½	ounces (2¾ cups) ATK Gluten-Free Flour Blend (page 13)
1	tablespoon baking powder (see page 20)
¼	teaspoon baking soda
½	teaspoon salt
⅛	teaspoon pepper
⅛	teaspoon cayenne pepper
4	ounces extra-sharp cheddar cheese, cut into ½-inch cubes (1 cup)
1¼	cups sour cream
3	tablespoons unsalted butter, melted and cooled
2	large eggs, lightly beaten

1. Adjust oven rack to middle position and heat oven to 350 degrees. Spray 8½ by 4½-inch loaf pan with vegetable spray, then sprinkle ½ cup Parmesan evenly in bottom of pan.

2. Whisk flour blend, baking powder, baking soda, salt, pepper, and cayenne together in large bowl. Stir in cheddar, breaking up any clumps, until coated with flour mixture. In separate bowl, whisk together sour cream, melted butter, and eggs until smooth. Using rubber spatula, stir sour cream mixture into flour mixture until thoroughly combined (batter will be heavy and thick).

3. Scrape batter into prepared pan, smooth top, and sprinkle remaining ½ cup Parmesan evenly over loaf. Bake until deep golden brown and toothpick inserted in center comes out clean, 40 to 45 minutes, rotating pan halfway through baking.

4. Transfer to wire rack and let bread cool in pan for 10 minutes. Remove loaf from pan and let cool on rack for at least 1 hour before serving. (Once cooled, bread can be wrapped in double layer of plastic wrap and stored at room temperature for up to 1 day. To serve, warm in 300-degree oven for 10 minutes.

TEST KITCHEN TIP

Use Two Cheeses for Cheese Bread

The secret to our cheese bread is using two different cheeses prepared two different ways. While most cheese bread recipes call for shredded cheese, we prefer the cheddar cheese cut into small cubes, which create cheesy pockets throughout the bread. Grating Parmesan on the large holes of a box grater and sprinkling it in the pan and on top of the loaf ensure a crunchy crust with good flavor.

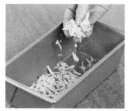

Spray 8½ by 4½-inch loaf pan with vegetable spray, then sprinkle ½ cup coarsely grated Parmesan evenly in bottom of pan.

Skillet Cornbread

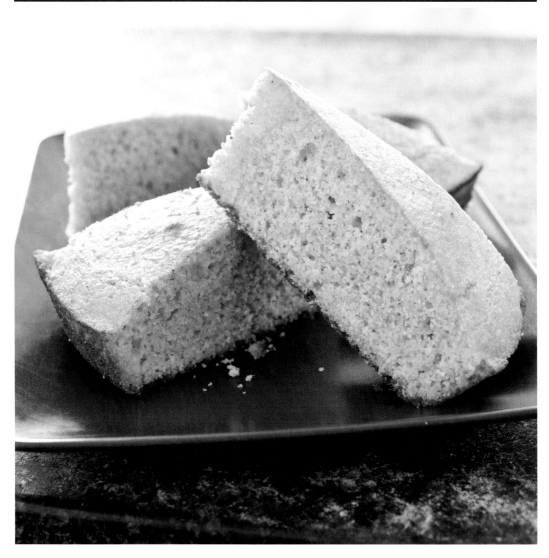

G-F TESTING LAB

CORNMEAL   The test kitchen's favorite cornmeal for baking is finely ground Whole-Grain Arrowhead Mills Cornmeal. This brand has been processed in a gluten-free facility, but not all brands are. Make sure to read the label. See page 149 for more details on cornmeal.

✅ WHY THIS RECIPE WORKS

Unlike its sweet, cakey Northern counterpart, Southern cornbread is thin, crusty, and decidedly savory. It is traditionally made with cornmeal and no flour or sugar, so it is naturally gluten-free from the start. We used yellow cornmeal for potent corn flavor (which we toasted first to bring out its flavor) and, veering from tradition, added a small amount of sugar to enhance the natural sweetness of the corn. Creating a cornmeal mush by moistening the toasted cornmeal with a combination of sour cream and milk (favored over the traditional buttermilk for extra richness) produced a fine, moist crumb. Baking the cornbread in a greased preheated cast-iron skillet gave it a seriously crunchy, golden crust. Using a combination of oil and butter for greasing the skillet (as well as in the batter) struck the perfect balance of flavor and performance—the butter added flavor while the oil raised the smoke point so the butter wouldn't burn. We prefer to use a cast-iron skillet here because it makes the best crust; however, any 10-inch ovensafe skillet will work for this recipe. Cornbread is best served warm.

Skillet Cornbread
SERVES 8 TO 10

11¼	ounces (2¼ cups) cornmeal
1½	cups sour cream
½	cup milk
¼	cup vegetable oil
4	tablespoons unsalted butter
2	tablespoons sugar
1	teaspoon baking powder (see page 20)
1	teaspoon baking soda
¾	teaspoon salt
2	large eggs

1. Adjust oven racks to lower-middle and middle positions and heat oven to 450 degrees. Place 10-inch cast-iron skillet on middle rack and heat for 10 minutes. Meanwhile, spread cornmeal over rimmed baking sheet and toast in oven on lower-middle rack until fragrant and lightly golden, about 5 minutes.

2. Carefully transfer toasted cornmeal to large bowl and whisk in sour cream and milk; set aside. When skillet is hot, add oil and continue to heat until just smoking, about 5 minutes.

3. Using potholders (skillet handle will be hot), remove skillet from oven, carefully add butter, and gently swirl to incorporate. Pour hot oil-butter mixture into cornmeal mixture and whisk to incorporate. Whisk in sugar, baking powder, baking soda, and salt, followed by eggs.

4. Quickly scrape batter into hot skillet and smooth top. Bake on middle rack until top begins to crack and sides are golden brown, 12 to 15 minutes, rotating skillet halfway through baking. Let bread cool in skillet on wire rack for 5 minutes. Remove bread from pan and let cool on rack for at least 10 minutes before serving.

TEST KITCHEN TIP
Ensuring a Well-Browned Bottom Crust

Pouring the batter into a hot, greased cast-iron skillet ensures a crisp crust. Remember the handle will be very hot, so use a potholder.

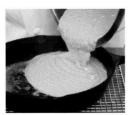

Working quickly, scrape batter into hot skillet, smooth top with rubber spatula, and return skillet to oven.

Light and Fluffy Biscuits

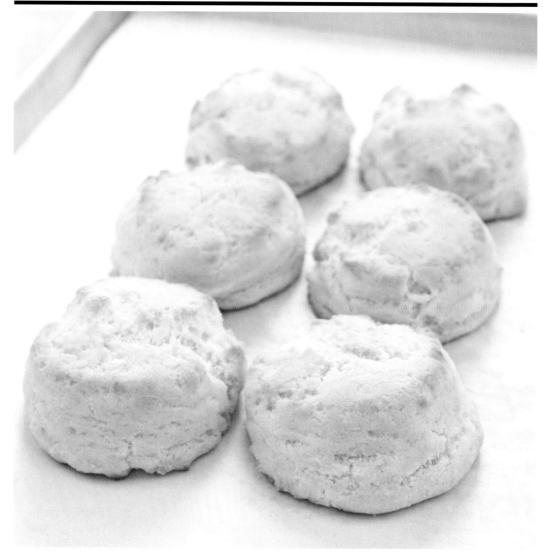

G-F TESTING LAB

FLOUR SUBSTITUTION	King Arthur Gluten-Free Multi-Purpose Flour 9 ounces = **1½ cups plus 2 tablespoons**	Bob's Red Mill All-Purpose GF Baking Flour 9 ounces = **1½ cups plus ⅓ cup**
	Note that biscuits made with King Arthur will be slightly sandy and a bit starchy and will spread more, and biscuits made with Bob's Red Mill will be coarser and will spread more and have a distinct bean flavor.	
PSYLLIUM HUSK	Do not omit the powdered psyllium husk; it is crucial to the structure of the biscuits. For more information, see page 16.	
RESTING TIME	Do not shortchange the 30-minute rest for the dough; if you do, the biscuits will be gritty and spread too much.	

WHY THIS RECIPE WORKS

While gluten development is less important in tender biscuits than in chewy bread, our gluten-free flour blend still fell short. As we did with other breads, we strengthened the protein network with psyllium and added an egg to boost the overall protein content. The biggest challenge was the fat. A biscuit must be buttery, but gluten-free flours just don't absorb fat all that well, and many early attempts were very greasy. A combination of butter and oil was key. (For more information on oil versus butter in baking, see page 306.) Gluten-free flours don't absorb liquid very well either, and we found that biscuits made with buttermilk spread way too much. Switching to thicker yogurt solved the problem. (We prefer whole-milk yogurt, but low-fat yogurt will work, producing slightly drier biscuits.) Tasters missed the tang of the buttermilk, but supplementing the yogurt with a little lemon juice fixed that problem. As with other chemically leavened quick breads and cookies, we found that biscuits were much improved by letting the dough rest for 30 minutes before baking. Not only did the resting time help to thicken the wet dough a bit (making it easier to shape), more importantly it allowed the starches in the flour blend to fully hydrate. If you skip this step the biscuits will have a slightly gritty, starchy texture. Placing the biscuits fairly close together on the baking sheet trapped a little extra steam, which made them just a bit lighter and more tender. Biscuits are best eaten the day they are baked, but they can be frozen (see page 209 for instructions).

Light and Fluffy Biscuits
MAKES 6 BISCUITS

9	ounces (2 cups) ATK Gluten-Free Flour Blend (page 13)
4	teaspoons baking powder (see page 20)
1½	teaspoons powdered psyllium husk
1	teaspoon sugar
½	teaspoon salt
¼	teaspoon baking soda
3	tablespoons unsalted butter, chilled and cut into ¼-inch pieces
¾	cup plain whole-milk yogurt
1	large egg, lightly beaten
2	tablespoons vegetable oil
2	teaspoons lemon juice

1. Whisk flour blend, baking powder, psyllium, sugar, salt, and baking soda in large bowl until combined. Add butter to flour blend mixture, breaking up chunks with fingertips until only small, pea-size pieces remain. In separate bowl, whisk together yogurt, egg, oil, and lemon juice until combined. Using rubber spatula, stir yogurt mixture into flour mixture until thoroughly combined and no flour pockets remain, about 1 minute. Cover bowl with plastic wrap and let batter rest at room temperature for 30 minutes.

2. Adjust oven rack to middle position and heat oven to 450 degrees. Line rimmed baking sheet with parchment paper and place inside of second baking sheet. Using greased ⅓-cup dry measure, scoop heaping amount of batter and drop onto prepared sheet. (Biscuit should measure about 2½ inches in diameter and 1½ inches high.) Repeat with remaining batter, spacing biscuits about ½ inch apart in center of prepared sheet.

3. Bake until golden and crisp, about 15 minutes, rotating sheet halfway through baking. Transfer sheet to wire rack and let cool for 5 to 10 minutes before serving.

VARIATION
Sweet Biscuits
Pair these biscuits with macerated fruit and whipped cream to make shortcakes.

Increase sugar in dough to 2 tablespoons. Sprinkle additional 2 tablespoons sugar evenly over biscuits just before baking.

Biscuits

We wanted a drop biscuit that would offer an easy and quick alternative to a traditional rolled biscuit, but with the same tender texture and buttery flavor. The classic recipe is nothing more than flour, baking powder, baking soda, sugar, and salt mixed with butter and buttermilk. In order to produce an equally tender biscuit with a light, fluffy crumb we had to rework the ingredient list quite extensively.

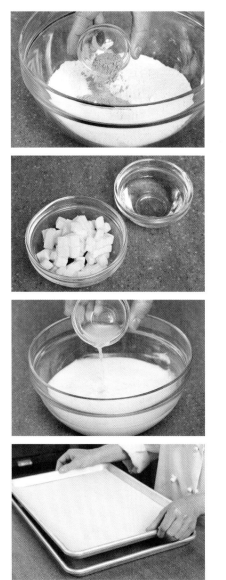

1. ADD PSYLLIUM AND EGG FOR STRUCTURE: While traditional biscuits rely on gluten for structure, we had to find another solution. Adding powdered psyllium husk (as we had done in bread recipes) helped strengthen the proteins in gluten-free flours so they could do a better job of trapping gas and steam during baking. However, using too much psyllium imparted an earthy flavor that was out of place in biscuits. An egg provided additional structure along with moisture and elasticity.

2. USE TWO FATS: Butter plays an important role in making biscuits tender and tasty. A batch of fluffy drop biscuits typically relies on at least a stick of butter. We found that our biscuit dough could absorb only 3 tablespoons of butter (the rest just leached out and made the biscuits greasy). With so little fat in the dough, the biscuits were very tough and dry. Two tablespoons of vegetable oil added back some richness, as did replacing the usual buttermilk with thicker, richer whole-milk yogurt.

3. THICKER DAIRY PLEASE: Biscuits are traditionally made with buttermilk. Because gluten-free flours don't absorb liquid well, we found the dough was very liquid-y and spread too much in the oven. Using less milk didn't work—the starches in the flour never hydrated, and they imparted a gritty texture to the baked biscuits. Switching to thicker yogurt (spiked with a little lemon juice for extra tang) produced a dough with the right consistency, and letting the dough rest for 30 minutes (as we had done with muffins and other chemically leavened bread) allowed the starches to hydrate before baking.

4. DOUBLE UP ON SHEET PANS: A biscuit is typically baked at a high temperature for a short time to achieve a golden crust and nice rise. We struggled to get a nice color on the tops of the biscuits without burning the bottoms. Lowering the oven temperature seemed like a natural solution, but we needed to bake them so long that the inside dried out. We had better luck staying with the high temperature but using a second baking sheet as insulation to keep the bottoms from burning.

Pizza

✔ WHY THIS RECIPE WORKS

The best pizza crusts are a study in contrasts: tender and airy on the inside, and crisp and pleasantly chewy on the exterior. The gluten-free pizza crusts we sampled were instead a study in compromise. Even when they were palatable (and many were not), most fell into one of two camps: dense and doughy, or thin and cracker-crunchy. We set out to make a gluten-free pizza crust that could stand alongside the best wheat-based crusts. To improve tenderness and produce an open crumb, we increased the amount of water in the dough until it resembled a thick batter; this allowed the dough to expand more fully during fermentation. (To open the crumb even further, we also added a second leavener in the form of baking powder.) But all the extra water required cooking off to avoid gumminess, necessitating the addition of a parbaking step. (When we topped and then baked the raw dough, the cheese and toppings burned before the crust cooked through.) To prevent the exterior of the crust from drying out before the interior was fully cooked during parbaking, we chose a low-and-slow approach: start with a cold oven followed by a long, gentle bake. In order to achieve a crisp exterior, we first tried adding more oil to the dough. This helped, but not enough, and pouring in even more oil just made the crust greasy. A more effective approach was to add richness and fat in the form of almond flour, which provided the crispness and delicate crunch we sought without adding obvious flavor or greasiness.

Pizza Crusts
MAKES 2 PARBAKED CRUSTS

- 16 ounces (3⅓ cups plus ¼ cup) ATK Gluten-Free Flour Blend (page 13)
- 2½ ounces (½ cup plus 1 tablespoon) almond flour
- 4½ teaspoons powdered psyllium husk
- 2½ teaspoons baking powder (see page 20)
- 2 teaspoons salt
- 1 teaspoon instant or rapid-rise yeast
- 2½ cups warm water (100 degrees)
- ¼ cup vegetable oil
  Vegetable oil spray

1. Using stand mixer fitted with paddle, mix flour blend, almond flour, psyllium, baking powder, salt, and yeast together on low speed until combined. Slowly add water and oil in steady stream until incorporated. Increase speed to medium and beat until sticky and uniform, about 6 minutes. (Dough will resemble thick batter.)

2. Remove bowl from mixer, cover with plastic wrap, and let stand until inside of dough is bubbly (use large spoon to peer inside dough), about 90 minutes.

3. Adjust oven racks to lower and middle positions. Line 2 baking sheets with parchment paper and spray liberally with vegetable oil spray. Transfer half of dough to center of one prepared sheet. Using oil-sprayed spatula, spread dough into 8-inch circle. Spray top of dough with vegetable oil spray, cover with large sheet of plastic, and, using hands, press dough out to 11½-inch round, about ¼ inch thick, leaving outer ¼ inch slightly thicker than center; remove plastic. Repeat with remaining dough and remaining prepared sheet.

4. Place sheets in oven and set oven temperature to 325 degrees. Bake dough until firm to touch, golden brown on underside, and just beginning to brown on top, 45 to 50 minutes, switching and rotating sheets halfway through baking. Transfer crusts to wire rack and let cool. (Baked and cooled crusts can sit at room temperature for up to 4 hours. Completely cooled crusts can be wrapped first with plastic and then with aluminum foil and frozen for up to 2 weeks. Frozen crusts can be topped and baked as directed in pizza recipes. Note that crusts do not need to thaw before topping and baking.)

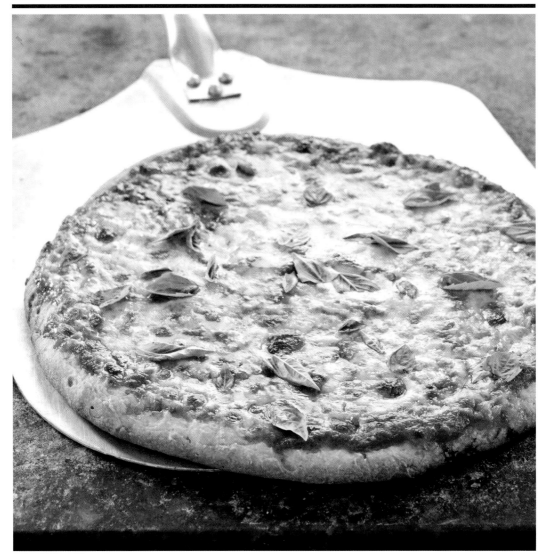

G-F TESTING LAB

FLOUR SUBSTITUTION	King Arthur Gluten-Free Multi-Purpose Flour 16 ounces = **2⅔ cups plus ¼ cup**	Bob's Red Mill GF All-Purpose Baking Flour 16 ounces = **2⅔ cups plus ½ cup**
	Note that pizza crust made with King Arthur will be slightly denser and not as chewy, and pizza crust made with Bob's Red Mill will be thicker and more airy and will have a distinct bean flavor.	
ALMOND FLOUR	If you do not have almond flour, you can process 2½ ounces blanched almonds in a food processor until finely ground, about 30 seconds.	
PSYLLIUM HUSK	Do not omit the powdered psyllium husk; it is crucial to the structure of the crust. For more information, see page 16.	

Reinventing Pizza Dough

THE PROBLEM Given that pizza dough does not have to rise as much as yeast breads, we figured this recipe would be fairly easy to transform. We'd replace the wheat flour with our flour blend and add some psyllium to help create a structural network in a dough capable of expanding around the gases produced during fermentation. We'd include the usual yeast, salt, oil, and water, and the dough would rise and bake up just fine, right? Unfortunately, our early tests were quite gummy, especially at the interface between the sauce and crust, and they weren't what you would call light and airy.

MORE LIFT, PLEASE We noticed that while the dough rose well during proofing, it didn't necessarily stay as open by the time it was baked. Rolling or pressing out the dough to make a crust expelled much of the gas, and it never seemed to recover from the handling, even when the dough was left to proof a second time, postshaping. The first thing we tried was adding more yeast, assuming it would help increase the amount of gas production in the dough and create an open crumb. Yet no matter how much we added, the dough refused to budge. In fact, the only noticeable difference it made was that, in high enough amounts, it gave the dough an unpleasantly yeasty, "overproofed" flavor.

If we couldn't get the crust to hold onto gas the whole time, maybe we could give it a little boost when it mattered most: during baking. To this end, we added a few teaspoons of baking powder to the dough. Sure enough, the leavener, activated by the heat of the oven, gave the dough a bit more of the lift it had been missing.

MORE WATER = GREATER ELASTICITY Traditional pizza dough can be rather stiff right after mixing and yet end up open and easily extensible once fully proofed, which leaves the finished product light and airy once baked. But in the case of our gluten-free pizza dough, things didn't work quite the same way. Even with psyllium in the mix and adding extra leavener, the proteins in the gluten-free flour didn't stretch enough. Maybe increasing the water (so that the dough started out looser) would help?

Even before we baked off the next batches, we could tell that we were onto something: The more water the dough contained, the more it rose during proofing. And as the amount of water increased, the finished crust became more tender and open. In fact, the dough seemed to benefit from the addition of far more water than we'd expected. The best results came when we added nearly double what you might use in a conventional recipe, making the "dough" more like a thick batter.

SHAPING A STICKY DOUGH Of course, more water presented a number of new problems. For one thing, it made shaping the crust rather challenging. Fixing this problem was easy: We went from shaping the dough by hand to spreading it on a baking sheet with a rubber spatula, much like spreading frosting on a cake, and then using a piece of plastic wrap to shape it into a pizza crust.

BAKING OFF EXCESS WATER All that water helped to make the dough more fluid and open during proofing, but it was an unwelcome guest in the oven. In order to remove the excess water, we began parbaking the crusts without sauce or cheese. We started by placing them in a hot oven until they'd dried out and begun to brown on the exterior, but that didn't really do the trick. This produced crusts that might look good on the exterior while remaining gummy inside. So we began lowering the oven temperature and increasing the baking time until the water had been driven off. In the end, we found it best to start the crusts in a cold oven and let them cook through slowly—this prevented the exterior of the crusts from overcooking before the interior was fully baked.

MORE FAT, FROM AN UNUSUAL SOURCE There remained one glaring flaw: the underside of the crust was more tough than crisp, even when parbaked as gently as possible. No problem, we thought, we would just add more oil to the dough. While this did help to crisp things up, it also left the pizza downright greasy. Even though more fat was the answer, the gluten-free flours couldn't absorb more oil. In the end, we achieved the desired crispness by adding almond flour, which boosted the overall fat content in the dough but didn't have the same greasy side effects as more oil. And, best of all, tasters couldn't detect any nut flavor in the finished pizza.

Classic Cheese Pizza
MAKES 2 PIZZAS, SERVING 4 TO 6

✔ **WHY THIS RECIPE WORKS**

Once our Pizza Crusts were parbaked and ready to go, we now needed to top and bake them. To keep things simple, we used a no-cook sauce that purees canned tomatoes, garlic, olive oil, red wine vinegar, and spices in the food processor. We supplemented the creamy, stretchy mozzarella with sharp, salty Parmesan for flavor. Using a baking stone helped to crisp the crust as it baked. If you do not have a baking stone, use a rimless or inverted baking sheet, heating it in the oven for 30 minutes. The sauce will yield more than needed in the recipe; extra sauce can be refrigerated for up to one week or frozen for up to one month.

1	(28-ounce) can whole peeled tomatoes, drained
1	tablespoon extra-virgin olive oil
1	teaspoon red wine vinegar
1	garlic clove, minced
1	teaspoon dried oregano
½	teaspoon salt
¼	teaspoon pepper
1	recipe Pizza Crusts (page 195)
1	ounce Parmesan cheese, finely grated (½ cup)
8	ounces whole-milk mozzarella cheese, shredded (2 cups)

1. One hour before baking pizza, adjust oven rack to upper-middle position, set baking stone on rack, and heat oven to 500 degrees. Process tomatoes, oil, vinegar, garlic, oregano, salt, and pepper in food processor until smooth, about 30 seconds. Transfer to bowl or container and refrigerate until ready to use.

2. Transfer 1 parbaked crust to pizza peel. Using back of spoon or ladle, spread ½ cup tomato sauce in thin layer over surface of dough, leaving ¼-inch border around edge. Sprinkle ¼ cup Parmesan evenly over sauce, followed by 1 cup mozzarella. Slide pizza carefully onto stone and bake until crust is well browned and cheese is bubbly and beginning to brown, 10 to 12 minutes. Transfer pizza to wire rack and let cool for 5 minutes before slicing and serving. Repeat with remaining crust, ½ cup tomato sauce, and remaining cheese.

VARIATION

Cheese Pizza with Prosciutto and Arugula

Toss 2 cups baby arugula with 2 teaspoons extra-virgin olive oil in bowl and season with salt and pepper to taste. Top each baked pizza with 2 ounces thinly sliced prosciutto cut into 1-inch strips, then top each with 1 cup dressed arugula. Let cool for 5 minutes before slicing and serving.

White Pizza with Ricotta, Sausage, and Bell Pepper
MAKES 2 PIZZAS, SERVING 4 TO 6

✔ **WHY THIS RECIPE WORKS**

For an altogether different take, we left out the red sauce and instead started with a combination of mozzarella and Pecorino as the base of our pizza. We then combined ricotta cheese with fresh herbs, seasonings, and a good dose of garlic and dolloped that over the top of our base. Italian sausage and red bell pepper—softened in the same skillet used to cook the sausage—added heft and color. If you do not have a baking stone, use a rimless or inverted baking sheet, heating it in the oven for 30 minutes.

4	ounces (½ cup) whole-milk ricotta cheese
2	tablespoons extra-virgin olive oil
2	tablespoons heavy cream
1	large egg yolk
2	garlic cloves, minced
1	teaspoon minced fresh oregano
½	teaspoon minced fresh thyme
⅛	teaspoon salt
⅛	teaspoon pepper
	Pinch cayenne pepper
1	pound hot or sweet Italian sausage, casings removed

1   **red bell pepper, stemmed, seeded, and cut into thin strips**
1   **recipe Pizza Crusts (page 195)**
1   **ounce Pecorino Romano cheese, finely grated (½ cup)**
8   **ounces whole-milk mozzarella cheese, shredded (2 cups)**

1. One hour before baking pizza, adjust oven rack to upper-middle position, set baking stone on rack, and heat oven to 500 degrees.

2. Whisk ricotta, oil, cream, egg yolk, garlic, oregano, thyme, salt, pepper, and cayenne together in bowl; refrigerate until ready to use. Cook sausage in 12-inch nonstick skillet over medium-high heat, breaking into small pieces with wooden spoon, until browned, about 5 minutes. Using slotted spoon, transfer sausage to paper towel–lined plate. Pour off all but 1 tablespoon fat from skillet, add bell pepper, and cook over medium heat until softened, about 5 minutes; set aside and cool to room temperature.

3. Transfer 1 parbaked crust to pizza peel. Sprinkle with ¼ cup Pecorino, followed by 1 cup mozzarella, leaving ¼-inch border around edge. Using 1 teaspoon measure, dollop half of ricotta cheese mixture evenly over pizza. Sprinkle with half of sausage and half of pepper. Slide pizza carefully onto stone and bake until crust is well browned and cheese is bubbly and beginning to brown, 10 to 12 minutes. Transfer pizza to wire rack and let cool for 5 minutes before slicing and serving. Repeat with remaining crust, remaining Pecorino and mozzarella, remaining ricotta mixture, and remaining sausage and pepper.

TEST KITCHEN TIP **Bake Before Topping**

Extra water in our dough helps it to rise and bake up tender, but all that water poses a problem during baking. The key is to parbake the crust before adding the toppings.

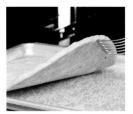

Bake dough until firm to touch, golden brown on underside, and just beginning to brown on top, 45 to 50 minutes. Cool crust before topping and baking again.

TEST KITCHEN TIP **Shaping Pizza Dough**

Our gluten-free pizza dough is much wetter than traditional pizza dough, so it does not double in size as it rises. To determine if the dough is ready for shaping, you must check that air bubbles have formed (meaning the yeast is doing its job). You will need the help of a greased rubber spatula to shape this wet, sticky dough.

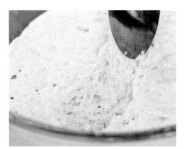 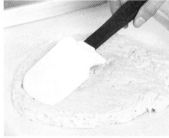 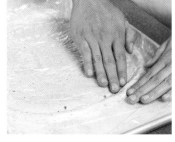

1. After dough has proofed for 90 minutes, check to determine if it is ready for shaping. Use large spoon to peer inside dough. If inside of dough is bubbly, it's ready.

2. Transfer half of dough to center of baking sheet lined with greased parchment. Using oil-sprayed spatula, spread dough into 8-inch circle, as though spreading frosting on cake.

3. Spray dough with vegetable oil spray, cover with plastic wrap, and press out to 11½-inch round, about ¼ inch thick, leaving outer ¼ inch slightly thicker than center.

Socca (Chickpea Flatbreads)

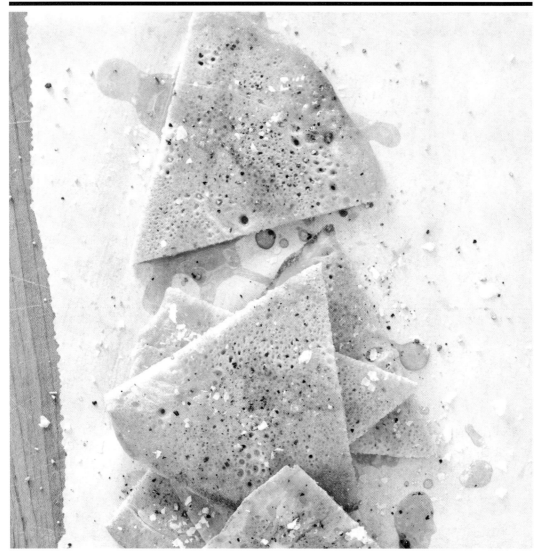

G-F TESTING LAB

CHICKPEA FLOUR As the name suggests, chickpea flour (also sold as garbanzo bean flour) is made from ground whole dried chickpeas. It is sold in most well-stocked supermarkets. See page 18 for more detail.

✓ WHY THIS RECIPE WORKS

Socca is a savory flatbread popular in southern France, where it is served as both an appetizer and a snack. The loose, pancakelike batter comes together in less than a minute—simply whisk together chickpea flour, water, olive oil, salt, and pepper—and it's naturally gluten-free. The biggest variables are the ratios of flour to water and the amount of oil. After several rounds of testing, we concluded that 1½ cups of both chickpea flour and water is best. Olive oil adds flavor, and more is better—up to a point. Any more than 3 tablespoons of oil will make the socca greasy. (More oil is used for cooking the socca.) Traditionally the batter is poured into a cast-iron skillet and baked in a large, often wood-burning oven. This method produces socca with a blistered top and a smoky flavor, but it doesn't really translate to the home oven. Instead of a crisp top, socca baked this way was dry and limp. After several more failed attempts, we ditched the oven and cast-iron skillet for the stovetop and a nonstick skillet. Up to this point, we had been filling the cast-iron skillet to create one large pancake. The ambient heat ensured the socca was cooked through. On the stovetop, however, the direct heat cooked only the bottom, leaving the top sticky and raw. And flipping the socca wasn't as easy as we'd hoped. We solved this problem by switching to a smaller skillet and using less batter to make several smaller flatbreads. As an added bonus, the smaller flatbreads now had a higher ratio of crunchy crust to tender interior. We loved the simplicity of this dish, and coming up with a few additions to our base proved easy enough. The combination of coriander and lemon highlighted the bright notes of the chickpea flour, while caramelized onions and rosemary gave the socca a more rounded, warm flavor. Serve warm socca drizzled with good olive oil and sprinkled with coarse salt and freshly ground black pepper.

Socca (Chickpea Flatbreads)
MAKES 5 FLATBREADS, SERVING 4 TO 6

- 6¾ ounces (1½ cups) chickpea (garbanzo bean) flour
- ½ teaspoon salt
- ½ teaspoon pepper
- 1½ cups water
- 6 tablespoons plus 1 teaspoon extra-virgin olive oil

1. Adjust oven rack to middle position and heat oven to 200 degrees. Set wire rack in rimmed baking sheet and place in oven. Whisk chickpea flour, salt, and pepper together in bowl. Slowly whisk in water and 3 tablespoons oil until combined and smooth.

2. Heat 2 teaspoons oil in 8-inch nonstick skillet over medium-high heat until shimmering. Add ½ cup batter to skillet, tilting pan to coat bottom evenly. Reduce heat to medium and cook until crisp at edges and golden brown on bottom, 3 to 5 minutes. Flip socca and continue to cook until second side is browned, 2 to 3 minutes. Transfer to wire rack in preheated oven. Repeat with remaining batter and oil. Cut each socca into wedges and serve.

VARIATIONS

Coriander-Lemon Socca

Add 1 teaspoon ground coriander and ½ teaspoon grated lemon zest to chickpea flour in step 1.

Caramelized Onion and Rosemary Socca

Heat 1 tablespoon olive oil in 8-inch nonstick skillet over medium-high heat until shimmering. Add ½ onion, sliced thin, reduce heat to medium, and cook, stirring often, until onion is softened and browned, about 10 minutes. Add 1½ teaspoons chopped fresh rosemary and cook until fragrant, about 30 seconds. Transfer to bowl and let cool slightly, then stir into chickpea flour batter. Wipe skillet clean and use in step 2.

Corn Tortillas

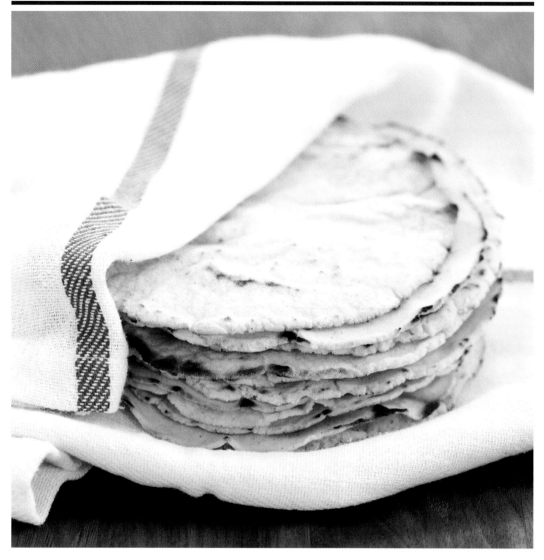

G-F TESTING LAB

MASA HARINA Maseca is the most widely available brand of masa harina. It is processed in a gluten-free facility. See page 18 for more detail on masa harina.

✓ WHY THIS RECIPE WORKS

Once you've tried homemade corn tortillas, you'll never want to buy the grocery store kind again. Fresh corn tortillas have a lightly sweet flavor and a soft, springy texture. Surprisingly, making tortillas is far easier than most people realize. Most of the recipes we researched were similar—masa harina and water are kneaded together to form a dough, then pressed into thin tortillas (either by hand or with a tortilla press) and toasted in a dry skillet. We then tested the few variables we found in our research, including whether to add salt (yes), and how long to rest the dough before pressing the tortillas (5 minutes so the masa is fully hydrated). Although you can press the dough into tortillas by hand or with a heavy skillet, we found it difficult to get the tortillas uniformly thin without lots of practice. We prefer to use a tortilla press. The dough was still a little finicky to work with, and we found that the addition of vegetable oil (a nontraditional ingredient) made the dough easier to handle. The oil also gave the cooked tortillas a softer texture that our tasters liked. When the tortilla puffs in the skillet after flipping, you know you've done it right: that's a sign that distinct layers are forming, and the finished product will be soft and tender. To reheat tortillas quickly we found it best to use the microwave. Simply stack the tortillas on a plate, sprinkle them with a little water, cover them with a paper towel, and microwave until warm and soft, 1 to 2 minutes. Tortillas can also be reheated one at a time in a skillet.

Corn Tortillas
MAKES ABOUT 22 SMALL TORTILLAS

- 10 **ounces (2 cups) masa harina**
- 2 **teaspoons vegetable oil**
- ¼ **teaspoon salt**
- 1¼ **cups warm water, plus more as needed**

1. Cut sides of sandwich-size zipper-lock bag but leave bottom seam intact so that bag folds open completely. Line tortilla press with 1 side of open bag. Line large plate with 2 damp kitchen towels.

2. Mix masa, 1 teaspoon oil, and salt together in medium bowl. Using rubber spatula, stir in water to form soft dough. Using hands, knead dough in bowl, adding more warm water, 1 tablespoon at a time, as needed, until dough is soft and tacky but not sticky, and has texture of Play-Doh. Cover and set dough aside for 5 minutes.

3. Meanwhile, heat remaining 1 teaspoon oil in 8-inch nonstick skillet over medium-high heat until shimmering. Using paper towel, wipe out skillet, leaving thin film of oil on bottom. Pinch off 1-ounce piece of dough (about 2 tablespoons) and roll into smooth 1¼-inch ball. Cover remaining dough with damp paper towel. Place ball in center of press on open bag, and fold other side of bag over dough. Press ball gently into ¹⁄₁₆-inch-thick tortilla (about 5 inches in diameter). Working quickly, gently peel plastic away from tortilla and carefully place tortilla in hot skillet.

4. Cook tortilla, without moving it, until tortilla moves freely when pan is shaken, about 30 seconds. Flip tortilla over and cook until edges curl and bottom is spotty brown, about 1 minute. Flip tortilla back over and continue to cook until first side is spotty brown and puffs up in center, 30 to 60 seconds. Lay toasted tortilla between damp kitchen towels; repeat shaping and cooking with remaining dough. (Tortillas can be transferred to zipper-lock bag and refrigerated for up to 5 days.)

TEST KITCHEN TIP **Shaping Tortillas**

Pressing the dough between a zipper-lock bag that has been cut open at the sides prevents the dough from sticking to the press and makes shaping these tortillas a breeze.

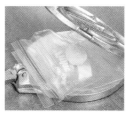

Place 1¼-inch ball of dough in center of tortilla press lined with open plastic bag. Fold other side of bag over dough. Press ball gently into ¹⁄₁₆-inch-thick tortilla.

Arepas (Corn Cakes)

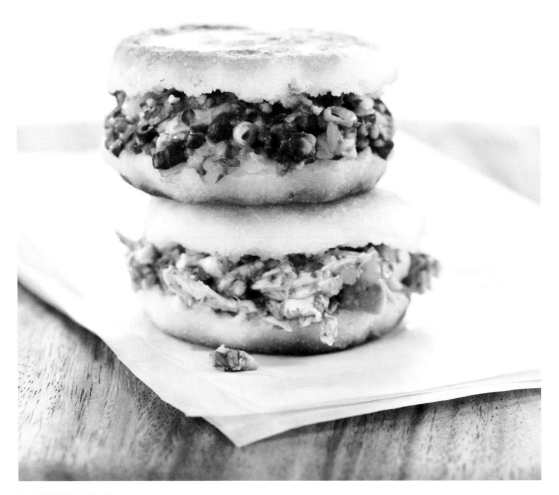

G-F TESTING LAB

MASAREPA This precooked corn flour is also known as harina precocida and masa al instante. It is prepared from starchier large kernel white corn (as opposed to the small kernel yellow corn familiar to most Americans). The germ is removed from the kernels during processing, and the kernels are dried and ground to a fine flour. Do not confuse masarepa with masa harina, which is used to make fresh Corn Tortillas (page 202) and Pupusas (page 206). Check labels carefully; not all brands are processed in a gluten-free facility.

✓ WHY THIS RECIPE WORKS

Arepas are a type of corn cake popular in Venezuela and Colombia, though iterations exist in other Latin countries. The Venezuelan variety is served as sandwiches that are split open and stuffed with anything from meat and cheese to corn, beans, or even fish. The arepa itself is made using masarepa (naturally gluten-free corn flour) along with water and salt. The dough is shaped into rounds, browned in a skillet with some oil, and finished in the oven. The cooking technique was straightforward enough and we were confident we could come up with a few delicious fillings, so we focused our attention on the ingredient list for the corn cakes. We started by testing the ratio of water to masarepa. Equal parts masarepa to warm water produced a dry, crumbly arepa, while adding significantly more water than masarepa produced a dough that was too loose to shape and fell apart during cooking. In the end, we found that using just a half cup more water than masarepa produced a dough that was easy to shape. Although moist and tender, the arepas were a little dense. A small amount of baking powder (an ingredient typically not used in arepas) lightened their texture just enough. Make either filling while the arepas are baking.

Arepas (Corn Cakes)
MAKES 8 CORN CAKES

10	ounces (2 cups) masarepa blanca
1	teaspoon salt
1	teaspoon baking powder (see page 20)
2½	cups warm water
¼	cup vegetable oil
1	recipe filling (see below)

1. Adjust oven rack to middle position and heat oven to 400 degrees. Whisk masarepa, salt, and baking powder together in bowl. Gradually add water and stir until combined. Using generous ⅓ cup dough, form eight 3-inch rounds, each about ½ inch thick.

2. Heat 2 tablespoons oil in 12-inch nonstick skillet over medium-high heat until shimmering.

Add 4 arepas and cook until golden on both sides, about 4 minutes per side. Transfer to wire rack set in rimmed baking sheet and repeat with remaining 2 tablespoons oil and remaining 4 arepas. (Fried arepas can be refrigerated in zipper-lock bag for up to 3 days or frozen for up to 1 month.)

3. Bake until arepas sound hollow when tapped on bottom, about 10 minutes. (If frozen, do not thaw before baking; increase baking time to 20 minutes.) Split hot arepas open using paring knife or 2 forks, and stuff each with generous 3 tablespoons of filling. Serve immediately.

Chicken and Avocado Filling
MAKES ENOUGH FOR 8 CORN CAKES

1	cup shredded rotisserie chicken
1	avocado, halved, pitted, and cut into ½-inch pieces
2	tablespoons minced fresh cilantro
2	scallions, sliced thin
1	tablespoon lime juice
¼	teaspoon chili powder
	Salt and pepper

Mix all ingredients together in bowl and season with salt and pepper to taste.

Black Bean and Cheese Filling
MAKES ENOUGH FOR 8 CORN CAKES

1	(15-ounce) can black beans, rinsed
4	ounces Monterey Jack cheese, shredded (1 cup)
2	tablespoons minced fresh cilantro
2	scallions, sliced thin
1	tablespoon lime juice
¼	teaspoon chili powder
	Salt and pepper

Using potato masher or fork, mash beans in bowl until most are broken. Stir in remaining ingredients and season with salt and pepper to taste.

Pupusas (Stuffed Corn Tortillas)

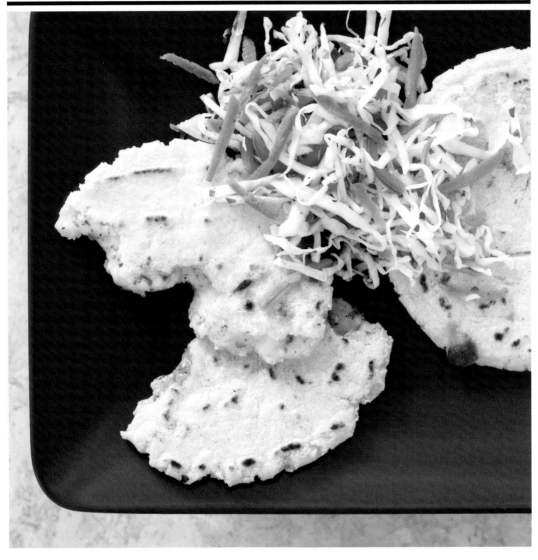

MASA HARINA   Maseca is the most widely available brand of masa harina. It is processed in a gluten-free facility. See page 18 for more detail on masa harina.

✓ WHY THIS RECIPE WORKS

Pupusas are the ultimate Salvadoran comfort food: a thick, handmade corn tortilla is stuffed with cheese and griddled until golden brown. The stuffed corn tortilla is traditionally topped with *curtido*, a tart cabbage slaw. While traditionally eaten as a side dish, we think pupusas make a great lunch or light dinner. The dough is similar to the one we use for thin corn tortillas, with a bit more water so it's more malleable and easy to stuff. For the filling, we stuck to the classic combination of cheese, spices, and cilantro. Monterey Jack cheese was the right choice here—just a few minutes in a hot skillet was all it took to melt, and its mild flavor didn't overpower the flavor of the corn flour. Make the curtido before you begin making the pupusas; as the slaw sits, the vinegar, salt, and sugar soften the cabbage and the flavor of the slaw improves.

Pupusas (Stuffed Corn Tortillas)
MAKES 10, SERVING 4 TO 6

TANGY CABBAGE SLAW
- 4 **cups shredded green cabbage**
- 1 **carrot, peeled and shredded**
- ¼ **cup cider vinegar**
- 2 **tablespoons water**
- 2 **tablespoons minced fresh cilantro**
- 1 **jalapeño chile, stemmed, seeded, and sliced thin**
- ⅛ **teaspoon minced fresh oregano**
- ½ **teaspoon sugar**
  Salt and pepper

PUPUSAS
- 6 **ounces Monterey Jack cheese, shredded (1½ cups)**
- 2 **tablespoons minced fresh cilantro**
- 2 **scallions, sliced thin**
- 1 **tablespoon lime juice**
- ¼ **teaspoon chili powder**
  Salt and pepper
- 10 **ounces (2 cups) masa harina**
- 2 **cups warm water**
- 1 **teaspoon vegetable oil**

1. FOR THE SLAW: Combine cabbage, carrot, vinegar, water, cilantro, jalapeño, oregano, sugar, and ½ teaspoon salt, and pepper to taste in bowl. Cover and refrigerate until cabbage wilts slightly, about 1 hour.

2. FOR THE PUPUSAS: Cut sides of small zipper-lock bag but leave bottom seam intact. Combine Monterey Jack, cilantro, scallions, lime juice, chili powder, and salt and pepper to taste in bowl.

3. Using rubber spatula, stir masa, water, and ¼ teaspoon salt together in medium bowl to form soft dough. Using hands, knead dough in bowl until soft and slightly tacky, but not sticky, about 1 minute.

4. Heat oil in 12-inch nonstick skillet over medium-high heat until shimmering. Using paper towel, wipe out skillet, leaving thin film of oil. Pinch off 2½-ounce piece of dough (heaping ¼ cup) and roll into ball. Cover remaining dough with damp paper towel. Using slightly wet hands, flatten into 4-inch-wide round and place 2 tablespoons of cheese mixture in center. Bring up sides of dough around filling and pinch top to seal. Press on pinched seal to flatten into 2½-inch round (about 1 inch thick). Place on 1 side of open zipper-lock bag and fold other side of bag over dough. Using large plate, press dough gently into ¼-inch-thick pupusa. Peel plastic away and place dough in hot skillet. Repeat shaping and filling, cooking 2 pupusas at a time. Cook pupusas until spotty brown on both sides, about 3 minutes per side. Transfer to platter and serve with slaw.

TEST KITCHEN TIP **Filling Pupusas**

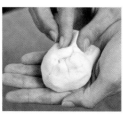

Wet hands slightly. Flatten dough ball into 4-inch patty and place 2 tablespoons of cheese mixture in center. Bring up sides of dough around filling and pinch top to seal.

Brazilian Cheese Bread Rolls

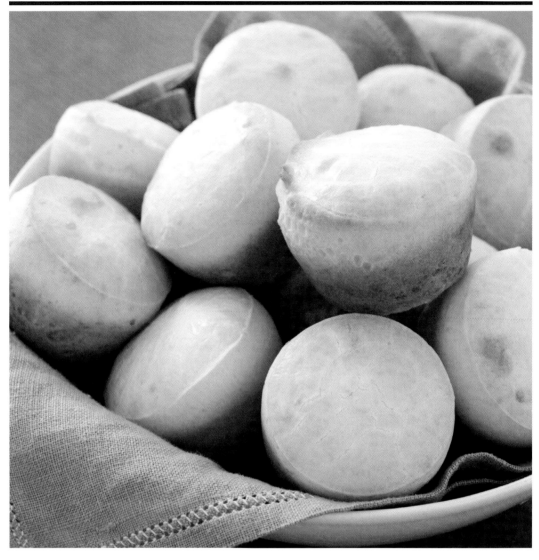

G-F TESTING LAB

TAPIOCA STARCH   Tapioca starch is often labeled tapioca flour. See page 20 for details on this ingredient.

✓ WHY THIS RECIPE WORKS

Brazilian cheese bread rolls (*pão de queijo*) are small rolls with a crunchy crust and a chewy center. They are typically made with tapioca starch, cheese, milk, oil, and eggs, so they are naturally gluten-free. There are many different approaches to the mixing method. Some recipes heat the batter on the stovetop and transfer it to a stand mixer before adding the eggs (much as you might make the dough for profiteroles or gougères). But we found that this method could be tricky. The heat made the tapioca starch quite gluey, and the dough became hard to handle. We preferred a simpler (and still traditional) approach that calls for making a looser dough (more like pancake batter) in a blender. Rather than shaping the dough by hand, we poured the resulting fluid batter into a greased mini muffin tin that we slid right into the oven. The high liquid content (from both milk and eggs) in the batter created a lot of steam in the oven that helped the rolls to rise. (There's no yeast or chemical leavener in this recipe.) We tested different types of cheese, and it was clear that these small rolls are best made with something potent, so they would pack a punch. We liked the combination of nutty Parmesan and tangy extra-sharp cheddar. These rolls are a fast snack or an accompaniment to dinner, ready in about 30 minutes (including time to heat the oven). They are best eaten warm, but leftovers can be frozen and reheated (see the instructions in sidebar at right).

Brazilian Cheese Bread Rolls
MAKES 24 SMALL ROLLS

- 8   ounces (2 cups) tapioca starch
- 4   ounces extra-sharp cheddar cheese, shredded (1 cup)
- 2   ounces Parmesan cheese, grated (1 cup)
- ⅔   cup whole milk
- ⅓   cup olive oil
- 2   large eggs
- 1   teaspoon salt

1. Adjust oven rack to middle position and heat oven to 375 degrees. Spray 24-cup mini muffin tin with vegetable oil spray. Process all ingredients together in blender until smooth, about 1 minute, scraping down sides of blender jar as needed.

2. Pour batter (about 2 tablespoons per muffin cup) into prepared muffin tin. (Each muffin cup will be nearly full.) Bake rolls until lightly golden and puffed, 17 to 20 minutes, rotating muffin tin halfway through baking. Let rolls cool in muffin tin on wire rack for 3 minutes, then remove rolls from pan. Serve warm.

TEST KITCHEN TIP
Making Cheese Bread Rolls

The "dough" for these Brazilian rolls is very loose and is easily prepared in a blender. Once combined, the batter is poured into a greased mini muffin tin and baked.

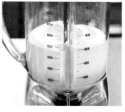 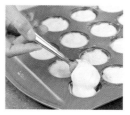

1. Process all ingredients in blender until smooth, about 1 minute, scraping down sides of blender jar as needed.

2. Pour batter (about 2 tablespoons per muffin cup) into prepared muffin tin.

TEST KITCHEN TIP
Freezing Biscuits, English Muffins, and Cheese Bread Rolls

Let biscuits, English muffins, and cheese bread rolls cool completely, then wrap individually in a double layer of plastic wrap and then a layer of aluminum foil before freezing. Biscuits can be reheated in a 425-degree oven for 10 minutes. A single English muffin, wrapped in a paper towel, can be microwaved for 20 seconds, then split and toasted. Cheese bread rolls can be reheated in a 375-degree oven for 10 minutes.

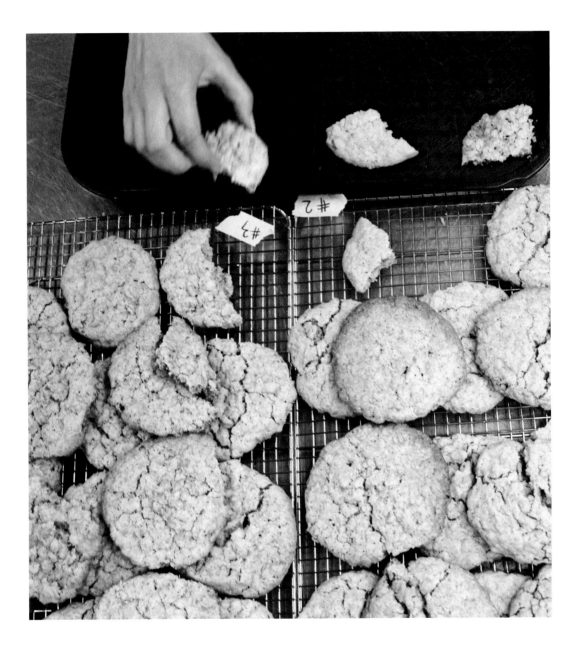

COOKIES AND BARS

Chocolate Chip Cookies

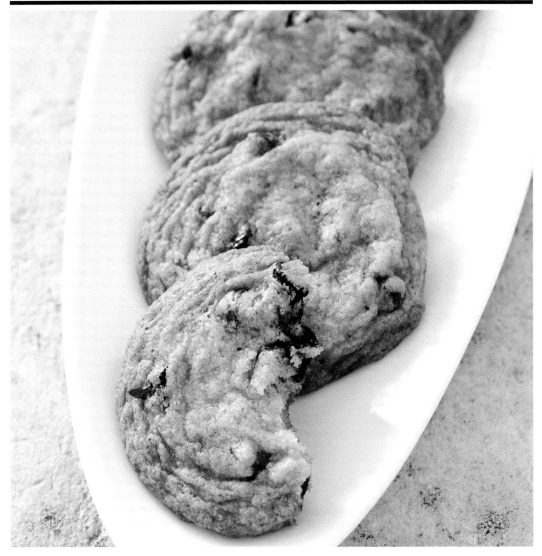

G-F TESTING LAB

FLOUR SUBSTITUTION	King Arthur Gluten-Free Multi-Purpose Flour 8 ounces = ¾ **cup plus** ⅔ **cup**	Bob's Red Mill GF All-Purpose Baking Flour 8 ounces = 1½ **cups plus 2 tablespoons**
	Note that cookies made with King Arthur will spread more and be more delicate, while cookies made with Bob's Red Mill will spread more and have a distinct bean flavor.	
XANTHAN GUM	Do not omit the xanthan gum; it is crucial to the structure of the cookies. For more information, see page 16.	
RESTING TIME	Do not shortchange the 30-minute rest for the dough; if you do, the cookies will spread too much.	

WHY THIS RECIPE WORKS

We started our testing by swapping in our flour blend for the all-purpose flour in a standard Toll House cookie recipe. It was no surprise that these cookies had problems: They were flat, sandy, and greasy. We'd discovered during our baked goods testing that gluten-free flour blends simply can't absorb as much fat as all-purpose flour can, so cutting back on the butter helped to minimize greasiness. Less butter, along with some xanthan gum, also helped alleviate the spread issue, so the cookies didn't bake up so flat. As for the sandiness, we knew from our gluten-free muffin testing (see Chapter 1) that fixing this problem required a two-step approach. The starches in our blend needed more liquid as well as more time to hydrate and soften, so we added a couple tablespoons of milk and let the dough rest for 30 minutes. This resting time also had a secondary benefit: It gave the sugar time to dissolve, which led to faster caramelization in the oven. And that meant a cookie not just with deeper flavor, but also with a chewier center and crisper edges. Finally, we wanted our cookies to be less cakey and more chewy. We realized creaming the butter, as the original Toll House recipe directs, was aerating the butter too much. Melting the butter instead, and changing the ratio of brown sugar to granulated sugar, gave our cookies the right chewy texture. The extra brown sugar also gave our cookies a more complex, toffeelike flavor. Bite for bite, this was a chocolate chip cookie that could rival the best versions of the classic. Not all brands of chocolate chips are processed in a gluten-free facility, so read labels carefully.

Chocolate Chip Cookies
MAKES ABOUT 24 COOKIES

- 8 ounces (1¾ cups) ATK Gluten-Free Flour Blend (page 13)
- 1 teaspoon baking soda
- ¾ teaspoon xanthan gum
- ½ teaspoon salt
- 8 tablespoons unsalted butter, melted
- 5¼ ounces (¾ cup packed) light brown sugar
- 2⅓ ounces (⅓ cup) granulated sugar
- 1 large egg
- 2 tablespoons milk
- 1 tablespoon vanilla extract
- 7½ ounces (1¼ cups) semisweet chocolate chips

1. Whisk flour blend, baking soda, xanthan gum, and salt together in medium bowl; set aside. Whisk melted butter, brown sugar, and granulated sugar together in large bowl until well combined and smooth. Whisk in egg, milk, and vanilla and continue to whisk until smooth. Stir in flour mixture with rubber spatula and mix until soft, homogeneous dough forms. Fold in chocolate chips. Cover bowl with plastic wrap and let dough rest for 30 minutes. (Dough will be sticky and soft.)

2. Adjust oven rack to middle position and heat oven to 350 degrees. Line 2 baking sheets with parchment paper. Using 2 soupspoons and working with about 1½ tablespoons of dough at a time, portion dough and space 2 inches apart on prepared sheets. Bake cookies, 1 sheet at a time, until golden brown and edges have begun to set but centers are still soft, 11 to 13 minutes, rotating sheet halfway through baking.

3. Let cookies cool on sheet for 5 minutes, then transfer to wire rack. Serve warm or at room temperature. (Cookies are best eaten on day they are baked, but they can be cooled and placed immediately in airtight container and stored at room temperature for up to 1 day.)

TEST KITCHEN TIP
Cooling and Storing Gluten-Free Cookies

Like their traditional counterparts, gluten-free cookies need to briefly cool on the baking sheet when they come out of the oven. This gives them time to set up, reducing the chance they'll break when you slide a spatula underneath. Once they've slightly cooled, move them to a wire rack to finish cooling according to the recipe.

But keep in mind that you don't want to let them sit out for an extended time. Like other gluten-free baked goods, these cookies have a shorter shelf life than cookies made with all-purpose flour. Gluten-free flour blends have a higher starch content, and that starch is very good at absorbing moisture. It continues to absorb the moisture in the cookies over time, making them taste drier and crumble more easily. Consequently, they are best eaten the day they are made.

However, if you do want to store leftover baked cookies, we have found that they will keep acceptably well in an airtight container for a day or two at room temperature. But don't refrigerate any of these cookies because that will make them only drier. And if you do store them, we recommend using a container instead of a zipper-lock bag, and stacking them in as few layers as possible, using parchment in between each layer, since the cookies become more delicate over time and fare better with sturdier protection.

TEST KITCHEN TIP
Freezing Cookie Dough

Given the fact gluten-free cookies don't store all that well—and that a fresh cookie, gluten-free or traditional, is better than an old one—we have found that freezing the cookie dough is a good option in some recipes. For the drop-style cookies, you can freeze portioned and shaped cookie dough as directed in the recipe, then bake off cookies straight from the freezer as you want them. This process applies to Chocolate Chip, Chocolate, Peanut Butter, and Chewy Sugar Cookies. Note that the dough for our Oatmeal-Raisin Cookies doesn't freeze well (the cookies become tough).

For the Holiday Cookies, after making the dough and shaping it into disks, you can wrap each disk in plastic and refrigerate for up to two days or freeze for up to two weeks. Just make sure to defrost frozen dough completely in the refrigerator overnight before rolling it out. The Shortbread dough does not freeze well.

Bars likewise are best eaten the day they are made. Between the starches in the flour blend and the additional moisture, the lemon and raspberry bars just don't keep more than a day; for this brief period you can store raspberry bars at room temperature, and lemon bars in the refrigerator. The brownies will hold well at room temperature for a couple of days.

To bake frozen cookie dough, arrange the dough balls (do not thaw) on parchment-lined baking sheet and bake as directed, increasing baking time by 2 to 5 minutes.

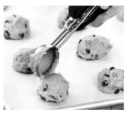 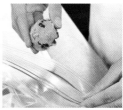

1. After portioning and shaping dough according to recipe, arrange unbaked cookies on baking sheet. Place sheet in freezer.

2. Freeze dough until completely firm, 2 to 3 hours, then transfer to zipper-lock freezer bag and freeze for up to 2 weeks.

Chocolate Chip Cookies

In the pantheon of cookies, chocolate chip cookies are just about everyone's favorite. But gluten-free versions are all too often overly cakey or gritty—a far cry from the classic. Here's how we made gluten-free chocolate chip cookies with a rich, buttery flavor, a crisp exterior, and a tender but not too cakey interior.

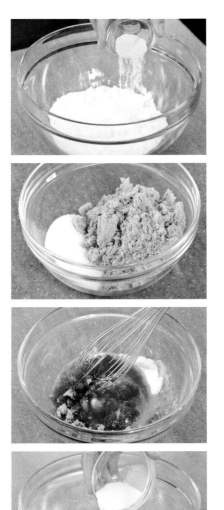

1. ADD XANTHAN GUM: Because starches are liquid when hot and don't set up until cool, and because the bonds between the proteins in gluten-free flour blends are weak and few in number, gluten-free cookies don't have the ability to hold their shape like traditional cookies, which have the power of gluten to provide structure, even when hot. To prevent the cookies from spreading all over the baking sheet, we needed to add something to reinforce the weak structure of our gluten-free flour. Just a small amount of xanthan gum did the trick.

2. GET THE SUGAR RATIO RIGHT: We wanted a cookie that was chewy in the center and slightly crisp on the outside. The Toll House cookie recipe calls for equal amounts of granulated sugar and brown sugar. Granulated sugar contributes to a caramelized, crisp texture and provides structure, while brown sugar adds moisture and rich caramel notes. We went up on brown sugar and down on granulated sugar to achieve a perfectly chewy center with crisp edges. Using more brown sugar than white also enhanced the butterscotch flavor notes in this classic cookie.

3. USE LESS BUTTER (AND MELT IT): A traditional chocolate chip cookie recipe has about 12 tablespoons of butter, but our gluten-free version couldn't handle this much fat. That's because our flour blend has more starch and less protein than all-purpose flour has, and it's the proteins that are compatible with fat. We found that 8 tablespoons of butter were the most our cookies could handle; any additional butter couldn't be absorbed and so made the cookies greasy. Creaming aerated the butter, which made the cookies too cakey; melting the butter got us closer to the texture we were after.

4. HYDRATE THE DOUGH: Because we had to decrease the amount of butter in our cookies, the dough had very little liquid to hydrate the flour (remember, butter is about 18 percent water) and we were left with gritty cookies. To solve this problem, we added a small amount of liquid to our dough in the form of milk, and then we let the dough rest to give the starches enough time to absorb the liquid. Two tablespoons of milk and a 30-minute rest hydrated the dough just enough to eliminate grittiness. Resting the dough also helped stiffen it, which improved structure and prevented spread.

Chocolate Cookies

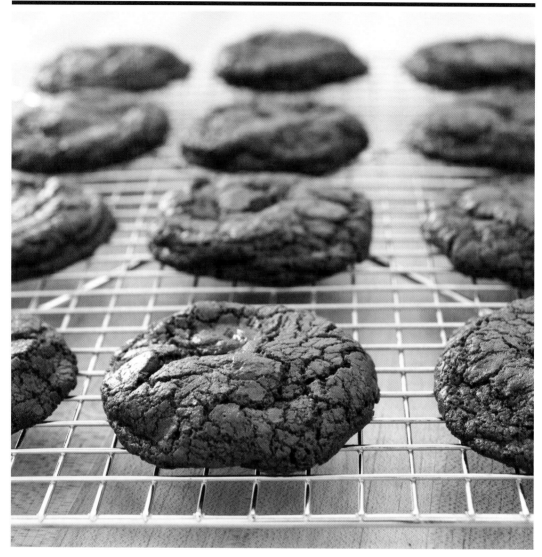

G-F TESTING LAB

FLOUR SUBSTITUTION	King Arthur Gluten-Free Multi-Purpose Flour 4 ounces = ¾ **cup**	Bob's Red Mill GF All-Purpose Baking Flour 4 ounces = ½ **cup plus** ⅓ **cup**
	Note that cookies made with King Arthur will be more cakey and slightly gritty, while cookies made with Bob's Red Mill will have a slight bean flavor.	
XANTHAN GUM	Do not omit the xanthan gum; it is crucial to the structure of the cookies. For more information, see page 16.	
CHOCOLATE	Not all brands of chocolate are processed in a gluten-free facility; read the label.	
RESTING TIME	Do not shortchange the 30-minute rest for the dough; if you do, the cookies will spread too much.	

WHY THIS RECIPE WORKS

There are two big issues with most gluten-free cookies (and, really, with gluten-free baking in general): off-flavors and dry, tough textures. But given the huge amount of flavor and moisture melted chocolate can provide, you'd think that making a great gluten-free chocolate cookie would be easy. Not so fast. Even the most promising recipes we tried failed us, with subpar chocolate flavor and a pervasive dry texture. So we started by amping up the chocolate flavor, adding not just melted chocolate but also chips, cocoa powder, and a little espresso powder (which is great for creating more complex chocolate flavor in baked goods). To address the texture, we began by tinkering with the sugar. Cookies made with all granulated sugar were too crisp, but those made with all brown sugar resulted in cookies that were so moist they were flimsy. A compromise was in order. To ensure sufficient structure, our cookies required ¼ cup of granulated sugar (along with xanthan gum). And ¾ cup of brown sugar brought the sweetness to the right level (and made the flavor more complex), while boosting the chewy texture. Still, they weren't chewy enough, so we turned to the butter. We'd just learned from developing our Fudgy Brownies recipe (page 236) that using both unsaturated fat (oil) and saturated fat (butter)—and a higher proportion of unsaturated to saturated—delivered chewier brownies. So wouldn't the same logic apply to our cookies? We switched out 5 tablespoons of butter for vegetable oil, and just as we'd suspected, we got the chewy cookies we were after. And finally, resting the dough for 30 minutes ensured the starches in our flour blend were fully hydrated, preventing any chance of a gritty texture. Dutch-processed or natural unsweetened cocoa powder will work in this recipe.

Chocolate Cookies
MAKES ABOUT 24 COOKIES

- 12 **ounces semisweet chocolate, chopped**
- 4 **ounces (¾ cup plus 2 tablespoons) ATK Gluten-Free Flour Blend (page 13)**
- ¾ **ounce (¼ cup) unsweetened cocoa powder**
- ½ **teaspoon baking soda**
- ½ **teaspoon salt**
- ¼ **teaspoon xanthan gum**
- 5¼ **ounces (¾ cup packed) light brown sugar**
- 1¾ **ounces (¼ cup) granulated sugar**
- 2 **large eggs**
- 5 **tablespoons vegetable oil**
- 2 **tablespoons unsalted butter, melted and cooled**
- 1 **teaspoon vanilla extract**
- ½ **teaspoon instant espresso powder**
- 9 **ounces (1½ cups) bittersweet chocolate chips**

1. Microwave semisweet chocolate in bowl at 50 percent power, stirring occasionally, until melted, 2 to 4 minutes; let cool slightly. In separate bowl, whisk together flour blend, cocoa, baking soda, salt, and xanthan gum; set aside.

2. Whisk brown sugar, granulated sugar, eggs, oil, melted butter, vanilla, and espresso powder together in large bowl until well combined and smooth, then whisk in cooled chocolate. Stir in flour mixture with rubber spatula until soft, homogeneous dough forms. Fold in chocolate chips. Cover bowl with plastic wrap and let dough rest for 30 minutes. (Dough will be sticky and soft.)

3. Adjust oven rack to middle position and heat oven to 350 degrees. Line 2 baking sheets with parchment paper. Working with 2 generous tablespoons of dough at a time, roll into balls and space 2 inches apart on prepared sheets. Bake cookies, 1 sheet at a time, until puffed and cracked and edges have begun to set but centers are still soft (cookies will look raw between cracks and seem underdone), 12 to 14 minutes, rotating sheet halfway through baking.

4. Let cookies cool on sheet for 5 minutes, then transfer to wire rack. Serve warm or at room temperature. (Cookies are best eaten on day they are baked, but they can be cooled and placed immediately in airtight container and stored at room temperature for up to 2 days.)

Oatmeal-Raisin Cookies

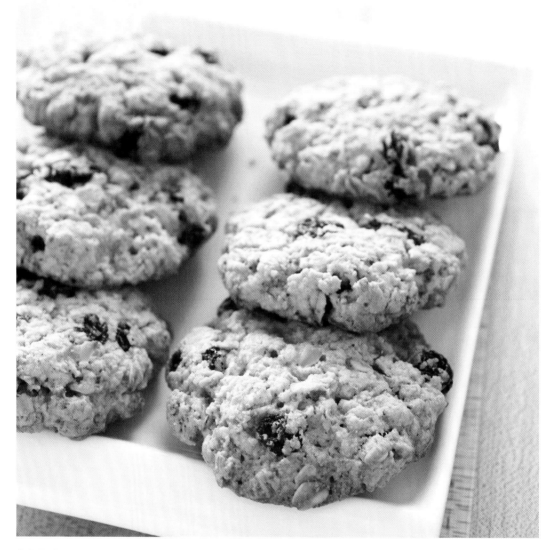

G-F TESTING LAB

FLOUR SUBSTITUTION	King Arthur Gluten-Free Multi-Purpose Flour 3 ounces = ⅓ **cup plus** ¼ **cup**	Bob's Red Mill GF All-Purpose Baking Flour 3 ounces = ½ **cup plus 2 tablespoons**
	Note that cookies made with King Arthur will be harder and drier, while cookies made with Bob's Red Mill will be stickier and will have a slight bean flavor.	
XANTHAN GUM	Do not omit the xanthan gum; it is crucial to the structure of the cookies. For more information, see page 16.	
RESTING TIME	Do not shortchange the 30-minute rest for the dough; if you do, the cookies will spread too much.	

WHY THIS RECIPE WORKS

You'd think creating a gluten-free oatmeal-raisin cookie would be easy. But our favorite test kitchen recipe, which calls for 3 cups of rolled oats, also requires a good amount of flour. When we swapped in our flour blend, we ended up with rock-hard pucks. Between the oats and all the starches in the flour blend, the moisture was getting soaked up entirely. We tried the simplest solution first—adding water to the dough—but this resulted in cookies that were thin and tough. Thinking of ways to add moisture and create a more tender cookie without the spread, we combined a portion of the oats (toasted first to enhance their flavor) with a small amount of water. Within 10 minutes, the oats had soaked up the liquid and softened. We stirred them into the dough, let the dough rest for 30 minutes to hydrate the starches in our flour blend and thus avoid grittiness, then baked off a batch. These cookies set up well and were more tender. But now we had a new problem: Our cookies were too cakey. We took a cue from our Chewy Sugar Cookies (page 221) and substituted almond flour for a few ounces of our flour blend. This gave our cookies richness, heft, and chew without any noticeable almond flavor. (See page 222 for instructions on making your own almond flour.) After portioning the dough onto the baking sheet, flatten the dough balls to ensure that the oats spread out evenly. Do not use quick oats in this recipe.

Oatmeal-Raisin Cookies
MAKES ABOUT 24 COOKIES

- 9 ounces (3 cups) gluten-free old-fashioned rolled oats
- ½ cup warm tap water
- 4 ounces (¾ cup plus 2 tablespoons) almond flour
- 3 ounces (⅔ cup) ATK Gluten-Free Flour Blend (page 13)
- ½ teaspoon salt
- ½ teaspoon baking powder (see page 20)
- ¼ teaspoon xanthan gum
- ⅛ teaspoon ground nutmeg
- 7 ounces (1 cup packed) brown sugar
- 3½ ounces (½ cup) granulated sugar
- 8 tablespoons unsalted butter, melted and cooled
- 1 large egg, plus 1 large yolk
- 2 tablespoons vegetable oil
- 1 teaspoon vanilla extract
- 1 cup raisins

1. Adjust oven rack to middle position and heat oven to 375 degrees. Spread oats evenly on rimmed baking sheet and bake until fragrant and lightly browned, about 10 minutes, stirring halfway through baking; cool on wire rack. Transfer half of cooled oats to bowl and stir in water. Cover bowl with plastic wrap and let sit until water is absorbed, about 10 minutes.

2. Whisk almond flour, flour blend, salt, baking powder, xanthan gum, and nutmeg together in medium bowl; set aside. Whisk brown sugar, granulated sugar, melted butter, egg and yolk, oil, and vanilla together in large bowl until well combined and smooth. Stir in flour mixture, oat-water mixture, and remaining toasted oats using rubber spatula until soft, homogeneous dough forms. Fold in raisins. Cover bowl with plastic and let dough rest for 30 minutes.

3. Adjust oven rack to middle position and heat oven to 325 degrees. Line 2 baking sheets with parchment paper. Working with 2 generous tablespoons of dough at a time, roll into balls and space 2 inches apart on prepared sheets. Press dough to ½-inch thickness using bottom of greased measuring cup. Bake cookies, 1 sheet at a time, until edges are set and beginning to brown but centers are still soft and puffy, 22 to 25 minutes, rotating sheet halfway through baking.

4. Let cookies cool on sheet for 5 minutes, then transfer to wire rack. Serve warm or at room temperature. (Cookies are best eaten on day they are baked, but they can be cooled and placed immediately in airtight container and stored at room temperature for up to 2 days.)

Oatmeal-Raisin Cookies

Great oatmeal-raisin cookies should be soft and chewy and have a lot of oat flavor, whether they're made with wheat flour or gluten-free flour. Unfortunately, substituting our flour blend, which is lower in protein and higher in starch compared with all-purpose flour, coupled with the addition of plenty of moisture-absorbing rolled oats, created a dry, tough cookie. To achieve the right balance of tender crumb and slight chew, here's what we did.

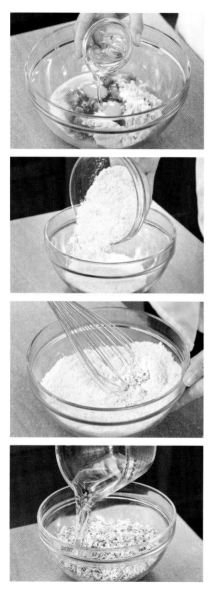

1. USE BUTTER AND OIL: A traditional oatmeal-raisin cookie uses butter, not oil. Butter provides good nutty flavor that complements oats, and it provides moisture. Butter (unlike oil) is not a pure fat: It contains about 18 percent water. During baking, that water turns to steam, which gives the cookie a little extra rise and also creates a more tender crumb. However, in our gluten-free version, we found that using only butter for the fat gave us a cookie that had a more cakelike than cookie-like texture. Swapping in some oil for butter (we settled on a 4:1 ratio of butter to oil) helped make our cookies less cakey.

2. ADD ALMOND FLOUR: The oil helped to make our cookies less cakey, but they needed to be chewier still, plus they baked up flat. We looked to our flour blend as the next ingredient to tweak. Just as with all-purpose flour, the proteins in the blend form an elastic structure around the starches. But the low protein content in the blend translates to less structure in the cookie. To boost the protein—and thus give our cookies more substance and chew—we swapped in 4 ounces of high-protein almond flour for a portion of our blend. With about three times as much protein, this substitution made a huge improvement.

3. SKIP THE SODA, ADD THE POWDER: Many cookie recipes contain baking powder and baking soda. Baking soda interferes with proteins in the flour (in both gluten-free and all-purpose flour) that create structure, causing the cookies to spread. We found baking soda didn't do our cookies any favors; the dough spread out into a thin layer around a clump of oats. For even spread and distribution of oats, we were better off omitting the soda and simply pressing each portion of dough into a ½-inch-thick cookie before baking. Baking powder was a keeper, giving our cookies the proper rise and a tender crumb.

4. SOAK THE OATS: The real key to making our cookies soft and tender lay in the amount of moisture in our dough and how it was incorporated. Starchy gluten-free flour blends soak up lots of moisture, as do oats, and the liquid from the eggs, butter, and sugar wasn't enough for this cookie dough. For a dough that was moist but not overly loose, we found the key was adding water to some of the oats and letting them sit for 10 minutes. Once the liquid was absorbed, we stirred the oats into the dough. This gave us just the right soft, tender cookie.

Chewy Sugar Cookies

✓ WHY THIS RECIPE WORKS

Sugar cookies usually rely on just a handful of ingredients—granulated sugar, flour, butter, leavener, and eggs. So when we plugged our flour blend into a recipe, we weren't surprised to find the gluten-free flour's starchy flavor and mouthfeel to be far too noticeable. Plus, these cookies were greasy and stale-tasting, and they spread too much. Fixing the greasiness was easy; we cut back on the butter. But this change made our cookies too lean-tasting. We often add dairy products to baked goods for richness and tenderness, so we tried adding heavy cream, but it was too thin and made our dough liquid-y. Likewise when we tried sour cream, we ended up with a soupy dough. Cream cheese, however, enriched the dough without making it loose and was a clear step in the right direction. Letting the dough rest helped avoid grittiness, but to mitigate the starchy flavor we eventually realized we needed to find something to replace a portion of the starchy flour blend. Scanning the long list of gluten-free flours, we realized most were off the table since they either were equally (if not more) starchy or had unwelcome off-flavors. But then we landed on nut flours. Almond flour had a neutral flavor and color that went unnoticed in our cookies. Replacing a portion of our blend with it not only broke up the starchiness, but it also gave our cookies a much-needed heft and chew because of the additional protein it contributed. For the leaveners, we found that our cookies needed both baking powder and baking soda. Baking powder provided the right amount of lift, while baking soda helped them spread just enough. Baking soda also gave our cookies the right crackly top, creating bubbles in the dough that rose to the top of each cookie during baking and left fissures behind. And finally, before baking we rolled each portion of dough in sugar for added texture, visual appeal, and a little extra sweetness, then flattened them with the bottom of a measuring cup to ensure even baking. The final dough will be softer than most cookie doughs. For the best results, handle the dough as briefly and as gently as possible when shaping the cookies.

Chewy Sugar Cookies
MAKES ABOUT 24 COOKIES

- 8 ounces (1¾ cups) ATK Gluten-Free Flour Blend (page 13)
- 4 ounces (¾ cup plus 2 tablespoons) almond flour
- 1 teaspoon baking powder (see page 20)
- ½ teaspoon baking soda
- ½ teaspoon salt
- ½ teaspoon xanthan gum
- 8¾ ounces (1¼ cups) sugar, plus ⅓ cup for rolling
- 3 ounces cream cheese, softened and cut into 8 pieces
- 8 tablespoons unsalted butter, melted and still warm
- 1 large egg
- 1 tablespoon vanilla extract

1. Whisk flour blend, almond flour, baking powder, baking soda, salt, and xanthan gum together in medium bowl; set aside. Place 1¼ cups sugar and cream cheese in large bowl. Place remaining ⅓ cup sugar in shallow dish and set aside. Pour warm butter over sugar and cream cheese and whisk to combine (some small lumps of cream cheese will remain but will smooth out later). Whisk in egg and vanilla and continue to whisk until smooth. Stir in flour mixture with rubber spatula and mix until soft, homogeneous dough forms. Cover bowl with plastic wrap and refrigerate until chilled, about 30 minutes. (Dough will be sticky and soft.)

2. Adjust oven rack to middle position and heat oven to 350 degrees. Line 2 baking sheets with parchment paper. Using 2 soupspoons and working with 2 tablespoons of dough at a time, portion 6 cookies and place in sugar to coat. Roll each ball in sugar, then space 2 inches apart on prepared sheets. Repeat with remaining dough in batches. Press dough to ½-inch thickness using bottom of measuring cup. Sprinkle tops of cookies evenly with sugar remaining

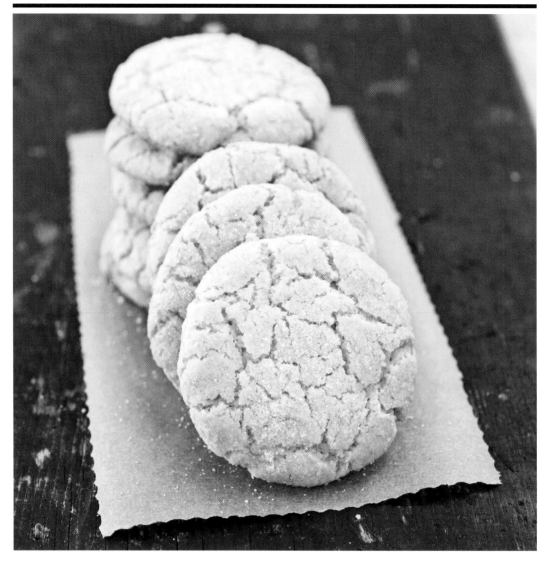

G-F TESTING LAB

FLOUR SUBSTITUTION	King Arthur Gluten-Free Multi-Purpose Flour 8 ounces = ¾ **cup plus** ⅔ **cup**	Bob's Red Mill GF All-Purpose Baking Flour 8 ounces = 1½ **cups plus 2 tablespoons**
	Note that cookies made with King Arthur will spread more and be more delicate, while cookies made with Bob's Red Mill will spread more and have a distinct bean flavor.	
ALMOND FLOUR	If you don't have almond flour, you can process 4 ounces blanched almonds in a food processor until finely ground, about 45 seconds.	
XANTHAN GUM	Do not omit the xanthan gum; it is crucial to the structure of the cookies. For more information, see page 16.	
RESTING TIME	Resting the dough for 30 minutes keeps the cookies from spreading too much.	

in shallow dish for rolling, using 2 teaspoons for each sheet. (Discard remaining sugar.)

3. Bake cookies, 1 sheet at a time, until edges are set and just beginning to brown, 12 to 14 minutes, rotating sheet halfway through baking. Let cookies cool on sheet for 5 minutes, then transfer to wire rack. Serve warm or at room temperature. (Cookies are best eaten on day they are baked, but they can be cooled and placed immediately in airtight container and stored at room temperature for up to 1 day.)

TEST KITCHEN TIP **Shaping Sugar Cookies**

Sugar-cookie dough is particularly sticky because of all the sugar it contains. Dropping balls of dough directly into the sugar, then rolling each ball in the sugar shapes them into rounds and gives them their sugary coating in a single, easy step.

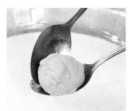 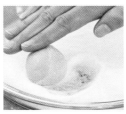

1. Using 2 soupspoons and working with 2 tablespoons of dough at a time, portion 6 cookies into shallow dish with sugar.

2. Roll each ball in sugar, then space 2 inches apart on prepared sheets.

TEST KITCHEN TIP **Portioning Drop Cookies**

In our drop-cookie recipes, we often call for portioning dough using soupspoons because we know everyone owns them. But gluten-free cookie dough is often quite sticky, so our preferred method is to use a spring-loaded scoop. It not only ensures consistent size and proper yield, but it makes the process faster and easier. We think it's well worth the small investment. The number stamped on the handle of these scoops corresponds to the number of level scoops needed to make 32 ounces. (Remember: 1 ounce equals 2 tablespoons.) Use a #40 scoop for our Chocolate Chip Cookies, and a #30 scoop for our Chocolate, Oatmeal-Raisin, Chewy Sugar, or Peanut Butter Cookies.

SMART SHOPPING
Baking Powder and Baking Soda

Leaveners are critical to gluten-free baking in general (see page 20 for more detail), but with cookies, traditional and gluten-free, they take on very distinct roles. You'll find both baking powder and baking soda used in many of our cookie recipes because together they help create cookies that not only rise but also spread to the right degree. Baking powder is responsible for lift, since it is engineered to produce most of its gas after the cookies go in the oven. But too much lift means humped cookies that bake unevenly. That's where baking soda comes in. It interferes with proteins in the dough and disrupts the structure, causing the cookies to spread. Baking soda also has an aesthetic effect: It delivers cookies with a crackly top.

TEST KITCHEN TIP
Pressing and Baking Cookies

To ensure even baking, we use the bottom of a flat-bottomed dry measuring cup to press each portion of dough for our Chewy Sugar, Oatmeal-Raisin, and Peanut Butter Cookies flat on baking sheets before moving the sheets to the oven. And since the doughs for our Oatmeal-Raisin and Peanut Butter Cookies are particularly moist (and don't have the barrier of a sugar coating like we use in our Chewy Sugar Cookies), in those recipes we also grease the bottom of the measuring cup to prevent sticking.

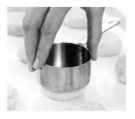

Using bottom of measuring cup, press each portion of dough to thickness indicated in specific recipe.

Peanut Butter Cookies

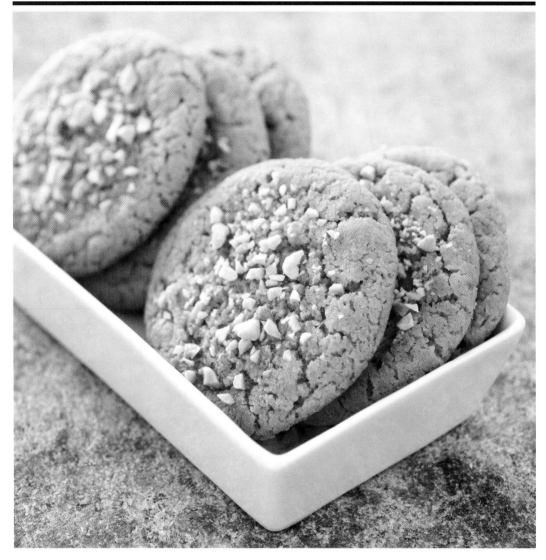

G-F TESTING LAB

FLOUR SUBSTITUTION	King Arthur Gluten-Free Multi-Purpose Flour 8 ounces = ¾ **cup plus** ⅔ **cup**	Bob's Red Mill GF All-Purpose Baking Flour 8 ounces = 1½ **cups plus 2 tablespoons**
	Note that cookies made with King Arthur will be denser and spread less, while cookies made with Bob's Red Mill will have a slight bean flavor.	
XANTHAN GUM	Do not omit the xanthan gum; it is crucial to the structure of the cookies. For more information, see page 16.	
RESTING TIME	Do not shortchange the 30-minute rest for the dough; if you do, the cookies will spread too much.	

✔ WHY THIS RECIPE WORKS

Gluten-free or not, most peanut butter cookies are either dry and sandy or overly cakey, and they all come up short on peanut butter flavor. We wanted a chewy, really peanut-buttery cookie that was also gluten-free. We started with the starring ingredient. We were surprised that we preferred commercial peanut butter (like Skippy) over natural-style peanut butters. The cookies made with the commercial varieties had a nice rise, a crisp edge, and a soft center; cookies made with all-natural options were sadly dry and crumbly. And smooth peanut butter won out over chunky since the latter gave the cookies an unappealing coarse texture. We found that we could pack a full cup of peanut butter into our cookies, but only as long as we kept the butter in check to avoid greasiness. To avoid cakey cookies, we used just enough flour to provide the necessary structure and volume. Even with less flour, we found we still needed to rest the dough for 30 minutes to ensure the starches in the flour blend were fully hydrated. Getting the sweeteners just right was key since we didn't want the sugars to overwhelm the peanut butter flavor, plus they were major players in the final texture. Granulated sugar was necessary for crisp edges and structure (along with xanthan gum), while brown sugar contributed chew and a nice molasses flavor that complemented the peanut butter. The cookies will look underdone after 12 to 14 minutes, but they will set up as they cool. The baking time is very important, and 2 minutes can be the difference between a soft, chewy cookie and a crisp cookie.

Peanut Butter Cookies
MAKES ABOUT 24 COOKIES

- 8 ounces (1¾ cups) ATK Gluten-Free Flour Blend (page 13)
- 1 teaspoon baking soda
- ½ teaspoon salt
- ¼ teaspoon xanthan gum
- 7 ounces (1 cup packed) light brown sugar
- 5¼ ounces (¾ cup) granulated sugar
- 1 cup creamy peanut butter
- 8 tablespoons unsalted butter, melted and still warm
- 2 large eggs
- 1 teaspoon vanilla extract
- ⅓ cup dry-roasted peanuts, chopped fine

1. Whisk flour blend, baking soda, salt, and xanthan gum together in medium bowl; set aside. Combine brown sugar, granulated sugar, and peanut butter in large bowl. Pour warm butter over sugar mixture and whisk to combine. Whisk in eggs and vanilla and continue to whisk until smooth. Stir in flour mixture with rubber spatula and mix until soft, homogeneous dough forms. Cover bowl with plastic wrap and let rest for 30 minutes. (Dough will be slightly shiny and soft.)

2. Adjust oven rack to middle position and heat oven to 325 degrees. Line 2 baking sheets with parchment paper. Working with 2 generous tablespoons of dough at a time, roll into balls and space 2 inches apart on prepared sheets. Press dough to ¾-inch thickness using bottom of greased measuring cup. Sprinkle tops evenly with peanuts.

3. Bake cookies, 1 sheet at a time, until puffed and edges have begun to set but centers are still soft (cookies will look underdone), 12 to 14 minutes, rotating sheet halfway through baking. Let cookies cool on sheet for 5 minutes, then transfer to wire rack. Serve warm or at room temperature. (Cookies are best eaten on day they are baked, but they can be cooled and placed immediately in airtight container and stored at room temperature for up to 1 day.)

Pignoli

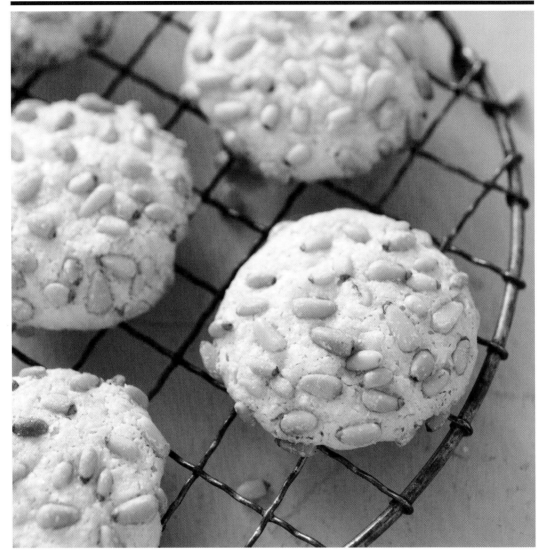

G-F TESTING LAB

ALMONDS   This recipe calls for slivered almonds, which are blanched during processing to remove the brown skin from the nuts. You can use sliced almonds if they have been blanched to remove the somewhat bitter skin.

WHY THIS RECIPE WORKS

With an appealingly light texture from egg whites (no yolks), and a nutty flavor profile that takes them beyond one-note macaroons and meringues, these classic Southern Italian cookies require only a few ingredients, are simple to make, and are also naturally gluten-free. For the base, most recipes we found rely on almond paste, and many call for both honey and granulated sugar for sweeteners. For a deeper, richer almond flavor and more controlled sweetness, we passed over the almond paste in favor of processing slivered almonds with our sweetener and egg whites. We found that granulated sugar alone was best here; honey was too intense and added flavors that tasters felt distracted from the otherwise clean, simple profile of the pignoli. Using slightly more almonds than sugar by volume also helped to keep the sweetness in check. Processing the almonds to a fine consistency was key to making cookies that held together, as any straggling bits of almond disrupted the texture. Some recipes we found added lemon or orange zest, but once again we found that these additions were more a distraction than an asset. Our base was a little sticky, but it was still easy enough to roll into balls, then coat in pine nuts for the classic finish to this Italian after-dinner cookie. There was no need to toast the pine nuts ahead of time since they toasted as the cookies baked. We let the baked cookies cool completely to room temperature to ensure they set up properly. These simple yet elegant cookies are perfect matched with dessert wine or coffee.

Pignoli
MAKES ABOUT 18 COOKIES

- 1⅔ cups slivered almonds
- 9⅓ ounces (1⅓ cups) sugar
- 2 large egg whites
- 1 cup pine nuts

1. Adjust oven racks to upper-middle and lower-middle positions and heat oven to 375 degrees. Line 2 baking sheets with parchment paper.

2. Process almonds and sugar in food processor until finely ground, about 30 seconds. Scrape down sides of bowl and add egg whites. Continue to process until smooth (dough will be wet), about 30 seconds; transfer mixture to bowl. Place pine nuts in shallow dish.

3. Working with 1 scant tablespoon dough at a time, roll into balls, roll in pine nuts to coat, and space 2 inches apart on prepared sheets.

4. Bake cookies until light golden brown, 13 to 15 minutes, switching and rotating sheets halfway through baking. Let cookies cool on sheets for 5 minutes, then transfer to wire rack. Let cookies cool to room temperature before serving. (Cookies can be stored in airtight container at room temperature for up to 4 days.)

SMART SHOPPING **Pine Nuts**

Also called piñons (Spanish) or pignoli (Italian), these diminutive nutlike seeds are actually harvested from pine cones. There are two main types of pine nuts: the delicately flavored, torpedo-shaped Mediterranean pine nuts and the more assertive corn kernel–shaped Chinese pine nuts. The less-expensive Chinese variety is more widely available, but both can be used interchangeably. Pine nuts have a mild taste and a slightly waxy texture. They need to be stored with care to prevent rancidity, and are best transferred to an airtight container as soon as their original packaging is opened. They will keep in the refrigerator for up to three months or in the freezer for up to nine months.

Shortbread

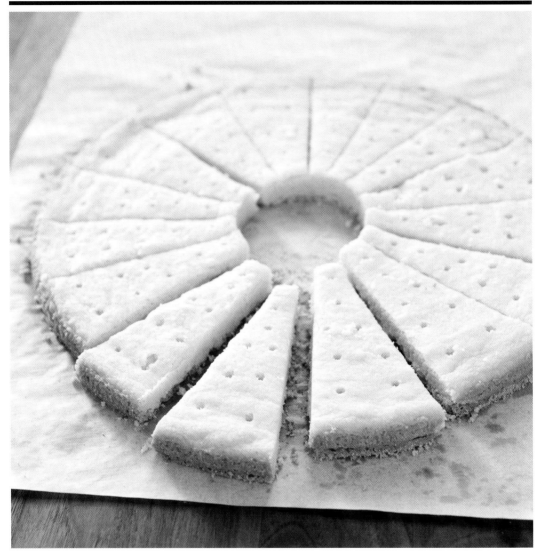

G-F TESTING LAB

FLOUR SUBSTITUTION	King Arthur Gluten-Free Multi-Purpose Flour 9 ounces = **1½ cups plus 2 tablespoons**	Bob's Red Mill GF All-Purpose Baking Flour 9 ounces = **1½ cups plus ⅓ cup**
	Note that shortbread made with King Arthur will be denser and slightly sandy, while shortbread made with Bob's Red Mill will be darker in color, drier, and more crumbly, and will have a distinct bean flavor.	
XANTHAN GUM	Do not omit the xanthan gum; it is crucial to the structure of the shortbread. For more information, see page 16.	

✓ WHY THIS RECIPE WORKS

With its short ingredient list—just flour, sugar, salt, and butter—a good shortbread should showcase a rich, buttery flavor, and it should have a dense, slightly sandy texture and a tawny, light brown color. For a traditional shortbread recipe using all-purpose flour, one of the biggest issues is trying to avoid gluten development, which makes the cookies tough. Obviously this wasn't going to be an issue with a gluten-free recipe, but without any gluten we had an entirely different problem: shortbread that was crumbly and had a coarse texture. Adding some xanthan gum provided structure so it wouldn't crumble, and to ensure the shortbread held its shape during cooking, we pressed the dough inside a springform pan collar and baked it in the collar with the clasp open at the start. Swapping in confectioners' sugar for the granulated gave the cookies the right sandy, rather than gritty, texture (resting the dough to hydrate the flour, as we'd done with several of our other cookies, wasn't an option since the shortbread dough contains so little moisture). We wanted to pack in as much butter as we could, and we found that 14 tablespoons was the most fat our flour blend could handle. As for the baking method, to ensure our cookies cooked through without browning too much, we got the best results by preheating the oven at a high temperature, then turning it down to 250 degrees when we put the cookies in. We baked them briefly, just until they were golden, and then cut them (at this stage, they could be cut without shattering). Then we returned the cookies to a turned-off oven, propping the door open to ensure they would simply dry out. Still, they baked slightly unevenly. Stamping a small circle of dough from the center with a biscuit cutter guaranteed even baking.

Shortbread
MAKES 16 WEDGES

- 9 **ounces (2 cups) ATK Gluten-Free Flour Blend (page 13)**
- 2⅔ **ounces (⅔ cup) confectioners' sugar**
- 1 **teaspoon xanthan gum**
- ½ **teaspoon salt**
- 14 **tablespoons unsalted butter, chilled and cut into ¼-inch-thick slices**

1. Adjust oven rack to middle position and heat oven to 450 degrees. Using stand mixer fitted with paddle, mix flour blend, sugar, xanthan gum, and salt on low speed until combined, about 5 seconds. Add butter and continue to mix until dough forms and pulls away from sides of bowl, 3 to 5 minutes.

2. Place collar of 9- or 9½-inch springform pan on parchment paper–lined baking sheet (do not use springform pan bottom). Press dough into collar in even ½-inch-thick layer, then smooth top of dough with back of spoon. Place 2-inch biscuit cutter in center of dough and cut out center. Discard extracted dough and replace cutter in center of dough. Open springform collar, but leave it in place.

3. Decrease oven temperature to 250 degrees and bake shortbread until top begins to turn pale golden and edges are golden, 15 to 20 minutes. Remove baking sheet from oven and turn off oven. Remove springform pan collar. Use chef's knife to score surface of shortbread into 16 even wedges, cutting halfway through shortbread. Using wooden skewer, poke 8 to 10 holes in each wedge. Return shortbread to oven and prop door open with handle of wooden spoon, leaving 1-inch gap at top. Allow shortbread to dry in turned-off oven until pale golden in center (shortbread should be firm but giving to touch), about 1 hour.

4. Transfer sheet to wire rack and let shortbread cool to room temperature, about 1 hour. Cut shortbread at scored marks to separate and serve. (Shortbread is best eaten on day it is baked, but it can be cooled and placed immediately in airtight container and stored at room temperature for up to 2 days.)

TEST KITCHEN TIP **Forming and Baking Shortbread**

Because of the significant amount of butter called for in the recipe, and the starches in our flour blend—both of which become molten in the oven—we bake the shortbread dough inside a springform pan collar to keep it from spreading. Once it has set up, we remove the collar, score the cookies, and continue baking in a turned-off oven to dry them out. To ensure even baking, we also cut a round out of the center of the dough using a biscuit cutter.

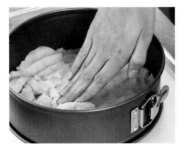

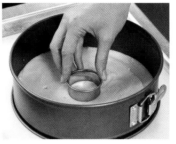

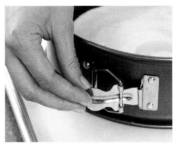

1. Press dough into closed upside-down springform pan collar on parchment-lined baking sheet to ½-inch thickness; smooth with back of spoon.

2. Cut hole in center of dough with 2-inch biscuit cutter; replace cutter in hole and discard extracted dough.

3. Open collar. Reduce oven temperature to 250 degrees, transfer sheet to oven, and bake shortbread until top begins to turn pale golden and edges are golden, 15 to 20 minutes.

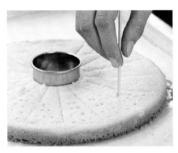

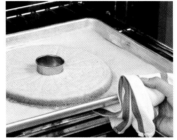

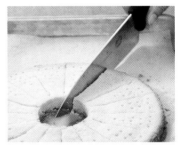

4. Remove springform pan collar. Score partially baked shortbread into 16 wedges, then poke 8 to 10 holes in each wedge.

5. Return shortbread to turned-off oven to dry; prop door open with wooden spoon or stick.

6. Transfer sheet to wire rack and let shortbread cool to room temperature. Cut shortbread at scored marks.

TEST KITCHEN TIP **Xanthan Gum in Gluten-Free Cookies**

We learned after developing a number of gluten-free muffins and quick breads that our low-protein flour blend needed reinforcement to deliver baked goods with the proper structure. When we started developing our cookie recipes, we found this to be even more important. In the case of our shortbread, the flour blend delivered a crumbly cookie that couldn't hold together, but a teaspoon of xanthan gum provided the necessary reinforcement and elasticity to produce the right texture. Xanthan gum proved even more critical in our drop cookies and Holiday Cookies. Unlike our shortbread, which we bake in a springform pan collar, and our bars, which have baking pans to keep them in check, drop cookies and Holiday Cookies are loose on the baking sheet. Xanthan gum was a must to ensure these cookies didn't spread all over the sheet. See page 16 for more information about xanthan and possible substitutions.

Florentine Lace Cookies

✔ WHY THIS RECIPE WORKS

With their toasty caramel-almond flavor, flecks of candied citrus, and chocolate drizzle finish, wafer-thin Florentine lace cookies are true showstoppers. And it's not surprising that most recipes are best left to the pros, with much of the process less like simple cookie baking and more like complicated candy making. But given their elegance (in both flavor and looks) and the fact they rely on such a small amount of flour, we agreed that figuring out how to make an approachable gluten-free Florentine was a must. Most recipes start by cooking butter, cream, and either corn syrup or honey in a saucepan until the mixture reaches 238 degrees to make the caramel base. We didn't want to futz around with the thermometer, and we found we didn't need to if we removed the saucepan from the heat when the mixture was consistently thick, bubbly, and a creamy tan color. At this point, we found that in batch after batch the target temp had been hit, and the resulting cookies were spot-on. Once the base was ready, the rest of the ingredients—typically flour, candied citrus, chopped almonds, vanilla, and a pinch of salt—are stirred in. We simplified things by swapping in orange marmalade for the candied citrus, and because chopped almonds interfered with the fine, lacy texture of the cookies, we ground them in the food processor before adding them to the batter. Flattening each portion before baking ensured evenly shaped, round cookies. For the finishing touch, we melted chocolate in the microwave, then quickly piped a drizzle onto each cookie with the help of a zipper-lock bag with the corner snipped off.

Florentine Lace Cookies
MAKES ABOUT 24 COOKIES

- 2 **cups slivered almonds**
- ¾ **cup heavy cream**
- 4 **tablespoons unsalted butter, cut into 4 pieces**
- 3½ **ounces (½ cup) sugar**
- ¼ **cup orange marmalade**
- 3 **tablespoons ATK Gluten-Free Flour Blend (page 13)**
- 1 **teaspoon vanilla extract**
- ¼ **teaspoon grated orange zest**
- ¼ **teaspoon salt**
- 4 **ounces bittersweet chocolate, chopped fine**

1. Adjust oven racks to upper-middle and lower-middle positions and heat oven to 350 degrees. Line 2 baking sheets with parchment paper. Process almonds in food processor until they resemble coarse sand, about 30 seconds.

2. Bring cream, butter, and sugar to boil in medium saucepan over medium-high heat. Cook, stirring frequently, until mixture begins to thicken, 5 to 6 minutes. Continue to cook, stirring constantly, until mixture begins to brown at edges and is thick enough to leave trail that doesn't immediately fill in when spatula is scraped along pan bottom, 1 to 2 minutes longer (some darker speckles may appear in mixture). Remove pan from heat and stir in ground almonds, marmalade, flour blend, vanilla, zest, and salt until combined.

3. Drop 6 level tablespoons of dough onto each prepared sheet spaced at least 3½ inches apart. When dough is cool enough to handle, use damp fingers to press each portion into 2½-inch circle.

4. Bake until deep brown from edge to edge, 15 to 17 minutes, switching and rotating sheets halfway through baking. Transfer baked cookies, still on parchment, to wire rack to cool. Let sheets cool for 10 minutes, line with fresh parchment, then repeat portioning and baking remaining dough.

5. Microwave 3 ounces chocolate in bowl at 50 percent power, stirring frequently, until about two-thirds of chocolate has melted, 1 to 2 minutes. Remove from microwave and add remaining 1 ounce chocolate and stir until melted, returning to microwave for no more than 5 seconds at a time to complete melting if necessary. Transfer chocolate

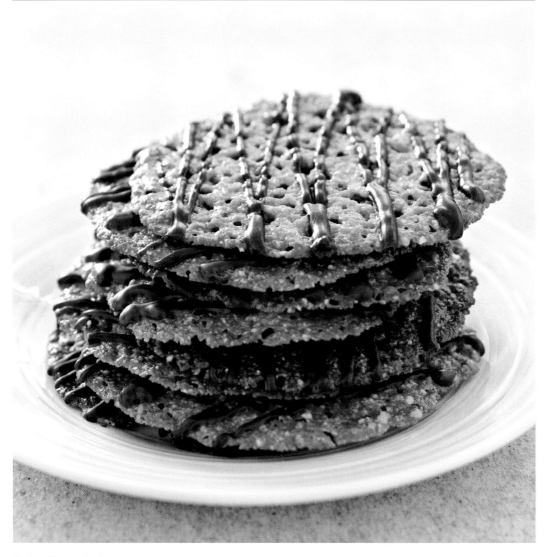

G-F TESTING LAB

FLOUR SUBSTITUTION	King Arthur Gluten-Free Multi-Purpose Flour **3 tablespoons**	Bob's Red Mill GF All-Purpose Baking Flour **3 tablespoons**
	Note that cookies made with King Arthur and Bob's Red Mill will need less time to bake; reduce the baking time by a few minutes. Cookies made with Bob's Red Mill will also be darker in color. Because so little flour blend is used in this recipe, there's no need to weigh it.	
CHOCOLATE	Not all brands of chocolate are processed in a gluten-free facility; make sure to read the label.	

to small zipper-lock bag and snip off corner to make hole no larger than ⅟₁₆ inch.

6. Transfer cooled cookies from parchment directly to wire racks. Pipe zigzag of chocolate over surface of each cookie, distributing chocolate evenly among all cookies. Refrigerate until chocolate is set, about 30 minutes. (Cookies can be stored in airtight container at cool room temperature for up to 4 days.)

TEST KITCHEN TIP **Making Florentines**

Most Florentine recipes are incredibly fussy. Our recipe simplifies things, and does so first by avoiding the need for a thermometer when making the caramel base. And for the chocolate drizzle, we found microwaving the chocolate at 50 percent power until it was mostly melted and then adding a little room-temperature chocolate delivered the same results as the involved process of tempering. And finally, we ditched the pastry bag in favor of an everyday zipper-lock bag with the corner snipped off to pipe on the chocolate.

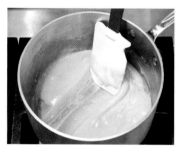

1. Bring cream, butter, and sugar to boil and cook, stirring, until mixture begins to brown at edges and leaves trail that doesn't immediately fill in when spatula is scraped along pan bottom.

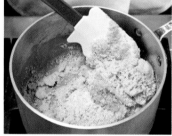

2. Off heat, stir in ground almonds, marmalade, flour blend, vanilla, orange zest, and salt until combined.

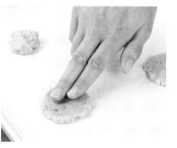

3. Drop 6 level tablespoons of dough onto 2 parchment-lined baking sheets, leaving at least 3½ inches in between. When dough is cool enough to handle, use damp fingers to press each portion into 2½-inch circle.

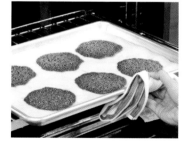

4. Bake cookies until uniformly brown; transfer on parchment paper to wire racks. Let sheets cool for 10 minutes, then repeat with remaining dough.

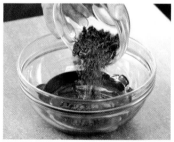

5. Microwave most of chocolate at 50 percent power, stirring frequently, until two-thirds melted. Stir in remaining chocolate until melted, microwaving as needed.

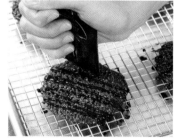

6. Pour chocolate into zipper-lock bag, snip off corner, and pipe onto cookies. Refrigerate for 30 minutes to set chocolate.

Holiday Cookies

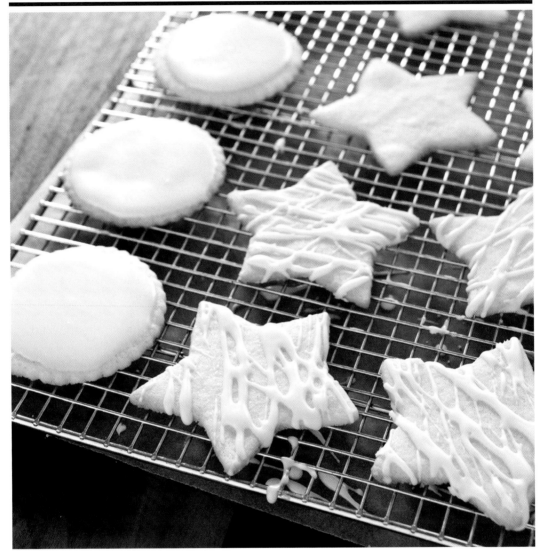

G-F TESTING LAB

FLOUR SUBSTITUTION	King Arthur Gluten-Free Multi-Purpose Flour 12½ ounces = **2¼ cups**	Bob's Red Mill GF All-Purpose Baking Flour 12½ ounces = **2½ cups**
	Note that cookies made with King Arthur will be very sandy, while cookies made with Bob's Red Mill will have a strong bean flavor. We don't recommend using store-bought flours in this recipe.	
XANTHAN GUM	Do not omit the xanthan gum; it is crucial to the structure of the cookies. For more information, see page 16.	
CHILLING TIME	Do not shortchange either of the chilling times for the dough; if you do, the cookies will spread too much.	

✓ WHY THIS RECIPE WORKS

To be suitable for decorating, holiday cookies must be thin and crisp. When we used our flour blend in our favorite recipe, we had a whole host of problems. The dough was incredibly sticky, and even when we managed to stamp out a few cookies, they turned out with an unappealing sandy, airy texture. They also lost their shape in the heat of the oven—not surprising given the gluten-free flour blend's high amount of starch, which doesn't set up until cool. Swapping out the granulated sugar in favor of superfine gave our cookies a more even crumb and a crisp texture. And unlike our drop cookies, where we used melted butter for a chewy texture, we opted to cream the butter here for a crisp texture. To make the dough easy to work with, we chilled it twice: before rolling it out, and again before stamping out the cookies. Chilling the dough wasn't enough to ensure cookies that held their shape through baking, so we added a small amount of xanthan gum for structure. If you do not have superfine sugar (which is sold in the baking aisle at most supermarkets), process granulated sugar in the food processor for 30 seconds.

Holiday Cookies
MAKES ABOUT 24 (3-INCH) COOKIES

COOKIES

12½	ounces (2¾ cups) ATK Gluten-Free Flour Blend (page 13)
½	teaspoon salt
¼	teaspoon xanthan gum
16	tablespoons unsalted butter, cut into 16 pieces and softened
7	ounces (1 cup) superfine sugar
1	large egg, plus 1 large yolk
2	teaspoons vanilla extract

GLAZE

1	tablespoon cream cheese, room temperature
2–3	tablespoons milk
6	ounces (1½ cups) confectioners' sugar

1. FOR THE COOKIES: Whisk flour blend, salt, and xanthan gum together in bowl; set aside. Using stand mixer fitted with paddle, beat butter and sugar at medium-high speed until pale and fluffy, about 3 minutes. Add egg, yolk, and vanilla and beat until well combined. Reduce speed to low, add flour mixture, and mix until flour is incorporated and dough comes together, 2 to 4 minutes. Divide dough into 4 even pieces. Press each piece into 4-inch disk, wrap each disk in plastic wrap, and refrigerate until dough is firm, about 1 hour. (Dough can be refrigerated up to 2 days or frozen for up to 2 weeks; defrost frozen dough in refrigerator before using.)

2. Working with 1 piece of dough at a time, roll ⅛ inch thick between 2 large sheets of parchment paper. Peel parchment from 1 side of dough and place back on dough. Flip dough over and repeat with second sheet of parchment. Slide dough, still between parchment, onto baking sheet and refrigerate until set, about 30 minutes.

3. Adjust oven rack to middle position and heat oven to 325 degrees. Line 2 baking sheets with parchment paper. Working with 1 sheet of dough at a time, peel parchment from 1 side of dough and cut into desired shapes using cookie cutters; space cookies 1½ inches apart on prepared sheets. Bake cookies, 1 sheet at a time, until firm to touch and edges are just beginning to brown, 12 to 14 minutes, rotating sheet halfway through baking. (Dough scraps can be patted together, chilled, and rerolled once.) Let cookies cool on sheet for 5 minutes, then transfer to wire rack. Let cookies cool to room temperature before glazing.

4. FOR THE GLAZE: Whisk cream cheese and 2 tablespoons milk together in medium bowl until no lumps remain. Add sugar and whisk until smooth, adding remaining 1 tablespoon milk as needed until glaze is thin enough to spread easily. Using back of spoon, drizzle or spread scant teaspoon of glaze onto each cooled cookie. Allow glazed cookies to dry at least 30 minutes. (Cookies are best eaten on day they are baked, but they can be stored in airtight container for up to 2 days.)

Fudgy Brownies

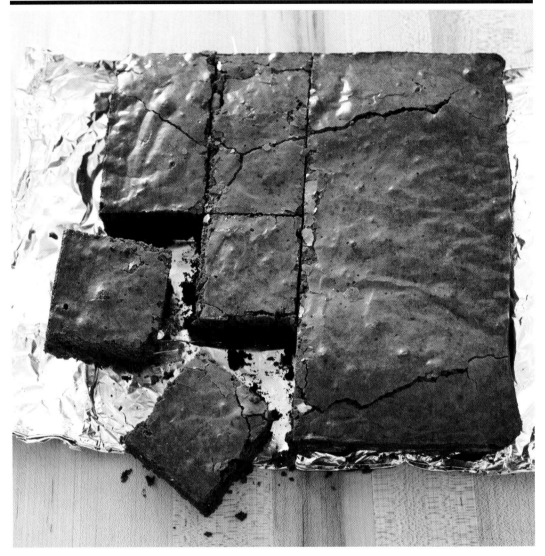

G-F TESTING LAB

FLOUR SUBSTITUTION	King Arthur Gluten-Free Multi-Purpose Flour 4 ounces = ¾ **cup**	Bob's Red Mill GF All-Purpose Baking Flour 4 ounces = ½ **cup plus** ⅓ **cup**
	Note that brownies made with King Arthur will have less structure and be slightly gritty, while brownies made with Bob's Red Mill will have a slight bean flavor.	
XANTHAN GUM	The xanthan gum can be omitted, but the brownies will be more crumbly, will not rise as well, and will sink somewhat in the middle.	
RESTING TIME	Do not shortchange the 30-minute rest for the batter; if you do, the brownies will be gritty.	

☑ WHY THIS RECIPE WORKS

Fudgy brownies contain less flour than cakey ones, so it made sense to start with our favorite recipe for fudgy brownies and use our flour blend instead. With cocoa powder, unsweetened chocolate, and bittersweet chocolate, this recipe delivers intense chocolate flavor. But when made with our flour blend, the brownies were a bit dry and dense (even for a fudgy brownie), and there was a subtle graininess. Cutting back on the amount of flour helped give the brownies the right moist, fudgy texture, and resting the batter for 30 minutes before baking gave the starches in our flour blend time to hydrate and soften. But reducing the amount of flour also had an unwanted side effect: The chocolate flavor fell out of balance. Now our brownies had a bitter edge. Both unsweetened chocolate and cocoa powder were candidates for elimination since they are on the more bitter end of the chocolate spectrum. Brownies made without cocoa lacked structure—so it had to stay. Dropping the unsweetened chocolate was a big step in the right direction, and switching the bittersweet out for semisweet chocolate eliminated the bitter flavor altogether. Not all brands of chocolate are processed in a gluten-free facility, so read labels carefully.

Fudgy Brownies
MAKES 16 BROWNIES

4	ounces (¾ cup plus 2 tablespoons) ATK Gluten-Free Flour Blend (page 13)
½	teaspoon salt
½	teaspoon xanthan gum
7	ounces semisweet chocolate, chopped coarse
8	tablespoons unsalted butter, cut into 8 pieces
3	tablespoons unsweetened cocoa powder
8¾	ounces (1¼ cups) sugar
3	large eggs
2	teaspoons vanilla extract

1. Make foil sling for 8-inch square baking pan by folding 2 long sheets of aluminum foil so each is 8 inches wide. Lay sheets of foil in pan perpendicular to each other, with extra foil hanging over edges of pan. Push foil into corners and up sides of pan, smoothing foil flush to pan; spray with vegetable oil spray.

2. Whisk flour blend, salt, and xanthan gum together in bowl; set aside. Microwave chocolate, butter, and cocoa in bowl at 50 percent power, stirring often, until melted and smooth, 1 to 3 minutes. Let mixture cool slightly.

3. Whisk sugar, eggs, and vanilla together in large bowl. Whisk in cooled chocolate mixture. Stir in flour mixture using rubber spatula and mix until well combined. Scrape batter into prepared pan and smooth top with spatula. Cover pan with plastic wrap and let batter rest for 30 minutes.

4. Adjust oven rack to middle position and heat oven to 350 degrees. Remove plastic and bake until toothpick inserted in center comes out with few moist crumbs attached, 45 to 55 minutes, rotating pan halfway through baking.

5. Let brownies cool completely in pan on wire rack, about 2 hours. Using foil overhang, lift brownies out of pan. Cut into squares and serve. (Brownies are best eaten on day they are baked, but they can be cooled and placed immediately in airtight container and stored at room temperature for up to 2 days.)

TEST KITCHEN TIP **Making a Foil Sling**

A foil sling makes removing bars tidy and easy. Make sure to grease foil sling to prevent sticking.

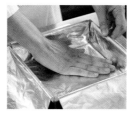

Lay two sheets of foil in pan perpendicular to each other, with extra foil hanging over edges of pan. Push foil into corners and up sides of pan, smoothing foil flush to pan.

Raspberry Streusel Bars

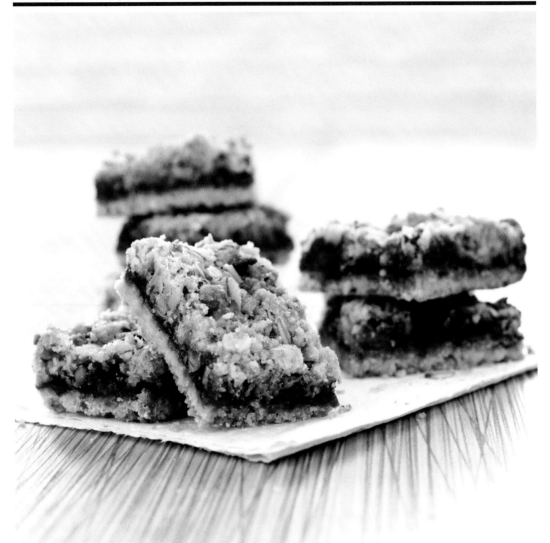

G-F TESTING LAB

FLOUR SUBSTITUTION	King Arthur Gluten-Free Multi-Purpose Flour 6 ounces = ¾ **cup plus ⅓ cup**	Bob's Red Mill GF All-Purpose Baking Flour 6 ounces = ⅔ **cup plus ½ cup**
	Note that bars made with King Arthur will be somewhat pasty, while bars made with Bob's Red Mill will have a bean flavor, be a bit more crumbly, and brown more quickly; if using Bob's Red Mill, you will need to reduce the baking time by a few minutes.	
OATS	Do not use quick oats; they have a dusty texture that doesn't work in this recipe. Make sure to buy old-fashioned rolled oats (see page 62).	
XANTHAN GUM	Do not omit the xanthan gum; it is crucial to the structure of the bars. For more information, see page 16.	

✓ WHY THIS RECIPE WORKS

A raspberry streusel bar should have a sturdy, buttery shortbreadlike base, a filling with bright raspberry flavor, and a rich streusel topping that lends texture and stays in place. For the base, we started with butter, our flour blend, and sugar (plus salt for a little flavor). By mixing pieces of softened butter into the dry ingredients using a stand mixer, we ensured the right fine crumb. The flavor was exactly what we wanted, but without gluten this base couldn't support the topping. Adding just ¼ teaspoon of xanthan gum gave the crust the structure it needed to hold up and slice neatly without crumbling. We also baked the crust before adding the fruit and streusel so that it could set up and wouldn't turn soggy from the moisture in the raspberry filling. For the streusel topping, we simply took a portion of our shortbread base mixture and added light brown sugar, pecans, and oats. The last component on our list was the fruit filling. Preserves seemed like a convenient option, but they lost a fair bit of flavor during the cooking process. Fresh berries alone, however, were too tart and loose. For a filling with just the right jammy consistency as well as bright flavor, a combination of preserves and fresh berries, plus a bit of lemon juice, did the trick. After baking the base, all we had to do was spread on the filling, crumble our streusel over the top, and return the pan to the oven for a short stint. See page 237 for details on how to make a foil sling.

Raspberry Streusel Bars

MAKES 16 BARS

- 6 ounces (1⅓ cups) ATK Gluten-Free Flour Blend (page 13)
- 2⅓ ounces (⅓ cup) granulated sugar
- ¼ teaspoon salt
- ¼ teaspoon xanthan gum
- 8 tablespoons unsalted butter, cut into ½-inch pieces and softened
- 2 tablespoons packed light brown sugar
- ⅓ cup pecans, chopped fine
- ¼ cup gluten-free old-fashioned rolled oats
- 6 ounces (½ cup) raspberry preserves
- 2½ ounces (½ cup) fresh raspberries
- 1½ teaspoons lemon juice

1. Adjust oven rack to middle position and heat oven to 375 degrees. Make foil sling for 8-inch square baking pan by folding 2 long sheets of aluminum foil so each is 8 inches wide. Lay sheets of foil in pan perpendicular to each other, with extra foil hanging over edges of pan. Push foil into corners and up sides of pan, smoothing foil flush to pan; spray with vegetable oil spray.

2. Using stand mixer fitted with paddle, mix flour blend, granulated sugar, salt, and xanthan gum on low speed until combined, about 5 seconds. Add butter, 1 piece at a time, and continue to mix until dough forms and pulls away from sides of bowl, 2 to 3 minutes.

3. Measure ½ cup dough into medium bowl and set aside. Distribute remaining dough evenly into prepared pan and press firmly into even layer using bottom of measuring cup. Bake until edges begin to brown, 14 to 18 minutes, rotating pan halfway through baking.

4. While crust is baking, add brown sugar, pecans, and oats to reserved dough; use hands to mix until well incorporated. Pinch mixture with fingers to create hazelnut-size clumps; set streusel aside.

5. Combine preserves, raspberries, and lemon juice in small bowl and mash with fork until combined but some berry pieces remain.

6. Spread filling evenly over hot crust; sprinkle streusel topping evenly over filling (do not press streusel into filling). Return pan to oven and bake until topping is golden brown and filling is bubbling, 22 to 25 minutes. Let bars cool completely in pan on wire rack, 1 to 2 hours. Using foil overhang, lift bars out of pan, cut into squares, and serve. (Bars are best eaten on day they are baked, but they can be cooled and placed immediately in airtight container and stored at room temperature for up to 1 day; crust and streusel will soften.)

Lemon Bars

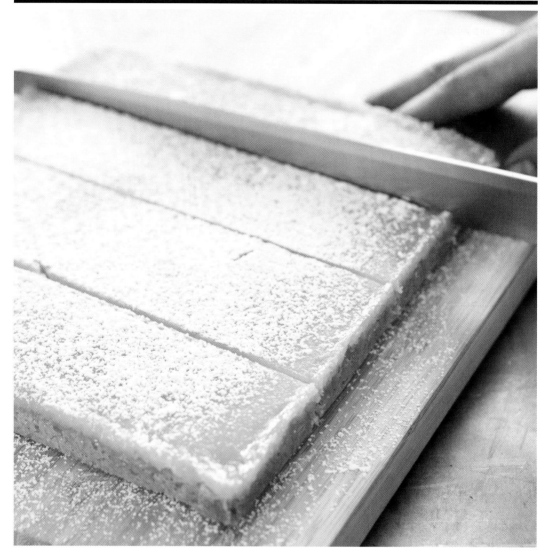

G-F TESTING LAB

FLOUR SUBSTITUTION	King Arthur Gluten-Free Multi-Purpose Flour 6 ounces = ¾ **cup plus** ⅓ **cup**	Bob's Red Mill GF All-Purpose Baking Flour 6 ounces = ⅔ **cup plus** ½ **cup**
	Note that bars made with King Arthur will be somewhat pasty, while bars made with Bob's Red Mill will have a distinct bean flavor and be a bit more crumbly.	
XANTHAN GUM	Do not omit the xanthan gum; it is crucial to the structure of the bars. For more information, see page 16.	

✓ WHY THIS RECIPE WORKS

For our gluten-free version of this classic, we started with the topping. Lemon juice plus zest ensured plenty of bright flavor, while butter and heavy cream added richness. This topping also needed some form of thickener so that it could set up and slice neatly. Some recipes rely on flour, but we found that eggs delivered better results. Seven yolks plus two whole eggs gave our topping a smooth, custardlike texture that set up just enough, and the lemon flavor was pure and clean. Next, we moved on to the base. We knew we wanted something similar to shortbread: a crisp, buttery crust that could support the topping yet slice neatly and easily. We'd just developed a simple shortbread crust using butter, sugar, our flour blend, and xanthan gum for our Raspberry Streusel Bars (page 238), and it worked perfectly here as well. To ensure the base didn't become soggy, we prebaked it just as we had with our Raspberry Streusel Bars, then topped it with the custard and returned the pan to the oven. Letting the bars cool for the full 2 hours was key to ensuring the custard topping set up. See page 237 for details on how to make a foil sling.

Lemon Bars
MAKES 16 BARS

CRUST
- 6 ounces (1⅓ cups) ATK Gluten-Free Flour Blend (page 13)
- 2⅓ ounces (⅓ cup) granulated sugar
- ¼ teaspoon salt
- ¼ teaspoon xanthan gum
- 8 tablespoons unsalted butter, cut into ½-inch pieces and softened

LEMON FILLING
- 2 large eggs, plus 7 large yolks
- 7 ounces (1 cup) plus 2 tablespoons granulated sugar
- ¼ cup grated lemon zest plus ⅔ cup juice (4 lemons)
- Pinch salt

- 4 tablespoons unsalted butter, cut into 4 pieces
- 3 tablespoons heavy cream
- Confectioners' sugar

1. Adjust oven rack to middle position and heat oven to 350 degrees. Make foil sling for 8-inch square baking pan by folding 2 long sheets of aluminum foil so each is 8 inches wide. Lay sheets of foil in pan perpendicular to each other, with extra foil hanging over edges of pan. Push foil into corners and up sides of pan, smoothing foil flush to pan; spray with vegetable oil spray.

2. FOR THE CRUST: Using stand mixer fitted with paddle, mix flour blend, granulated sugar, salt, and xanthan gum on low speed until combined, about 5 seconds. Add butter, 1 piece at a time, and continue to mix until dough forms and pulls away from sides of bowl, 2 to 3 minutes. Distribute mixture evenly into prepared pan and press firmly into even layer using bottom of measuring cup. Bake crust until fragrant and beginning to brown, 25 to 30 minutes, rotating pan halfway through baking. Transfer to wire rack and let cool before adding filling, about 30 minutes (do not turn off oven).

3. FOR THE FILLING: Whisk eggs and yolks together in medium saucepan. Whisk in granulated sugar until combined, then whisk in lemon zest and juice, and salt. Add butter and cook over medium heat, stirring constantly, until mixture thickens slightly and registers 170 degrees, about 5 minutes. Strain mixture immediately into bowl and stir in cream.

4. Pour filling over cooled crust. Bake until filling is shiny and opaque and center jiggles slightly when shaken, 15 to 20 minutes, rotating pan halfway through baking.

5. Let bars cool completely in pan on wire rack, about 2 hours. Using foil overhang, lift bars out of pan, cut into squares, and dust with confectioners' sugar before serving. (Bars are best eaten on day they are baked, but they can be cooled and refrigerated for up to 2 days.)

Granola Bars

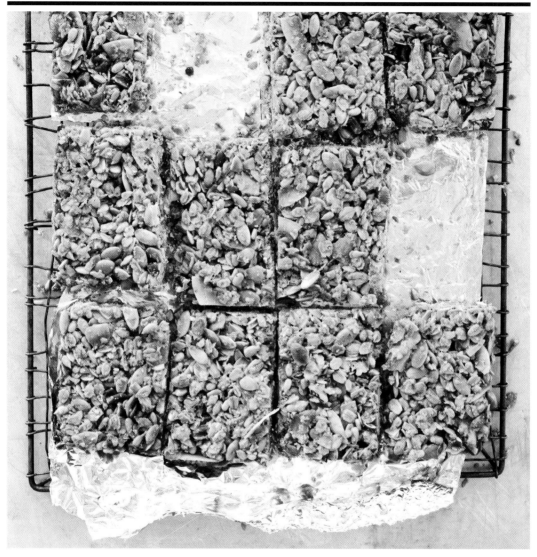

G-F TESTING LAB

OATS   Do not use quick oats; they have a dusty texture that doesn't work in this recipe. Make sure to buy old-fashioned rolled oats (see page 62) that have been processed in a gluten-free facility.

✓ WHY THIS RECIPE WORKS

Almost always too sugary and as dry as cardboard, most store-bought granola bars aren't worth the few bucks they cost, so we set out to make our own version of this naturally gluten-free treat. For plenty of flavor and texture, we started by adding sunflower seeds, pepitas, pecans, and coconut flakes to the usual oat base. For our sweetener (as well as some binding power), a combination of brown sugar and maple syrup provided a more complex flavor than granulated sugar alone, and they weren't as cloying as honey. To temper the sweetness further and also help create a crisp texture, we found that stirring in a surprising ingredient—extra-virgin olive oil—was the secret. The flavor and texture in our granola bars were great at this point, but they weren't holding together well enough. We didn't want to add any more sugar or syrup, so we had to consider more creative options. We eventually discovered that we could process some of the oats into a flour, then combine it with the oil and sugars to create a sticky paste that held our bars together. A little flaky sea salt elevated the flavors of our bars to the next level. We discovered the granola mixture shattered if we waited until it was cool before cutting the bars. So we cut the bars, still in the pan, shortly after they came out of the oven. They fused back together a bit and required a second cut once cool, but this time they cut cleanly and neatly. You can add ¼ teaspoon table salt if you don't have flaked sea salt. See page 237 for details on how to make a foil sling.

Granola Bars
MAKES 16 BARS

- ⅓ **cup maple syrup**
- 1¾ **ounces (¼ cup packed) light brown sugar**
- ¾ **teaspoon flaked sea salt**
- ⅓ **cup extra-virgin olive oil**
- 6 **ounces (2 cups) gluten-free old-fashioned rolled oats**
- ½ **cup pecans, chopped fine**
- ½ **cup raw pepitas**
- ½ **cup raw sunflower seeds**
- ½ **cup unsweetened flaked coconut**

1. Adjust oven rack to middle position and heat oven to 300 degrees. Make foil sling for 13 by 9-inch baking pan by folding 2 long sheets of aluminum foil; first sheet should be 13 inches wide and second sheet should be 9 inches wide. Lay sheets of foil in pan perpendicular to each other, with extra foil hanging over edges of pan. Push foil into corners and up sides of pan, smoothing foil flush to pan; spray with vegetable oil spray.

2. Whisk maple syrup, sugar, and salt together in large bowl. Whisk in oil.

3. Process ½ cup oats in food processor until finely ground, 30 to 40 seconds. Transfer to bowl with maple syrup mixture and stir in remaining 1½ cups oats, pecans, pepitas, sunflower seeds, and coconut until all dry ingredients are thoroughly coated.

4. Transfer oat mixture to prepared pan and spread into thin, even layer. Generously spray large metal spatula with oil spray, then firmly compress oat mixture with spatula until very compact. Bake granola bars until deeply golden, about 45 minutes, rotating pan halfway through baking.

5. Let bars cool in pan on wire rack for 15 minutes, then cut, still in pan, into 16 bars. Let cool to room temperature, about 1 hour. Using foil overhang, lift bars out of pan and transfer to cutting board. Using sharp knife, carefully recut bars following original cuts. (Granola bars can be stored at room temperature in airtight container for up to 1 week.)

TEST KITCHEN TIP
Making Crunchy Granola Bars

To make thin, crisp bars, firmly pack the granola mixture in the pan before baking it.

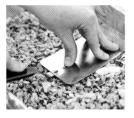

Grease wide metal spatula with vegetable oil spray. Transfer granola bar mixture to prepared pan and press into compact, even layer using spatula.

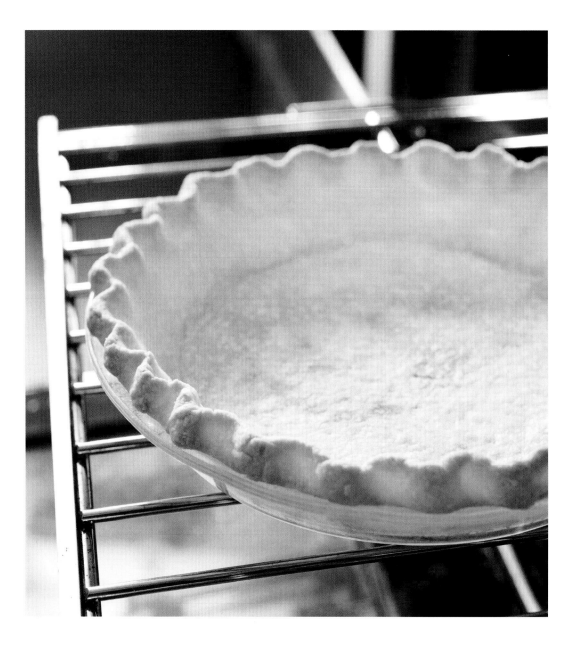

PIES, FRUIT DESSERTS, AND TARTS

Pie Dough

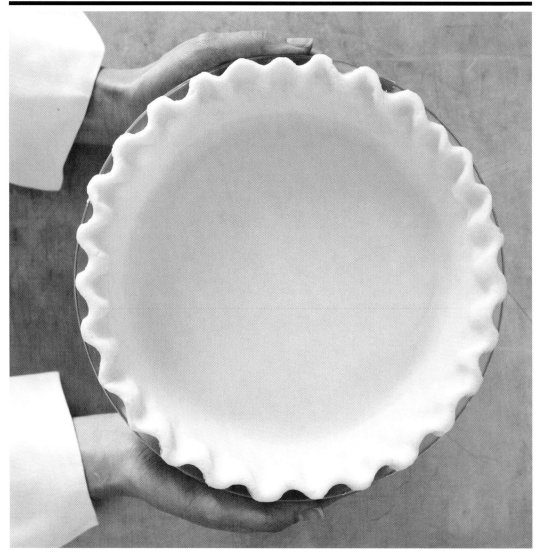

G-F TESTING LAB

FLOUR SUBSTITUTION	King Arthur Gluten-Free Multi-Purpose Flour 13 ounces (for double crust) = **2¼ cups plus 2 tablespoons** 6½ ounces (for single crust) = **⅔ cup plus ½ cup**	Bob's Red Mill GF All-Purpose Baking Flour 13 ounces (for double crust) = **2½ cups plus 2 tablespoons** 6½ ounces (for single crust) = **1⅓ cups**
	Note that pie dough made with King Arthur will be less sturdy, and pie dough made with Bob's Red Mill will be darker in color, drier, and slightly rubbery and will have a slight bean flavor.	
XANTHAN GUM	Do not omit the xanthan gum; it is crucial to the structure of the pie dough. For more information, see page 16.	

✔ WHY THIS RECIPE WORKS

Perfect pie dough has just the right balance of tenderness and structure. The former comes from fat, the latter from the long protein chains, called gluten, that form when flour mixes with water. Too little gluten and the dough won't stick together; too much and the crust turns tough. So presumably we would face mostly a structural issue with a gluten-free dough, since gluten-free flours are naturally low in protein. As our first step, we swapped in our gluten-free flour blend for the wheat flour in all the pie dough recipes the test kitchen has developed over the years. We produced workable doughs in every case, but an all-butter dough (which includes sour cream for tenderness) had the necessary richness to stand up to the starchiness of the gluten-free flour blend and was clearly the best starting point. Although we weren't surprised to find that the dough was still too soft and lacked structure, we were taken aback by how tough it was; on its own, the sour cream was not sufficient to tenderize a gluten-free dough. We solved the structural problem easily with the addition of a modest amount of xanthan gum, but flakiness and tenderness were still elusive. In an effort to further tenderize our dough, we tested ingredients that are known to tenderize: baking soda, lemon juice, and vinegar. Vinegar was the clear winner, producing a pie crust that was not only tender, but also light and flaky. Like conventional recipes, this pie dough can be prepared in advance and refrigerated for 2 days; however, it is not sturdy enough to withstand freezing.

Double-Crust Pie Dough
MAKES ENOUGH FOR ONE 9-INCH PIE

- 5 tablespoons ice water
- 3 tablespoons sour cream
- 1 tablespoon rice vinegar
- 13 ounces (2¾ cups plus 2 tablespoons) ATK Gluten-Free Flour Blend (page 13)
- 1 tablespoon sugar
- 1 teaspoon salt
- ½ teaspoon xanthan gum
- 16 tablespoons unsalted butter, cut into ¼-inch pieces and frozen for 10 to 15 minutes

1. Combine ice water, sour cream, and vinegar together in bowl. Process flour blend, sugar, salt, and xanthan gum together in food processor until combined, about 5 seconds. Scatter butter over top and pulse mixture until butter is size of large peas, about 10 pulses.

2. Pour half of sour cream mixture over flour mixture and pulse until incorporated, about 3 pulses. Pour remaining sour cream mixture over flour mixture and pulse until dough just comes together, about 6 pulses.

3. Divide dough into 2 even pieces. Turn each piece of dough onto sheet of plastic wrap and flatten each into 5-inch disk. Wrap each piece tightly in plastic and refrigerate for 1 hour. Before rolling out dough, let it sit on counter to soften slightly, about 15 minutes. (Dough can be wrapped tightly in plastic and refrigerated for up to 2 days.)

Single-Crust Pie Dough
MAKES ENOUGH FOR ONE 9-INCH PIE

- 2½ tablespoons ice water
- 1½ tablespoons sour cream
- 1½ teaspoons rice vinegar
- 6½ ounces (¾ cup plus ⅔ cup) ATK Gluten-Free Flour Blend (page 13)
- 1½ teaspoons sugar
- ½ teaspoon salt
- ¼ teaspoon xanthan gum
- 8 tablespoons unsalted butter, cut into ¼-inch pieces and frozen for 10 to 15 minutes

1. Combine ice water, sour cream, and vinegar together in bowl. Process flour blend, sugar, salt, and xanthan gum together in food processor until combined, about 5 seconds. Scatter butter over top and pulse mixture until butter is size of large peas, about 10 pulses.

2. Pour half of sour cream mixture over flour mixture and pulse until incorporated, about 3 pulses. Pour remaining sour cream mixture over flour mixture and pulse until dough just comes together, about 6 pulses.

3. Turn dough onto sheet of plastic wrap and flatten into 5-inch disk. Wrap tightly in plastic and refrigerate for 1 hour. Before rolling out dough, let it sit on counter to soften slightly, about 15 minutes. (Dough can be wrapped tightly in plastic and refrigerated for up to 2 days.)

TEST KITCHEN TIP **Making a Single-Crust Pie**

Because gluten-free pie dough is so soft, fitting it properly into a pie plate requires some finesse—you can't just pick up the dough or wrap it around the rolling pin to move it. The steps below will show you how to fit it into the pie plate successfully. Our gluten-free pie dough must be chilled before baking (like traditional pie dough), but then it can go from freezer to oven without first covering with parchment or foil and lining with pie weights because it does not puff up while baking. For recipes that call for a partially baked pie shell, preheat the oven to 375 degrees and place the chilled pie shell on the middle rack and bake for 20 to 25 minutes, until light golden brown, rotating the shell halfway through baking. For a fully baked pie shell, bake it an additional 5 minutes, until golden brown.

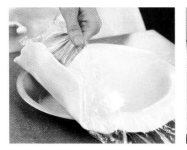

1. After rolling dough between two sheets of plastic, remove top sheet of plastic from dough and gently invert dough over 9-inch pie plate.

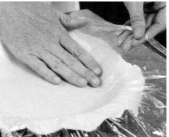

2. Working around circumference, ease dough into plate by gently lifting plastic wrap with one hand while pressing dough into plate bottom with other hand. Let excess dough hang over rim.

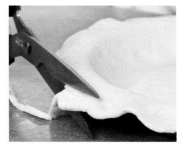

3. Remove plastic wrap. Trim excess dough with kitchen shears, leaving ½-inch overhang beyond lip of pie plate.

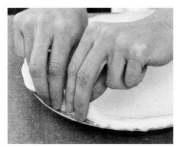

4. Tuck overhang underneath itself to form tidy, even edge that sits on lip of pie plate.

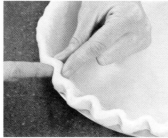

5. Using index finger of one hand and thumb and index finger of other hand, create fluted ridges perpendicular to edge of pie plate.

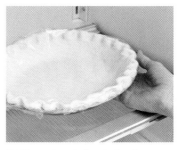

6. Wrap dough-lined pie plate loosely in plastic and place in freezer until fully chilled and firm, at least 15 minutes or up to 1 hour.

Pie Dough

Our low-protein gluten-free flour blend was an asset in some aspects of developing our pie dough recipe since less protein means less chance for turning out a tough dough that is hard to roll out. That said, we still needed to strike a balance between adding structure to our dough so it wouldn't crumble and creating the flaky layers that are the hallmark of great pie crust. Here is what we learned.

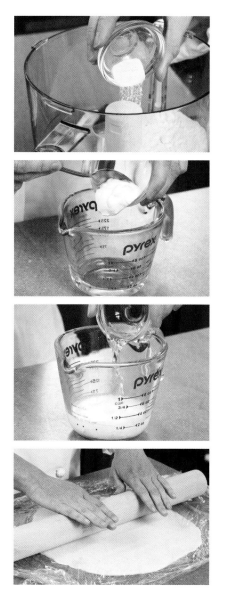

1. ADD XANTHAN GUM FOR STRUCTURE: In traditional pie dough, you do not want a lot of gluten development because it makes the dough tough, but you do need a little bit for structure. In contrast to all-purpose flour, gluten-free flour blends have less protein, and those proteins also form weaker bonds, resulting in pie dough that has a hard time holding together. The dough needed reinforcement to provide structure and elasticity. To prevent the pie crust from crumbling we added a small amount of xanthan gum, which acts similarly to gluten, and it helped bind the proteins, creating a sturdy network.

2. ADD SOUR CREAM FOR WORKABILITY: The test kitchen's all-butter pie dough includes sour cream for the tenderizing and workability that shortening traditionally adds. In our testing we explored alternatives to the sour cream to see if they would make a difference in any way. We tried adding cream cheese and yogurt. Cream cheese turned our crust tough and rubbery while yogurt added a tang that tasters didn't like. Sour cream added richness that complemented the butter flavor, while keeping the dough workable.

3. ADD VINEGAR FOR FLAKINESS AND TENDERNESS: In our quest for a flaky, tender gluten-free crust, we tested ingredients that are known to tenderize dough, namely baking soda, lemon juice, and vinegar. Baking soda produced a crust that was too crumbly and overly browned. Lemon juice and vinegar produced crusts that were indeed tender, but the crust made with vinegar was also light and flaky. Adding vinegar lowered the pH of the dough, which weakened the bonds just enough to produce a pie crust that was tender with flaky layers.

4. ROLL BETWEEN SHEETS OF PLASTIC WRAP: Our gluten-free dough was a lot softer than regular pie dough, but we knew that using extra flour blend to roll it out would work against us; this additional flour would have no opportunity to hydrate, which meant, as we learned from our testing of muffins and other baked goods, that we'd end up with a gritty texture. Instead, we simply rolled out the dough between two sheets of plastic wrap to prevent sticking and allow for easy transfer to the pie plate.

Pumpkin Pie

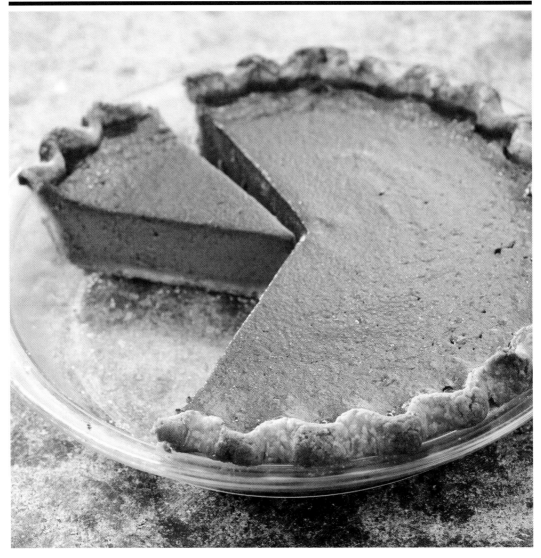

FLOUR SUBSTITUTION	See page 246 for information about using various brands of gluten-free flour in the pie dough.

✓ WHY THIS RECIPE WORKS

Pumpkin pie filling is naturally gluten-free, so we weren't worried about changing it, but when we used our favorite recipe to bake one in a gluten-free pie crust, we found that the loose, liquid-y filling turned our once-flaky crust gummy and raw-tasting. We needed to start with a thicker mixture that would not readily soak into the crust. Cooking the pumpkin mixture briefly on the stovetop drove off some of the moisture that had ruined the crust in the first round of testing. As an added bonus, this stint on the stovetop also helped to bloom the spices and intensify their warmth, resulting in the most flavorful pumpkin pie filling we had ever tasted. Next, we made sure that both shell and filling were hot when we assembled the pie, so the custard could begin to firm up almost immediately rather than soaking into the pastry. Finally, we baked the pie quickly, in the lower half of the oven, exposing the bottom of the crust to more intense heat and thus keeping it crisp and flaky. We avoided curdling by taking the pie out of the oven as soon as the center thickened to the point where it no longer sloshed but instead wiggled like gelatin when the pie plate was gently shaken. Timing is important here, as the filling must be prepared while the crust bakes. Be sure to use pumpkin puree, not pumpkin pie filling. The pie may be served slightly warm, chilled, or at room temperature. This pie is best the day it is made.

Pumpkin Pie
SERVES 8

- 1   recipe Single-Crust Pie Dough (page 247)
- 1   (15-ounce) can pumpkin puree
- 7   ounces (1 cup packed) dark brown sugar
- 2   teaspoons ground ginger
- 2   teaspoons ground cinnamon
- 1   teaspoon ground nutmeg
- ½   teaspoon salt
- ¼   teaspoon ground cloves
- ⅔   cup heavy cream
- ⅔   cup whole milk
- 4   large eggs

1. Adjust oven rack to middle position and heat oven to 375 degrees. Roll dough into 12-inch circle between 2 large sheets of plastic wrap. Remove top plastic, gently invert dough over 9-inch pie plate, and ease dough into plate. Remove remaining plastic and trim dough ½ inch beyond lip of pie plate. Tuck overhanging dough under itself to be flush with edge of pie plate. Crimp dough evenly around edge using your fingers.

2. Cover dough loosely in plastic and freeze until chilled and firm, about 15 minutes. Remove plastic and bake until crust is light brown in color, 20 to 25 minutes, rotating pie plate halfway through baking. Transfer pie plate to wire rack. (Crust must still be warm when filling is added.) Adjust oven rack to lower position and increase oven temperature to 425 degrees.

3. While crust bakes, process pumpkin puree, sugar, ginger, cinnamon, nutmeg, salt, and cloves together in food processor until combined, about 1 minute. Transfer pumpkin mixture to medium saucepan (do not clean processor bowl) and bring to simmer over medium-high heat. Cook pumpkin mixture, stirring constantly, until thick and shiny, about 5 minutes. Whisk in cream and milk, return to simmer briefly, then remove from heat.

4. Process eggs in food processor until uniform, about 5 seconds. With machine running, slowly add about half of hot pumpkin mixture through feed tube. Stop machine, add remaining pumpkin, and continue processing mixture until uniform, about 30 seconds longer.

5. Immediately pour warm filling into warm, partially baked pie crust. (If you have any extra filling, ladle it into pie after 5 minutes of baking, by which time filling will have settled.) Bake until filling is puffed and lightly cracked around edges and center wiggles slightly when jiggled, about 25 minutes. Let pie cool on wire rack until filling has set, about 2 hours; serve slightly warm or at room temperature.

Deep-Dish Apple Pie

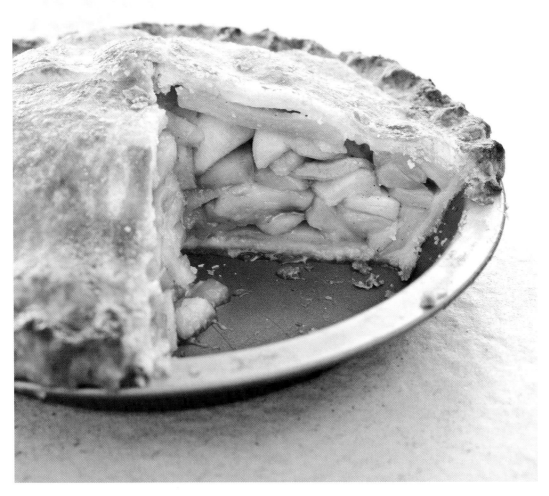

G-F TESTING LAB

FLOUR SUBSTITUTION	See page 246 for information about using various brands of gluten-free flour in the pie dough.

✓ WHY THIS RECIPE WORKS

The simplest recipes call for piling sliced apples, tossed with sugar and spices, between two layers of pie dough and baking. This method spelled disaster for our gluten-free pie crust, which absorbed juices shed by the apples. Precooking the apples prevented a flood of juices from ruining the crust. To guarantee a crisp bottom crust, we baked the pie in a metal pie plate on a preheated baking sheet. We like a mix of tart and sweet apples, such as Granny Smiths and Golden Delicious, but you can also use Empires or Cortlands (tart) and Fuji, Jonagolds, or Braeburns (sweet). It's not safe to place a glass (Pyrex) pie plate on a preheated baking sheet. If you must use a glass pie plate, do not preheat the baking sheet; your crust will not be as crisp. This pie is best served the day it is made.

Deep-Dish Apple Pie
SERVES 8

- 2½ pounds Granny Smith apples, peeled, cored, and sliced ¼ inch thick
- 2½ pounds Golden Delicious apples, peeled, cored, and sliced ¼ inch thick
- 3½ ounces (½ cup) plus 1 teaspoon granulated sugar
- 1¾ ounces (¼ cup packed) light brown sugar
- ½ teaspoon grated lemon zest plus 1 tablespoon juice
- ¼ teaspoon salt
- ⅛ teaspoon ground cinnamon
- 1 recipe Double-Crust Pie Dough (page 247)
- 1 large egg white, lightly beaten

1. Toss apples, ½ cup granulated sugar, brown sugar, lemon zest, salt, and cinnamon together in Dutch oven. Cover and cook over medium heat, stirring often, until apples are tender when poked with fork but still hold their shape, 15 to 20 minutes. (Apples and juices should gently simmer during cooking.) Transfer apples and juices to rimmed baking sheet

and let cool to room temperature, about 30 minutes. Drain apples thoroughly in colander.

2. Adjust oven rack to lowest position, place foil-lined rimmed baking sheet on rack, and heat oven to 425 degrees. Roll 1 disk of dough into 12-inch circle between 2 large sheets of plastic wrap. Remove top plastic, gently invert dough over 9-inch metal pie plate, and ease dough into plate; remove remaining plastic. Roll other disk of dough into 12-inch circle between 2 large sheets of plastic; remove top plastic.

3. Spread apples into dough-lined pie plate, mounding slightly in middle, and drizzle with lemon juice. Gently invert top crust over filling and remove plastic. Trim dough ½ inch beyond lip of pie plate, pinch dough edges together, and tuck under itself to be flush with edge of pie plate. Crimp dough evenly around edge using your fingers. Cut four 2-inch slits in top crust. Brush pie with egg white and sprinkle with remaining teaspoon sugar.

4. Place pie on preheated baking sheet and bake until crust is dark golden brown, 45 to 55 minutes, rotating sheet halfway through baking. Let pie cool on wire rack to room temperature, about 2 hours; serve slightly warm or at room temperature.

TEST KITCHEN TIP
Topping a Double-Crust Pie

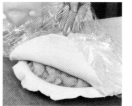 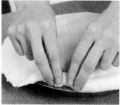

1. Invert top crust over filling and remove plastic; trim excess dough with shears, leaving ½-inch overhang to line up with bottom dough.

2. Pinch top and bottom layers of dough together and fold dough under itself so that edge of fold is flush with outer rim of pie plate.

Blueberry Pie

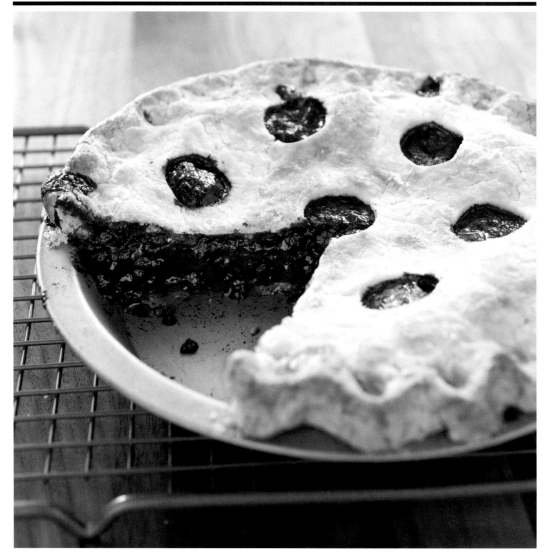

G-F TESTING LAB

FLOUR SUBSTITUTION	See page 246 for information about using various brands of gluten-free flour in the pie dough.
TAPIOCA STARCH	Tapioca starch is often labeled tapioca flour. See page 20 for more details on this ingredient. If you do not have tapioca starch, you can substitute instant tapioca or pearl tapioca in the filling; you will need to grind the tapioca to a powder in a spice grinder or mini food processor. If using pearl tapioca, reduce the amount to 5 teaspoons.

WHY THIS RECIPE WORKS

We wanted a pie that had a firm, juicy filling full of fresh blueberry flavor with still plump berries, and we also wanted a crisp, flaky crust. To thicken the pie, we tried cornstarch as well as our gluten-free flour blend but preferred tapioca starch, which was subtle enough to allow the berry flavor to shine through. Too much of it, though, created a congealed mess. Cooking some of the blueberries down to a saucy consistency helped us reduce the amount of tapioca required, as did adding a peeled Granny Smith apple that we shredded on the large holes of a box grater. Rich in pectin, the apple helped thicken the berries naturally. Since gluten-free pie crusts can easily turn soggy, we found that preheating a sheet pan in the oven and baking the pie on the lower rack helped keep the crust crisp. It's not safe to place a glass (Pyrex) pie plate on a preheated baking sheet. If you must use a glass pie plate, do not preheat the baking sheet; note, however, that your crust will not be as crisp. This pie is best served the day it is made.

Blueberry Pie
SERVES 8

- 30 ounces (6 cups) blueberries
- 1 Granny Smith apple, peeled, cored, and shredded
- 5¼ ounces (¾ cup) sugar
- 2 tablespoons tapioca starch
- 2 teaspoons grated lemon zest plus 2 teaspoons juice
- Pinch salt
- 1 recipe Double-Crust Pie Dough (page 247)
- 1 large egg white, lightly beaten

1. Cook 3 cups blueberries in medium saucepan over medium heat, mashing occasionally with potato masher to help release juices, until half of berries have broken down and mixture is thickened and measures 1½ cups, about 8 minutes. Let cool slightly.

2. Place shredded apple in clean kitchen towel and wring dry. Combine apple, cooked berry mixture, remaining 3 cups uncooked berries, sugar, tapioca starch, lemon zest and juice, and salt in large bowl.

3. Adjust oven rack to lowest position, place foil-lined rimmed baking sheet on rack, and heat oven to 425 degrees. Roll 1 disk of dough into 12-inch circle between 2 large sheets of plastic wrap. Remove top plastic, gently invert dough over 9-inch metal pie plate, and ease dough into plate; remove remaining plastic. Roll other disk of dough into 12-inch circle between 2 large sheets of plastic. Remove top plastic. Using 1¼-inch round cookie cutter, cut hole in center of dough, then cut out 6 more holes, about 1½ inches from hole in center, evenly spaced around center hole.

4. Spread blueberry mixture evenly into dough-lined pie plate. Gently invert top crust over filling and remove remaining plastic. Trim dough ½ inch beyond lip of pie plate, pinch dough edges together, and tuck under itself to be flush with edge of pie plate. Crimp dough evenly around edge using your fingers. Brush pie with egg white.

5. Place pie on preheated baking sheet and bake until crust is light golden brown, about 25 minutes. Reduce oven temperature to 350 degrees, rotate baking sheet, and continue to bake until juices are bubbling and crust is deep golden brown, 30 to 40 minutes longer. Let pie cool on wire rack to room temperature, about 4 hours. Serve.

TEST KITCHEN TIP **A Pretty Top Crust**

An easy way to make a pretty double-crust blueberry pie is to precut holes in the crust before placing it on the pie. These holes also help with evaporation during baking.

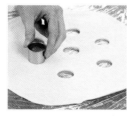

Using 1¼-inch round cookie cutter, cut round from center of dough. Cut another 6 rounds from dough, 1½ inches from edge of center hole and equally spaced around center hole.

Fresh Strawberry Pie

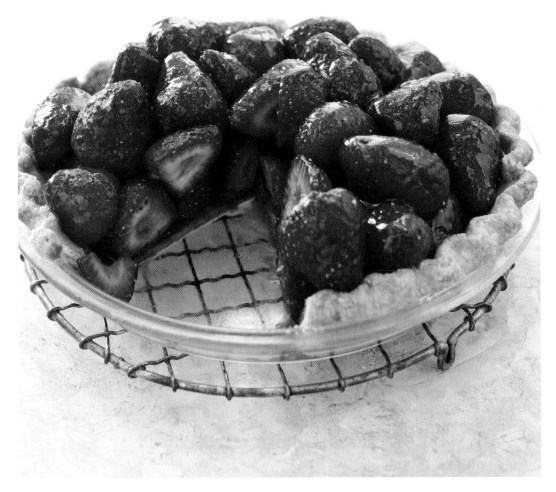

G-F TESTING LAB

FLOUR SUBSTITUTION See page 246 for information about using various brands of gluten-free flour in the pie dough.

✓ WHY THIS RECIPE WORKS

To make the glazy filling that would hold our ripe berries in place, we first simmered pureed strawberries with sugar and cornstarch. We tossed this thickened puree with whole, fresh berries and piled them into a baked pie crust, but after a short time the filling became a gloppy mess atop a soggy crust. Increasing the amount of cornstarch dulled the fresh strawberry flavor. Gelatin produced a bouncy filling, while arrowroot and tapioca produced overly thin fillings. Next, we tried tossing the berries with jarred strawberry jam. This offered a reasonably thick texture, but the sweetness was cloying. The solution: Make our own "jam" from fresh berries, sugar, and pectin so that we could control the sweetness. This version was better, but pectin alone was still too firm. We remembered the looser texture of our original cornstarch test and decided to combine the two. This method produced just the right supple, lightly clingy glaze that coated the strawberries without sogging out the crust. To account for any imperfect strawberries, the ingredient list calls for more berries than you will need. Make sure the strawberries are at room temperature and dried well so the glaze will adhere properly. For the fruit pectin, we recommend both Sure-Jell for Less or No Sugar Needed Recipes and Ball RealFruit Low or No-Sugar Needed Pectin. The pie is at its best after 2 or 3 hours of chilling; the glaze becomes softer and wetter as it continues to chill, and the crust will become soggy if the pie is refrigerated for more than 5 hours. Serve with whipped cream.

Fresh Strawberry Pie
SERVES 8

- 1   recipe Single-Crust Pie Dough (page 247)
- 3   pounds strawberries, hulled (9 cups)
- 5¼ ounces (¾ cup) sugar
- 2   tablespoons cornstarch
- 1½ teaspoons low-sugar or no-sugar-needed fruit pectin
-     Pinch salt
- 1   tablespoon lemon juice

1. Adjust oven rack to middle position and heat oven to 375 degrees. Roll dough into 12-inch circle between 2 large sheets of plastic wrap. Remove top plastic, gently invert dough over 9-inch pie plate, and ease dough into plate. Remove remaining plastic and trim dough ½ inch beyond lip of pie plate. Tuck overhanging dough under itself to be flush with edge of pie plate. Crimp dough evenly around edge using your fingers.

2. Cover dough loosely in plastic and freeze until chilled and firm, about 15 minutes. Remove plastic and bake until crust is golden brown, 25 to 30 minutes, rotating pie plate halfway through baking. Let crust cool completely on wire rack, at least 1 hour or up to 3 hours.

3. Select 6 ounces misshapen, underripe, or otherwise unattractive berries, halving those that are large; you should have about 1½ cups. Process strawberries in food processor to smooth puree, 20 to 30 seconds, scraping down bowl as needed (you should have about ¾ cup puree).

4. Whisk sugar, cornstarch, pectin, and salt together in medium saucepan. Stir in berry puree, making sure to scrape corners of pan. Cook over medium-high heat, stirring constantly with heatproof rubber spatula, and bring to full boil. Boil, scraping bottom and sides of pan to prevent scorching, for 2 minutes to ensure that cornstarch is fully cooked (mixture will appear frothy when it first reaches boil, then will darken and thicken with further cooking). Transfer glaze to large bowl and stir in lemon juice. Let cool until slightly warm.

5. Meanwhile, pick over remaining strawberries and measure out 2 pounds of most attractive ones; halve or quarter any berries larger than 1½ inches. Add strawberries to bowl with glaze and fold in gently with rubber spatula until evenly coated. Scoop strawberry mixture into pie shell, piling into mound. If any cut strawberry sides face up on top, turn them face down. If necessary, rearrange berries so that holes are filled and mound looks attractive. Refrigerate pie until chilled, about 2 hours. Serve.

Individual Blueberry-Almond Buckles

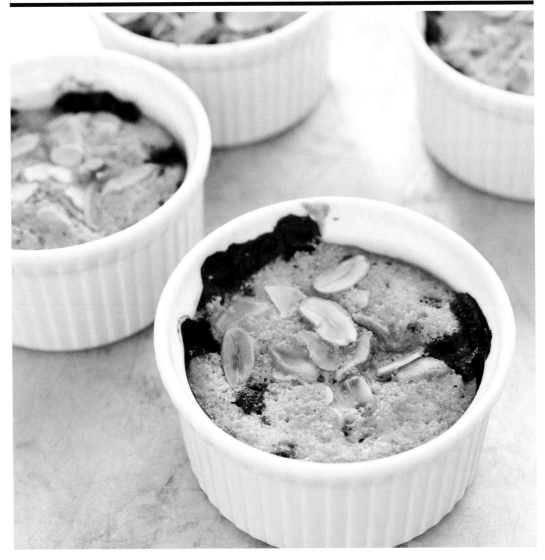

G-F TESTING LAB

FLOUR SUBSTITUTION	King Arthur Gluten-Free Multi-Purpose Flour 3½ ounces = ½ cup plus 2 tablespoons	Bob's Red Mill GF All-Purpose Baking Flour 3½ ounces = ⅔ cup

Note that buckles made with Bob's Red Mill will have a distinct bean flavor.

✓ WHY THIS RECIPE WORKS

These individual fruit-packed cakes are an easy make-ahead dessert that is especially handy when entertaining. We made the simple batter for these buckles in the food processor, folding in the berries at the end, which kept prep work and dishes to a minimum. This recipe requires very little flour because we grind up nuts to give the batter both flavor and structure; as a result, our gluten-free flour blend worked easily here. It helps too that these buckles are laden with fresh fruit and are meant to be moist and dense and not firm and cakey. Plus the ramekins help these buckles cook evenly, and we didn't have to worry about soggy centers or even about unmolding. For a nice finishing touch, we topped the buckles with a portion of the nuts before baking. Coating the ramekins with vegetable oil spray prevented the buckles from sticking. Do not substitute frozen berries here. Serve warm with vanilla ice cream or whipped cream.

Individual Blueberry-Almond Buckles
SERVES 8

- 5¼ ounces (¾ cup) sugar
- ½ cup sliced almonds, toasted and chopped coarse
- 4 tablespoons unsalted butter, softened
- ¼ teaspoon salt
- ⅓ cup heavy cream
- 2 large eggs
- ½ teaspoon almond extract
- 3½ ounces (¾ cup) ATK Gluten-Free Flour Blend (page 13)
- ½ teaspoon baking powder (see page 20)
- 15 ounces (3 cups) fresh blueberries

1. Adjust oven rack to middle position and heat oven to 375 degrees. Spray eight 6-ounce ramekins with vegetable oil spray and place on rimmed baking sheet.

2. Process sugar, ¼ cup almonds, butter, and salt together in food processor until finely ground, 10 to 15 seconds. With processor running, add cream, eggs, and almond extract and continue to process until smooth, about 5 seconds. Add flour blend and baking powder and pulse until incorporated, about 5 pulses.

3. Transfer batter to large bowl and gently fold in blueberries. Spoon batter into prepared ramekins and sprinkle evenly with remaining ¼ cup almonds. (Buckles can sit at room temperature, covered with plastic wrap, for up to 2 hours.)

4. Bake buckles until golden and beginning to pull away from sides of ramekins, 25 to 30 minutes, rotating sheet halfway through baking. Let buckles cool on wire rack for 10 minutes before serving.

VARIATIONS
Individual Raspberry-Pistachio Buckles
Don't use frozen raspberries here.

Substitute shelled pistachios for almonds, 1 teaspoon vanilla extract for almond extract, and fresh raspberries for blueberries.

Individual Blackberry-Walnut Buckles
Substitute walnuts for almonds, 1 teaspoon vanilla extract for almond extract, and fresh blackberries for blueberries.

Individual Fresh Berry Gratins with Zabaglione

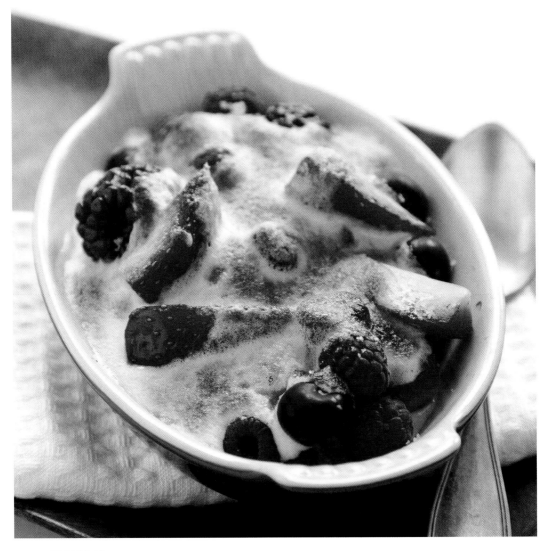

G-F TESTING LAB

BERRIES   We prefer to make this recipe with a variety of berries but you can use just one type of fruit if you prefer. Do not use frozen berries.

✓ WHY THIS RECIPE WORKS

Berry gratins can be a very humble affair in which fresh fruit is simply dressed up with sweetened bread crumbs and baked, or they can be a bit more sophisticated, as when they are topped with the foamy Italian custard called zabaglione. Since zabaglione, made with egg yolks, sugar, and wine, is naturally gluten-free, we decided to choose this approach. But making the zabaglione takes a little finesse. It requires constant watching so that the mixture doesn't overcook. It also needs to be whisked until it's the ideal thick, creamy texture. We were after a foolproof method for this topping for a gratin that could serve as an elegant finale to a summer meal. We chose to make individual gratins and settled on a mix of berries, which we tossed with sugar and salt to draw out their juices. To prevent a custard with scrambled eggs, we kept the heat low; for the right texture, we whisked until the custard was somewhat thick. As for flavor, traditional Marsala wine gave us an overly sweet zabaglione; crisp, dry Sauvignon Blanc provided a clean flavor that worked better with the berries. Whipped cream worked well as a thickening agent. We spooned our zabaglione over the berries and sprinkled a mixture of brown and granulated sugars on top before broiling for a crackly, caramelized crust.

Individual Fresh Berry Gratins with Zabaglione
SERVES 4

BERRY MIXTURE
- 15 ounces (3 cups) mixed blackberries, blueberries, raspberries, and strawberries (strawberries hulled and halved lengthwise if small, quartered if large)
- 2 teaspoons granulated sugar
  Pinch salt

ZABAGLIONE TOPPING
- 3 large egg yolks
- 3 tablespoons granulated sugar
- 3 tablespoons dry white wine such as Sauvignon Blanc
- 2 teaspoons packed light brown sugar
- 3 tablespoons heavy cream, chilled

1. FOR THE BERRY MIXTURE: Line rimmed baking sheet with aluminum foil. Toss berries, granulated sugar, and salt together in bowl. Divide berry mixture evenly among 4 shallow 6-ounce gratin dishes set on prepared sheet; set aside.

2. FOR THE ZABAGLIONE: Whisk egg yolks, 2 tablespoons plus 1 teaspoon granulated sugar, and wine together in medium bowl until sugar is dissolved, about 1 minute. Set bowl over saucepan of barely simmering water and cook, whisking constantly, until mixture is frothy. Continue to cook, whisking constantly, until mixture is slightly thickened, creamy, and glossy, 5 to 10 minutes (mixture will form loose mounds when dripped from whisk). Remove bowl from saucepan and whisk constantly for 30 seconds to cool slightly. Transfer bowl to refrigerator and chill until egg mixture is completely cool, about 10 minutes.

3. Meanwhile, adjust oven rack 6 inches from broiler element and heat broiler. Combine remaining 2 teaspoons granulated sugar and light brown sugar in bowl.

4. Whisk heavy cream in large bowl until it holds soft peaks, 30 to 90 seconds. Using rubber spatula, gently fold whipped cream into cooled egg mixture. Spoon zabaglione over berries and sprinkle sugar mixture evenly over zabaglione; let stand at room temperature for 10 minutes, until sugar dissolves.

5. Broil until sugar is bubbly and caramelized, 1 to 4 minutes. Serve immediately.

VARIATION
Individual Fresh Berry Gratins with Lemon Zabaglione
Replace 1 tablespoon wine with equal amount lemon juice, and add 1 teaspoon grated lemon zest to egg yolk mixture in step 2.

Individual Pavlovas with Tropical Fruit

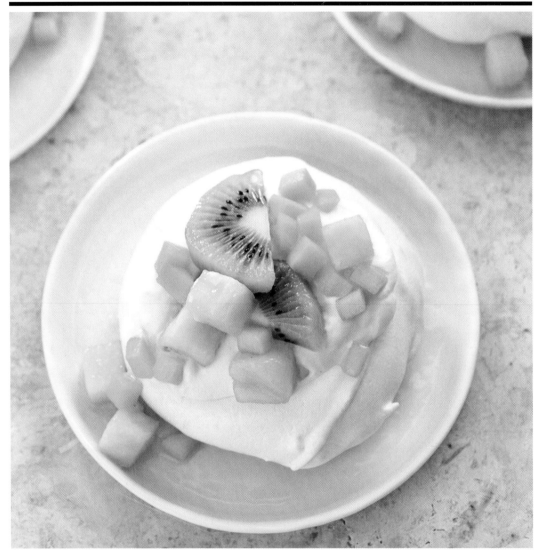

G-F TESTING LAB

CREAM OF TARTAR   This white powder sold in the spice aisle ensures that the whipped eggs are both stable and glossy. See page 21 for details on this ingredient.

✓ WHY THIS RECIPE WORKS

These naturally gluten-free meringue shells filled with whipped cream and topped with fresh fruit make a light ending to a meal. The key to this recipe is successfully making the meringues. Individual meringues are easier to shape than one large meringue and easier to serve because there's no slicing required. We portion out the mixture into small mounds on a baking sheet and use the back of a spoon to create a concave center for holding the whipped cream and fruit. Baking the meringues at 200 degrees for 1½ hours yielded perfectly dry, crisp white shells, but they required gradual cooling off in a turned-off oven to ensure crispness. Adding a tablespoon of sugar to the fruit was necessary to extract some of their juices and create a flavorful syrup that soaked into the meringue and whipped cream. The fruit is the garnish here, so it's worth taking time to cut it into tidy pieces. Avoid making pavlovas on humid days or the meringue shells will turn out sticky.

Individual Pavlovas with Tropical Fruit
SERVES 6

MERINGUES AND FRUIT
- 4   large egg whites, room temperature
- ¾   teaspoon vanilla extract
- ¼   teaspoon cream of tartar
- 7   ounces (1 cup) plus 1 tablespoon sugar
- 1   mango, peeled, pitted, and cut into ¼-inch pieces
- 2   kiwis, peeled, halved lengthwise, and sliced thin
- 1½ cups ½-inch pineapple pieces

WHIPPED CREAM
- 1   cup heavy cream, chilled
- 1   tablespoon sugar
- 1   teaspoon vanilla extract

1. FOR THE MERINGUES: Adjust oven rack to middle position and heat oven to 200 degrees. Line baking sheet with parchment paper.

2. Using stand mixer fitted with whisk, whip egg whites, vanilla, and cream of tartar on medium-low speed until foamy, about 1 minute. Increase speed to medium-high and whip whites to soft, billowy mounds, about 1 minute. Gradually add 1 cup sugar and whip until glossy, stiff peaks form, 1 to 2 minutes.

3. Using ½-cup measure, scoop six ½-cup mounds of meringue onto prepared sheet, spacing them about 1 inch apart. Gently make small, bowl-shaped indentation in each meringue using back of spoon. Bake until meringues are smooth, dry, and firm, about 1½ hours. Turn oven off and leave meringues in oven until completely dry and hard, about 2 hours. (Meringue shells can be stored in airtight container at room temperature for up to 2 weeks.)

4. Gently toss fruit with remaining 1 tablespoon sugar in bowl. Let sit at room temperature until sugar has dissolved and fruit is juicy, about 30 minutes.

5. FOR THE WHIPPED CREAM: Using clean, dry mixer bowl and whisk attachment, whip cream, sugar, and vanilla on medium-low speed until foamy, about 1 minute. Increase speed to high and whip until soft peaks form, 1 to 3 minutes. (Whipped cream can be refrigerated for up to 8 hours; rewhisk before serving.)

6. To assemble, place meringue shells on individual plates and spoon about ⅓ cup whipped cream into each. Top with about ½ cup fruit (some fruit and juice will fall onto plate). Serve immediately.

VARIATIONS

Individual Pavlovas with Mixed Berries
Substitute 1½ cups each raspberries and blueberries and 1 cup blackberries for mango, kiwi, and pineapple.

Individual Pavlovas with Strawberries, Blueberries, and Peaches
Substitute 1 cup strawberries, sliced thin, 1 cup blueberries, and 2 peaches, peeled, halved, pitted, and sliced ¼ inch thick, for mango, kiwi, and pineapple.

Peach Cobbler with Cornmeal Biscuits

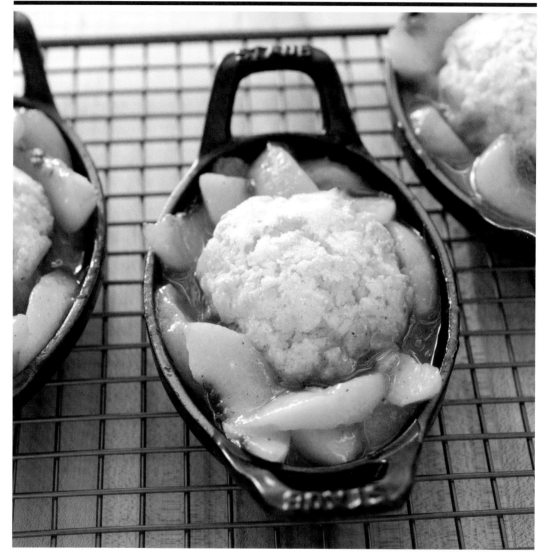

G-F TESTING LAB

FLOUR SUBSTITUTION	King Arthur Gluten-Free Multi-Purpose Flour 4½ ounces = ½ **cup plus** ⅓ **cup**	Bob's Red Mill GF All-Purpose Baking Flour 4½ ounces = ¾ **cup plus 2 tablespoons**

Note that biscuits made with King Arthur will be a bit pasty, and biscuits made with Bob's Red Mill will be darker in color and more crumbly, will not rise as well, and will have a slight bean flavor.

CORNMEAL The test kitchen's favorite cornmeal for baking is finely ground Whole-Grain Arrowhead Mills Cornmeal. This brand has been processed in a gluten-free facility, but not all brands are. Make sure to read the label. See page 149 for more details on cornmeal.

✔ WHY THIS RECIPE WORKS

Our first attempts at trying to marry our gluten-free biscuits with peach cobbler filling proved right away that a sturdier biscuit would be in order. Our gluten-free biscuits softened dramatically when paired with the hot filling. Clearly a biscuit that was not made with all flour blend would be a better bet, and the less time it spent atop a hot filling, the better. For this reason, we decided to take another route for our cobbler topping: cornmeal biscuits. Cornmeal paired with an equal amount of our flour blend would make a sturdier biscuit, and we thought the corn flavor would pair well with the peach filling. We started with an old yet beloved cornmeal biscuit recipe, which had very little sugar and baking powder. Increasing both and adding a little baking soda gave us the lift and sturdiness needed for this recipe, while the extra sugar tilted the biscuit to the sweet rather than the savory side—perfect for our cobbler. The baking powder gave us the lift that we needed to form traditional-looking biscuits. We parbaked these biscuits as well as the filling, so they needed to spend only about 5 minutes together in the oven for the perfect cobbler.

Peach Cobbler with Cornmeal Biscuits
SERVES 8

5	ounces (1 cup) cornmeal
4½	ounces (1 cup) ATK Gluten-Free Flour Blend (page 13)
2⅓	ounces (⅓ cup) plus 3 tablespoons sugar, plus extra as needed
2	teaspoons baking powder (see page 20)
¼	teaspoon baking soda
	Salt
8	tablespoons unsalted butter, cut into ¼-inch pieces and chilled
¾	cup buttermilk, chilled
4	pounds ripe but firm peaches, peeled, halved, pitted, and cut into ½-inch wedges
¼	teaspoon ground ginger
⅛	teaspoon ground cinnamon
5	teaspoons lemon juice
1½	teaspoons cornstarch

1. Adjust oven rack to middle position and heat oven to 375 degrees. Line baking sheet with parchment paper. Pulse cornmeal, flour blend, 2 tablespoons sugar, baking powder, baking soda, and ½ teaspoon salt together in food processor until combined, about 5 pulses. Scatter butter pieces over top and pulse until mixture resembles coarse cornmeal with few slightly larger butter lumps, about 10 pulses.

2. Transfer cornmeal mixture to medium bowl, add buttermilk, and stir with fork until dough gathers into moist clumps. Using greased ¼-cup dry measure, scoop out and drop 8 mounds of dough onto prepared baking sheet, spaced about 1 inch apart. Sprinkle 1 tablespoon sugar over top and bake until biscuits are puffed and lightly browned, 25 to 30 minutes. Let biscuits cool slightly on wire rack. (Cooled biscuits can be held at room temperature in sealed zipper-lock bag for up to 2 hours.)

3. Meanwhile, combine peaches, remaining ⅓ cup sugar, ginger, cinnamon, and pinch salt together in Dutch oven. Cover and cook over medium-low heat until peaches have softened and release their juices, 10 to 15 minutes.

4. Whisk lemon juice and cornstarch together in bowl, then stir into peaches and continue to cook, uncovered, until liquid has thickened, 2 to 5 minutes. Season with extra sugar to taste. Transfer to deep-dish pie plate or into 8 individual gratin dishes. (Fruit can be covered with plastic wrap and held at room temperature for up to 1½ hours.)

5. To serve, arrange biscuits on top of peach mixture and bake until heated through, 3 to 5 minutes. Serve immediately.

Apple Crisp

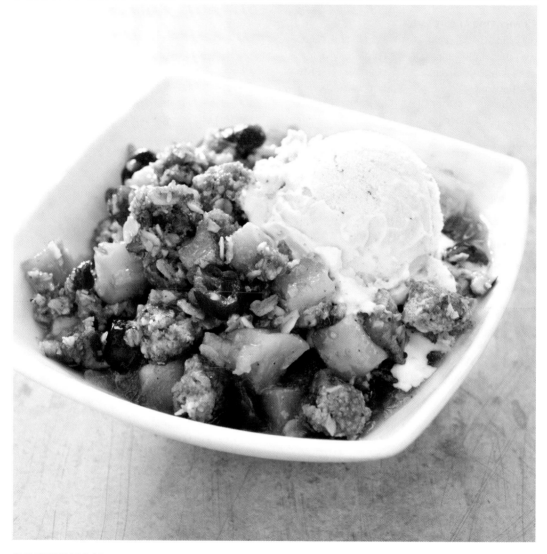

FLOUR SUBSTITUTION	King Arthur Gluten-Free Multi-Purpose Flour 1½ ounces = ¼ **cup**	Bob's Red Mill GF All-Purpose Baking Flour 1½ ounces = **5 tablespoons**
	Note that topping made with King Arthur will be slightly softer, and topping made with Bob's Red Mill will have a slight bean flavor.	
OATS	Do not use quick oats; they have a dusty texture that doesn't work in this recipe. Make sure to buy old-fashioned rolled oats (see page 62) that have been processed in a gluten-free facility.	

✅ WHY THIS RECIPE WORKS

Thinking this recipe would be easy to make gluten-free since only the topping contains flour, we started by making our classic recipe, which calls for parbaking the topping and the fruit separately and then combining them for a short stint in the oven. When we swapped out all-purpose flour for our gluten-free blend, the topping spread over the baking sheet. The low protein content in our flour blend meant it wasn't able to hold the topping together to form the desired crumbly bits. Recognizing that using less flour would work to our advantage, we experimented with larger amounts of oats and nuts, toasting them and then finely grinding nearly half of them to a flourlike consistency. In the end, we needed just ⅓ cup of flour blend. Given the stability of our new topping, we found that we did not need to parbake it. However, it was critical to parbake the apples because the time they required to cook through was far longer than the time needed to crisp the topping. For just the right, saucy consistency, we grated one apple, which broke down during cooking. We liked the way Golden Delicious apples worked in this recipe, as some broke down and created a saucy filling. You can use pecans or walnuts instead of sliced almonds in the topping. The baked crisp can be kept at room temperature for up to 4 hours; warm crisp in oven before serving.

Apple Crisp
SERVES 6

TOPPING

- ¾ cup gluten-free old-fashioned rolled oats
- ¾ cup sliced almonds
- 1½ ounces (⅓ cup) ATK Gluten-Free Flour Blend (page 13)
- 1¾ ounces (¼ cup packed) brown sugar
- 2 tablespoons granulated sugar
- 2 teaspoons vanilla extract
- 1 teaspoon water
- ⅛ teaspoon salt
- 6 tablespoons unsalted butter, cut into 6 pieces and softened

FILLING

- 4 teaspoons lemon juice
- ¾ teaspoon cornstarch
- 3 pounds Golden Delicious apples (about 6 medium), 5 peeled and cut into ½-inch cubes, 1 peeled and grated
- 2⅓ ounces (⅓ cup) granulated sugar
  Pinch salt
  Pinch ground cinnamon
  Pinch ground nutmeg

1. FOR THE TOPPING: Adjust oven rack to middle position and heat oven to 400 degrees. Place oats and nuts in two piles on parchment paper–lined baking sheet, and bake until lightly toasted, 3 to 5 minutes. Remove from oven and cool completely.

2. Pulse ½ cup oats, flour blend, brown sugar, granulated sugar, vanilla, water, and salt in food processor until combined, about 5 pulses. Sprinkle butter and half of almonds over top and process until mixture clumps together into large, crumbly balls, about 30 seconds, stopping halfway through to scrape down bowl. Sprinkle remaining almonds and remaining ¼ cup oats over mixture and combine with 2 quick pulses. Transfer mixture to bowl.

3. FOR THE FILLING: Whisk lemon juice and cornstarch in large bowl until cornstarch is dissolved. Stir in apples, sugar, salt, cinnamon, and nutmeg. Transfer mixture to 8-inch square baking dish, cover tightly with aluminum foil, and bake for 20 minutes.

4. Remove baking dish from oven, uncover, and stir filling well. Pinch topping into grape-size pieces (with some smaller loose bits) and sprinkle over filling. Bake until topping is well browned and fruit is tender and bubbling around edges, 20 to 25 minutes, rotating dish halfway through baking. Let crisp cool on wire rack until warm, about 15 minutes. Serve.

VARIATION
Apple-Cranberry Crisp
Substitute pecans for almonds and add ½ cup dried cranberries to filling along with apples in step 3.

Creating a Crisp Topping

THE PROBLEM The test kitchen's original apple crisp features a rich topping made with flour, two kinds of sugar, butter, and nuts atop tender apples. To ensure a crisp topping and perfectly cooked apples, we bake both separately and then marry them together at the end for a brief stint in the oven. The fruit filling needed no changes for our gluten-free version, so we focused our attention on the topping.

CRISPY, NOT CAKEY Simply swapping in gluten-free flour for the all-purpose flour in our traditional apple crisp recipe delivered a solid, cakelike layer of topping that, when crumbled, fell into the apples and created unappealing pockets of wet cake in the crisp. We tried adding the topping raw, but it sank into the filling and never cooked all the way through. We were missing the gluten proteins from all-purpose flour, which trap gas, creating structure in baked goods. Our goal was to find a substitute: We needed to add some bulk.

MORE NUTS AND OATS, LESS FLOUR To create more structure, we tried omitting the flour altogether, using ground oats as a substitute. The result was a sweet, granola-like topping that felt disconnected from the filling. Clearly some flour was needed. Decreasing the amount of flour to 1½ ounces from the original recipe's 5 ounces and upping the amount of nuts and oats was our next strategy. Finely grinding more than half of the oats allowed us to use less flour. We then added half the nuts when adding the butter, effectively grinding them as well. This topping was more cookielike, with the appealing crunch and texture of granola. Finally, we were getting somewhere.

TOAST AND GRIND Satisfied with the general direction of the topping, we continued to play with variables to perfect it. Parbaking the topping was still not working (it melted and burned in the oven), but toasting the nuts and oats before making the topping really amplified the flavor. We tried cutting back on butter to allow the nut and oat flavor to shine, but that made the topping too lean. We then discovered that the 6 tablespoons of butter we were using in the topping was not enough to hold it together as well as we hoped. We tried using brown sugar alone and then granulated sugar alone to solve this problem, but neither delivered the texture we were after. The topping of the crisp made with all granulated sugar was too grainy, while all brown sugar made it too chewy; we found that a mixture of ¼ cup brown sugar and 2 tablespoons granulated sugar was the right mix, while adding just a little water to the topping helped it clump together and kept the nuts and oats in the forefront.

A TWO-PART SOLUTION Our topping seemingly solved, we needed a method for perfectly cooking the apples and browning the topping. Knowing the topping was going on raw, we tried starting the whole crisp raw in the oven. The apples were not only undercooked, but unevenly cooked as well. Covering the apples with foil and parbaking them trapped steam and helped the apples soften properly, and stirring them before adding the topping allowed the apples to cook more evenly. We added the topping in crumbly bits to the parbaked apples to make the dish cohesive, and then baked it for 25 minutes. By the time the topping was nicely browned, the apples were pleasantly tender and sweet, and we had our perfect crisp.

Tart Shell

✓ WHY THIS RECIPE WORKS

While pie crust is tender and flaky, classic tart crust should be fine-textured, buttery-rich, crisp, and crumbly—it is often described as being similar to shortbread. We began experimenting with our classic recipe (which combines flour, confectioners' sugar, an egg yolk, heavy cream, and a stick of butter), substituting our gluten-free flour blend for the all-purpose flour, but found the crust too sweet and fragile. Adding xanthan gum helped reinforce the structure, but our tart shell was still too crumbly and too sweet (since rice flours, unlike all-purpose flour, have a distinct sweetness). Our next step was to go down on sugar and test adding another egg, egg yolks, and more cream. But still the crust was sandy and overly sweet. Our traditional tart crust uses confectioners' sugar to make the crust more shortbreadlike, but since our working recipe was leaning too far in the shortbread direction, so much so that the crust was almost powdery, we decided to try granulated sugar. Unfortunately, the granulated sugar produced a hard, candied shell. In the end we found that reducing the amount of sugar and using a mix of confectioners' sugar and brown sugar did the trick. We also learned that we didn't need the cream at all—just a very small amount of water was all that was required to bind the dough together. Refer to pages 270–271 when making this recipe.

Tart Shell

MAKES ONE 9-INCH TART SHELL

- 1 **large egg yolk**
- ½ **teaspoon vanilla extract**
- 7 **ounces (1⅓ cups plus ¼ cup) ATK Gluten-Free Flour Blend (page 13)**
- 2⅓ **ounces (⅓ cup packed) light brown sugar**
- 1 **ounce (¼ cup) confectioners' sugar**
- 1 **teaspoon xanthan gum**
- ¼ **teaspoon salt**
- 8 **tablespoons unsalted butter, cut into ¼-inch pieces and chilled**
- 2 **teaspoons ice water**

1. Whisk egg yolk and vanilla together in bowl. Process flour blend, brown sugar, confectioners' sugar, xanthan gum, and salt together in food processor until combined, about 5 seconds. Scatter butter over top and pulse until mixture resembles coarse cornmeal, about 10 pulses.

2. With processor running, add egg yolk mixture and continue to process until dough just comes together around processor blade, about 15 seconds. Add 1 teaspoon ice water and pulse until dough comes together. If dough does not come together, add remaining 1 teaspoon ice water and pulse until dough comes together.

3. Turn dough onto sheet of plastic wrap and flatten into 6-inch disk. Wrap dough tightly in plastic and refrigerate for 1 hour. (Dough can be refrigerated for up to 2 days or frozen for up to 2 months. If frozen, let dough thaw completely on counter before rolling out.)

4. Let dough sit on counter to soften slightly, about 10 minutes. Spray 9-inch tart pan with removable bottom with vegetable oil spray. Roll dough into 12-inch circle between 2 large sheets of plastic wrap, then slide onto baking sheet and remove top sheet of plastic. Place tart pan, bottom side up, in center of dough, press gently into dough to cut, making sure to hold tart pan firmly in place. Using both hands, carefully flip over sheet pan with dough and tart pan, setting tart pan right side up on counter. Remove sheet pan and peel off remaining plastic.

5. Run rolling pin over edges of tart pan to finish cutting dough. Gently press dough into bottom of tart pan, reserving scraps. Roll dough scraps into ½-inch rope. Line edge of tart pan with rope and gently press into fluted sides. Line tart pan with plastic and, using measuring cup, gently smooth dough to even thickness (sides should be about ¼ inch thick). Using paring knife, trim any excess dough above rim of tart pan. Freeze until chilled and firm, about 15 minutes. Bake and fill as directed in specific recipes.

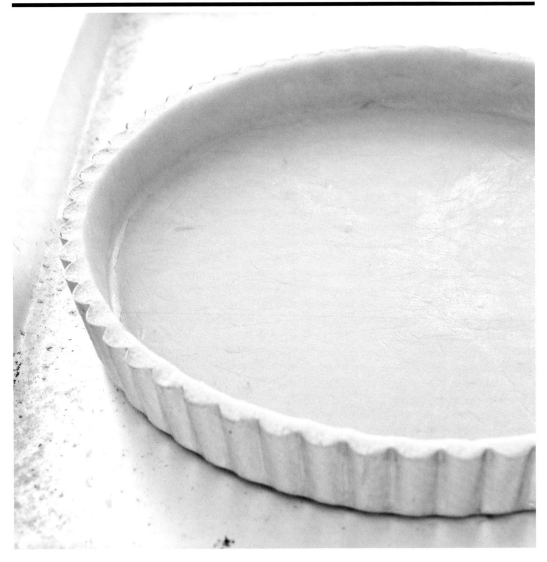

G-F TESTING LAB

FLOUR SUBSTITUTION	King Arthur Gluten-Free Multi-Purpose Flour 7 ounces = **1¼ cups**	Bob's Red Mill GF All-Purpose Baking Flour 7 ounces = **1¼ cups plus 2 tablespoons**
	Note that a tart shell made with King Arthur will be more crumbly and grainy, and a tart shell made with Bob's Red Mill will have a strong bean flavor.	
XANTHAN GUM	Do not omit the xanthan gum; it is crucial to the structure of the tart dough. For more information, see page 16.	

TEST KITCHEN TIP **Making a Tart Shell**

Because our gluten-free tart dough is softer than traditional dough, you need to roll it out between sheets of plastic wrap. We also discovered a super-easy method for getting this dough into the pan: We pressed the tart pan into the dough to cut it, and then inverted the baking sheet along with the tart pan so that the dough fell right into the pan. Make sure to chill the dough before starting this process. If at any point the dough becomes too soft to work with, slip the dough onto a baking sheet and refrigerate it until workable. Note that this dough needs to be lined with greased parchment or foil and weighted with pie weights before baking, or else it will puff up in the oven and the sides will shrink down.

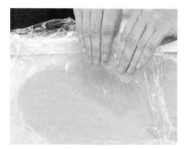

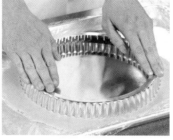

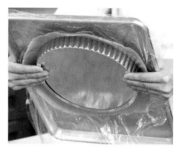

1. Roll dough into 12-inch circle between 2 sheets of plastic wrap. Slide onto baking sheet, then carefully remove top sheet of plastic.

2. Place tart pan, bottom side up, in center of dough and press gently so that sharp edge of tart pan cuts dough.

3. Holding tart pan in place, pick up sheet pan and carefully flip it over so that tart pan is right side up on counter. Remove sheet pan and peel off remaining plastic.

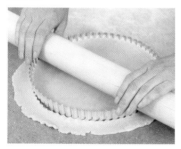

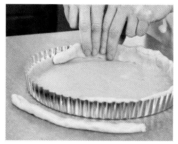

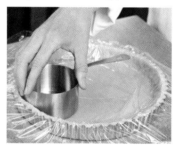

4. Run rolling pin over edges of tart pan to cut dough completely. Gently ease and press dough into bottom of pan, reserving scraps.

5. Roll dough scraps into ½-inch rope, line edge of tart pan with rope, and gently press into fluted sides.

6. Line tart pan with plastic wrap and, using measuring cup, gently press and smooth dough to even thickness (sides should be ¼ inch thick). Trim any excess dough with paring knife.

Rustic Walnut Tart

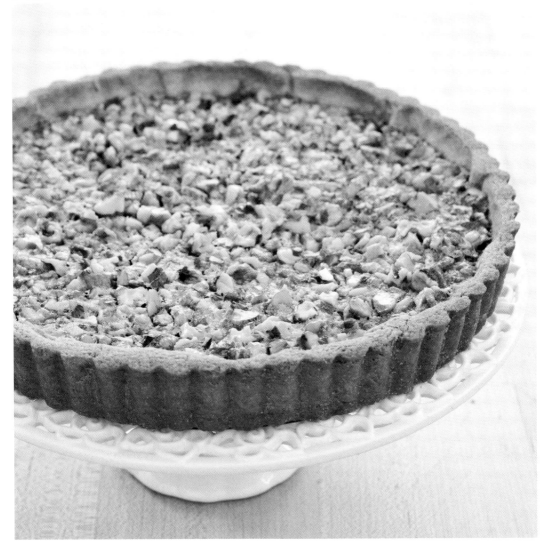

G-F TESTING LAB

FLOUR SUBSTITUTION   See page 270 for information about using various brands of gluten-free flour in the tart shell.

✔ WHY THIS RECIPE WORKS

This rustic yet beautiful tart features our gluten-free tart shell and a simple nut filling made with corn syrup and brown sugar as its base. A hefty amount of vanilla and a hit of bourbon pair nicely with the walnuts. Parbaking the shell ensures that it will be crisp. We also found that it was necessary to line the dough with greased parchment and fill the pan with pie weights, as the shell otherwise puffed up during baking because of the sugar and egg in the dough. The crust also shrank away from the sides of the pan if it was not baked with pie weights. Once filled, the tart should be baked until the filling is just firm enough to slice neatly. Pecans can be substituted for the walnuts if desired. There's no need to toast the nuts before chopping them; the tart bakes long enough to bring out their full flavor. Serve with whipped cream.

Rustic Walnut Tart
SERVES 8 TO 10

    1   recipe Tart Shell (page 269), chilled in
        freezer for 15 minutes
  3½   ounces (½ cup packed) light brown sugar
    ⅓   cup light corn syrup
    4   tablespoons unsalted butter, melted and
        cooled
    1   tablespoon bourbon or dark rum
    2   teaspoons vanilla extract
    ½   teaspoon salt
    1   large egg
  1¾   cups walnuts, chopped coarse

1. Adjust oven rack to middle position and heat oven to 375 degrees. Set chilled, dough-lined tart pan on rimmed baking sheet. Press greased parchment paper or greased double layer of aluminum foil into tart shell, covering edges to prevent burning, and fill with pie weights. Bake until tart shell is just set, about 15 minutes, rotating sheet halfway through baking.

2. Carefully remove weights and parchment and continue to bake tart shell until lightly golden, about 5 minutes. Transfer baking sheet with tart shell to wire rack and let cool while making filling. (Tart shell can be either slightly warm or completely cool when you add filling.)

3. Whisk sugar, corn syrup, melted butter, bourbon, vanilla, and salt together in large bowl until sugar dissolves. Whisk in egg until combined. Pour filling into prebaked tart shell and sprinkle evenly with walnuts. Bake tart on baking sheet until filling is set and walnuts begin to brown, 30 to 40 minutes, rotating sheet halfway through baking.

4. Transfer baking sheet with tart to wire rack and let cool to room temperature, about 2 hours. (Tart can be refrigerated for up to 1 day; bring to room temperature before serving.)

5. To serve, remove outer ring of tart pan, slide thin metal spatula between tart and tart pan bottom, and carefully slide tart onto serving platter or cutting board. Slice tart into wedges and serve.

TEST KITCHEN TIP **Prebaking Tart Dough**

Pie weights prevent the dough from melting out of shape or puffing up on the bottom as the tart shell bakes.

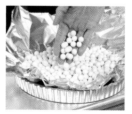

Set dough-lined tart pan on large baking sheet. Line with greased parchment paper or double layer of foil and fill shell with pie weights. (Pennies will work in a pinch.)

Nutella Tart

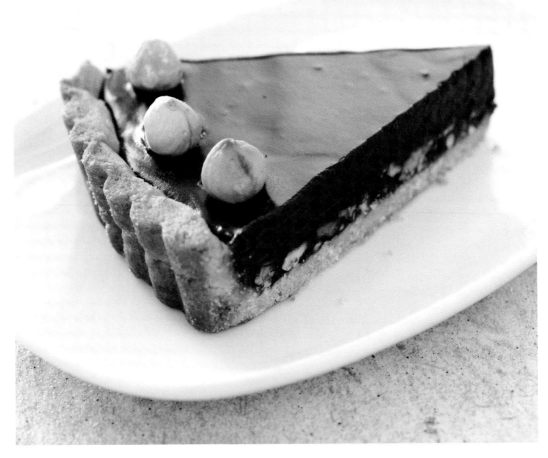

G-F TESTING LAB

FLOUR SUBSTITUTION	See page 270 for information about using various brands of gluten-free flour in the tart shell.

WHY THIS RECIPE WORKS

For an incredibly easy, incredibly irresistible dessert, we started with a flavor-packed base: Nutella. For a dense and velvety filling, we stirred Nutella into a simple ganache made of chocolate and cream. Nutella and cream alone made a filling that was too soft and didn't set up, but the addition of bittersweet chocolate helped the tart firm up, deepened the chocolate flavor, and tempered the sweetness level. Adding a little butter to the mixture proved important because it ensured the tart was easy to slice once it was chilled. To cook the filling, we turned to the microwave. Using low power and stirring the mixture often were key; when the power was too high, the filling became grainy. A bottom layer of chopped toasted hazelnuts sprinkled over our fully baked gluten-free tart shell contributed more nutty flavor and a nice crunch. Garnishing this easy tart with whole toasted hazelnuts amped up the elegance factor. If the ganache mixture looks curdled when whisking, add boiling water, 1 tablespoon at a time, and whisk until smooth. Make sure to serve with a dollop of whipped cream to cut the richness of the tart.

Nutella Tart
SERVES 8 TO 10

- 1 **cup hazelnuts**
- 1 **recipe Tart Shell (page 269), chilled in freezer for 15 minutes**
- 1½ **cups heavy cream**
- 1¼ **cups Nutella**
- 2 **ounces bittersweet chocolate, chopped fine**
- 4 **tablespoons unsalted butter, cut into 4 pieces**

1. Adjust oven rack to middle position and heat oven to 375 degrees. Toast hazelnuts on rimmed baking sheet until skins begin to blister and crack, 15 to 20 minutes. Wrap warm nuts in dish towel and rub gently to remove skins. Reserve 24 whole nuts for garnish, then chop remaining nuts coarsely.

2. Set chilled, dough-lined tart pan on rimmed baking sheet. Press greased parchment paper or greased double layer of aluminum foil into tart shell, covering edges to prevent burning, and fill with pie weights. Bake until tart shell is light golden brown and set, about 25 minutes, rotating sheet halfway through baking.

3. Carefully remove weights and parchment and continue to bake tart shell until golden, about 10 minutes. Transfer baking sheet with tart shell to wire rack and let cool while making filling. (Tart shell can be either slightly warm or completely cool when you add filling.)

4. Combine cream, Nutella, chocolate, and butter in bowl. Cover and microwave at 30 percent power, stirring often, until mixture is smooth and glossy, about 1 minute (do not overheat). Sprinkle chopped hazelnuts into prebaked tart shell. Pour warm Nutella mixture over nuts and smooth top. Refrigerate until filling is just set, about 15 minutes. Arrange reserved whole hazelnuts around edge of tart and continue to refrigerate until filling is firm, at least 1½ hours or up to 1 day.

5. To serve, remove outer ring of tart pan, slide thin metal spatula between tart and tart pan bottom, and carefully slide tart onto serving platter or cutting board. Slice tart into wedges and serve.

TEST KITCHEN TIP **Topping a Nutella Tart**

To ensure the decorative hazelnuts do not sink to the bottom of the tart, you must first chill the filled tart.

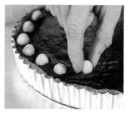

Refrigerate until filling is just set, about 15 minutes. Arrange reserved whole hazelnuts around edge of tart and continue to refrigerate until filling is firm, about 1½ hours.

Lemon Tart

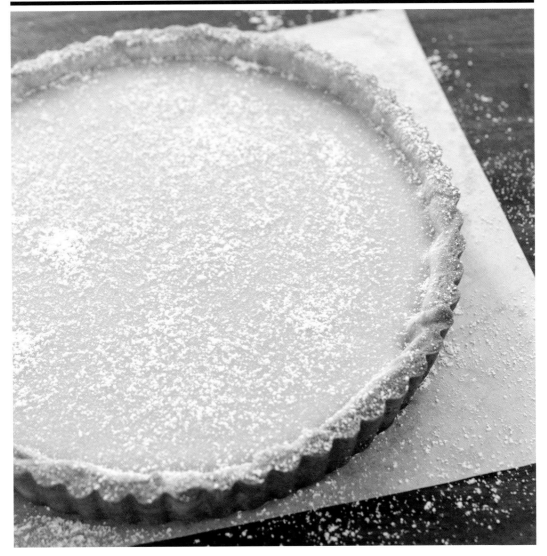

G-F TESTING LAB

FLOUR SUBSTITUTION   See page 270 for information about using various brands of gluten-free flour in the tart shell.

WHY THIS RECIPE WORKS

The filling for lemon tart, normally a simple stovetop lemon curd, is easy to make and naturally gluten-free, so with our gluten-free tart dough in hand, we thought this recipe would be an easy addition to our gluten-free dessert repertoire. Despite its simplicity, however, there is much that can go wrong with lemon tart: it can slip over the edge of sweet and become cloying; its tartness can grab at your throat; and it can be gluey or eggy or, even worse, metallic-tasting. For a balanced lemon curd with just enough sugar to offset the acidity of the lemons, we used 3 parts sugar to 2 parts lemon juice, plus a whopping ¼ cup of lemon zest for a bright, lemony flavor. To achieve a curd that was creamy and dense with a vibrant yellow color, we used a combination of whole eggs and egg yolks. A few pats of butter, whisked in as we cooked the curd over gentle heat, contributed more richness. For a smooth, light texture, we strained the curd, then stirred in heavy cream before pouring the filling into the prebaked tart shell and baking it until set. Once the lemon curd ingredients have been combined, cook the curd immediately; otherwise, it will have a grainy finished texture. The shell should still be warm when the filling is added. Dust with confectioners' sugar before serving, if desired. This tart is best served on the day it is made.

Lemon Tart
SERVES 8 TO 10

- **1 recipe Tart Shell (page 269), chilled in freezer for 15 minutes**
- **2 large eggs plus 7 large yolks**
- **7 ounces (1 cup) sugar**
- **¼ cup grated lemon zest plus ⅔ cup juice (4 lemons)**
  Pinch salt
- **4 tablespoons unsalted butter, cut into 4 pieces**
- **3 tablespoons heavy cream**

1. Adjust oven rack to middle position and heat oven to 375 degrees. Set chilled, dough-lined tart pan on rimmed baking sheet. Press greased parchment paper or greased double layer of aluminum foil into tart shell, covering edges to prevent burning, and fill with pie weights. Bake until tart shell is light golden brown and set, about 25 minutes, rotating sheet halfway through baking.

2. Carefully remove weights and parchment and continue to bake tart shell until golden, about 10 minutes. Transfer baking sheet with tart shell to wire rack and let cool while making filling.

3. Whisk eggs and yolks together in medium saucepan. Whisk in sugar until combined, then whisk in lemon zest and juice and salt. Add butter and cook over medium-low heat, stirring constantly, until mixture thickens slightly and registers 170 degrees. Immediately pour mixture through fine-mesh strainer into bowl and stir in cream.

4. Pour warm lemon filling into warm prebaked tart shell. Bake tart on baking sheet until filling is shiny and opaque and center jiggles slightly when shaken, 10 to 15 minutes, rotating sheet halfway through baking. Transfer baking sheet with tart to wire rack and let cool to room temperature, about 2 hours.

5. To serve, remove outer ring of tart pan, slide thin metal spatula between tart and tart pan bottom, and carefully slide tart onto serving platter or cutting board. Slice tart into wedges and serve.

Fresh Fruit Tart

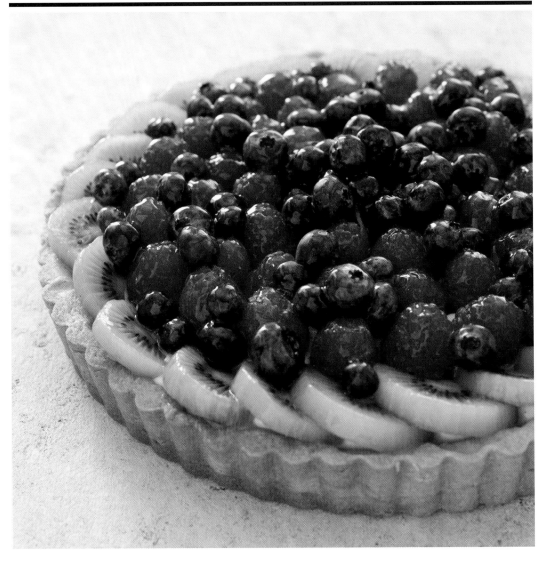

G-F TESTING LAB

FLOUR SUBSTITUTION	See page 270 for information about using various brands of gluten-free flour in the tart shell.

✅ WHY THIS RECIPE WORKS

Fresh fruit tarts usually offer little substance beyond their dazzling beauty, with rubbery or puddinglike fillings, soggy crusts, and underripe, flavorless fruit. We started by baking the crust until it was golden brown. We then filled the tart with pastry cream, made with half-and-half that was enriched with butter and thickened with just enough cornstarch to keep its shape without becoming gummy. For the fruit, we chose a combination of sliced kiwis, raspberries, and blueberries. The finishing touch: a drizzle of jelly glaze for a glistening presentation. Do not fill the prebaked tart shell until just before serving. Once filled, the tart should be topped with fruit, glazed, and served within 30 minutes.

Fresh Fruit Tart
SERVES 8 TO 10

2	cups half-and-half
3½	ounces (½ cup) sugar
	Pinch salt
½	vanilla bean, halved lengthwise, seeds removed and reserved
5	large egg yolks
3	tablespoons cornstarch
4	tablespoons unsalted butter, cut into ½-inch pieces and chilled
1	recipe Tart Shell (page 269), chilled in freezer for 15 minutes
2	large kiwis, peeled, halved lengthwise, and sliced ⅜ inch thick
10	ounces (2 cups) raspberries
5	ounces (1 cup) blueberries
½	cup red currant or apple jelly

1. Bring half-and-half, 6 tablespoons sugar, salt, and vanilla bean and seeds to simmer in medium saucepan over medium-high heat, stirring occasionally. As half-and-half mixture begins to simmer, whisk egg yolks, cornstarch, and remaining 2 tablespoons sugar together in medium bowl until smooth. Slowly whisk 1 cup of simmering half-and-half mixture into yolk mixture to temper, then slowly whisk tempered yolk mixture back into pan. Reduce heat to medium and cook, whisking vigorously, until mixture is thickened and few bubbles burst on surface, about 30 seconds.

2. Off heat, remove vanilla bean and whisk in butter. Transfer mixture to clean bowl, lay sheet of plastic wrap directly on surface, and refrigerate until chilled and firm, about 3 hours. (Pastry cream can be refrigerated for up to 2 days.)

3. Meanwhile, adjust oven rack to middle position and heat oven to 375 degrees. Set chilled, dough-lined tart pan on rimmed baking sheet. Press greased parchment paper or greased double layer of aluminum foil into tart shell, covering edges to prevent burning, and fill with pie weights. Bake until tart shell is light golden brown and set, about 25 minutes, rotating sheet halfway through baking.

4. Carefully remove weights and parchment and continue to bake tart shell until golden, about 10 minutes. Transfer baking sheet with tart shell to wire rack and let cool completely, at least 1 hour or up to 3 hours.

5. Spread chilled pastry cream evenly over bottom of cooled tart shell. Shingle kiwi slices around edge of tart, then arrange three rows of raspberries inside kiwi. Finally, arrange mound of blueberries in center, and scatter remaining over raspberries.

6. Melt jelly in small saucepan over medium-high heat, stirring occasionally to smooth out any lumps. Using pastry brush, dab melted jelly over fruit. To serve, remove outer ring of tart pan, slide thin metal spatula between tart and tart pan bottom, and carefully slide tart onto serving platter or cutting board. Slice tart into wedges and serve.

VARIATION
Mixed Berry Tart
Omit kiwi and add 2 cups extra berries (including blackberries and/or hulled and quartered strawberries). Combine berries in large zipper-lock bag and toss gently to mix. Carefully spread berries in even layer over filled tart. Glaze and serve as directed.

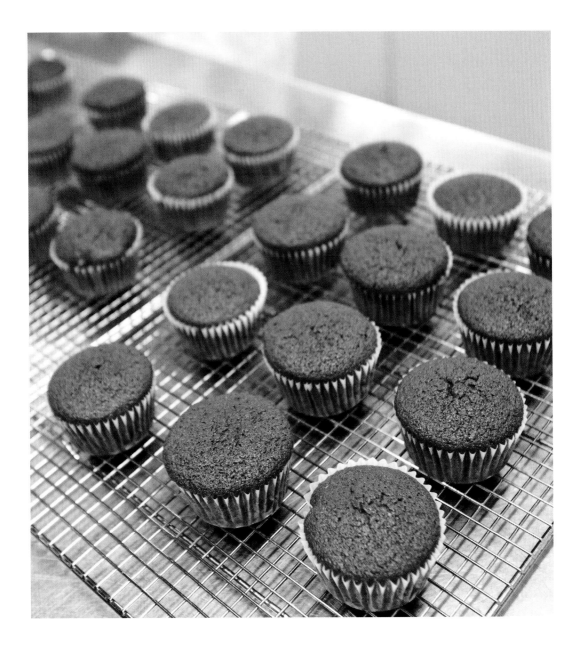

CAKES

Yellow Layer Cake

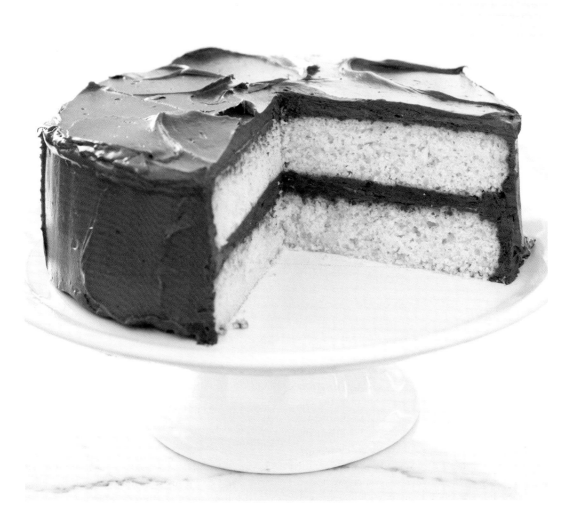

G-F TESTING LAB

FLOUR SUBSTITUTION	King Arthur Gluten-Free Multi-Purpose Flour 11 ounces = **2 cups**	Bob's Red Mill GF All-Purpose Baking Flour 11 ounces = **1⅔ cups plus ½ cup**
	Note that cake made with King Arthur will not rise as well and will have a somewhat grainy, pasty texture, and cake made with Bob's Red Mill will be darker in color and will have a coarser crumb and a distinct bean flavor.	
CHOCOLATE	Not all brands of chocolate are processed in a gluten-free facility; make sure to read the label.	
XANTHAN GUM	Do not omit the xanthan gum; it is crucial to the structure of the cake. For more information, see page 16.	

✔ WHY THIS RECIPE WORKS

A good yellow layer cake should melt in the mouth and taste of butter and vanilla. But many of the gluten-free layer cake recipes we tried tasted overly sweet, and most came out dense and gummy. If those problems weren't daunting enough, all of the initial recipes we tried were terribly greasy. The standard amount of butter in a traditional yellow layer cake (two sticks) was way too much. As we have learned time and time again, the starches in gluten-free flour just don't absorb fat (especially butter) all that well. We dramatically reduced the amount of butter in our working recipe, but predictably that left the cake too lean and dry. Replacing the milk or buttermilk used in classic recipes with sour cream was a step in the right direction, but we needed more richness. In the end, we borrowed a trick that works for chocolate cakes—melted chocolate—to help solve this problem. Rather than using unsweetened or bittersweet chocolate (neither acceptable in a yellow cake), we turned to white chocolate, and it worked like a charm, boosting richness without making the cake greasy. With one big problem solved, we now focused on lightening up the crumb. Adding extra baking powder and a bit of baking soda helped give our cake better rise and a tender texture. To create a really fluffy texture, we needed to whip the egg whites with some sugar to create a stable meringue-like mixture that could provide greater lift in the oven. Whipping the egg yolks with a bit more sugar ensured that sufficient air was in the batter. Note the relatively low oven temperature, which we found allows the layers to cook through without excessive browning. These lofty layers were tender yet sturdy enough to stand up to a thick coating of frosting. Use the Creamy Chocolate Frosting on page 284 or any of the easy frostings on page 290. See detailed frosting instructions on page 291. Once frosted, serve the cake within a few hours.

Yellow Layer Cake
SERVES 10 TO 12

6	ounces white chocolate, chopped
8	tablespoons unsalted butter, cut into 8 pieces
11	ounces (1¾ cups plus ⅔ cup) ATK Gluten-Free Flour Blend (page 13)
1	tablespoon baking powder (see page 20)
1¼	teaspoons xanthan gum
1	teaspoon salt
¼	teaspoon baking soda
4	large eggs, separated
	Pinch cream of tartar
7	ounces (1 cup) sugar
1½	tablespoons vanilla extract
⅔	cup sour cream
4	cups frosting

1. Adjust oven rack to middle position and heat oven to 325 degrees. Grease two 9-inch round cake pans, line bottoms with parchment paper, and grease parchment.

2. Microwave chocolate and butter together in bowl at 50 percent power, stirring occasionally, until melted, about 2 minutes. Whisk mixture until smooth, then set aside to cool slightly. In separate bowl, whisk flour blend, baking powder, xanthan gum, salt, and baking soda until combined.

3. Using stand mixer fitted with whisk, whip egg whites and cream of tartar on medium-low speed until foamy, about 1 minute. Increase speed to medium-high and whip whites to soft, billowy mounds, about 1 minute. Gradually add ½ cup sugar and whip until glossy, stiff peaks form, 2 to 3 minutes; transfer to bowl.

4. Return now-empty bowl to mixer, add egg yolks and vanilla, and whip on medium speed until well blended, about 30 seconds. Gradually add remaining ½ cup sugar, increase mixer speed to high, and whip until very thick and pale yellow, about 2 minutes. Reduce mixer speed to medium, add chocolate mixture and sour cream, and whip until combined, about 30 seconds. Reduce speed to low, slowly add flour blend mixture, and mix until thoroughly combined, about 1 minute.

5. Using rubber spatula, stir one-third of whipped egg whites into batter to lighten. Gently fold in remaining whites until no white streaks remain. Divide batter evenly between prepared pans and smooth tops. Bake until cakes begin to pull away from sides of pans and spring back when pressed lightly, 30 to 32 minutes, switching and rotating pans halfway through baking.

6. Let cakes cool in pans on wire rack for 10 minutes. Run knife around edge of cakes to loosen. Remove cakes from pans, discard parchment, and let cool completely on rack, about 1½ hours. (Cake layers can be wrapped tightly in plastic wrap and stored at room temperature for up to 1 day.)

7. Place 1 cake layer on platter and spread 1½ cups frosting evenly over top using small icing spatula or butter knife. Top with second cake layer, press lightly to adhere, then spread remaining 2½ cups frosting evenly over top and sides. Serve.

VARIATION
Yellow Sheet Cake
Four cups of frosting is enough to generously frost the top and sides of the cake.

Grease 13 by 9-inch baking pan, line bottom with parchment paper, and grease parchment. Scrape all of batter into prepared pan; baking time will not change. Let cake cool completely in pan on wire rack, about 2 hours. Run knife around edge of cake to loosen. Remove cake from pan, discard parchment, transfer to platter, and frost.

Creamy Chocolate Frosting
MAKES 4 CUPS
This not-too-sweet frosting relies on egg whites and sugar heated over a double boiler until thickened and foamy. Knobs of softened butter are then added, and the mixture is beaten until silky and light. Cool the chocolate to between 85 and 100 degrees before adding it as the final step in this recipe.

- 4⅔ ounces (⅔ cup) sugar
- 4 large egg whites
  Pinch salt
- 24 tablespoons (3 sticks) unsalted butter, cut into 24 pieces and softened
- 12 ounces bittersweet chocolate, melted and cooled
- 1 teaspoon vanilla extract

1. Combine sugar, egg whites, and salt in bowl of stand mixer; place bowl over pan of simmering water. Whisking gently but constantly, heat mixture until slightly thickened and foamy and it registers 150 degrees, 2 to 3 minutes.

2. Place bowl in stand mixer fitted with whisk. Beat mixture on medium speed until it has consistency of shaving cream and has cooled slightly, about 5 minutes. Add butter, 1 piece at a time, until smooth and creamy. (Frosting may look curdled after half of butter has been added; it will smooth out with additional butter.)

3. Once all butter is added, add cooled melted chocolate and vanilla and mix until combined. Increase speed to medium-high and beat until light and fluffy, about 30 seconds, scraping beater and sides of bowl with rubber spatula as necessary. If frosting seems too soft after adding chocolate, chill it briefly in refrigerator, then rewhip until creamy.

VARIATION
Creamy Chocolate Frosting for Cupcakes
This variation will yield enough for 12 cupcakes.

Cut all ingredient amounts by half; follow procedure as directed.

Yellow Layer Cake

Although the aim of most traditional cakes is minimal gluten development, eliminating gluten altogether presents myriad problems of its own. To achieve the tall, fluffy layers of a classic yellow layer cake without gluten, we had to take a different approach to both ingredients and mixing method.

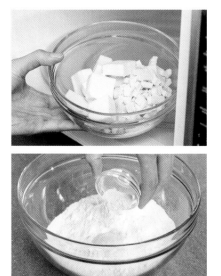

1. INCORPORATE MELTED WHITE CHOCOLATE: It was essential to reduce the fat in our gluten-free cake in order to combat greasiness, but simply using less butter left the layers tasting a bit too lean and dry. To replace some of the fat and moisture without leaving a greasy texture, we melted white chocolate with the butter in the microwave and then whisked the mixture until smooth and incorporated it into the batter. This emulsified combination added flavor and richness to the cake without turning it greasy.

2. ADD XANTHAN GUM FOR STRUCTURE: Because there was no gluten development to support the cake as it baked, we needed help creating structure. Xanthan gum proved essential to giving the cake the support and structure it needed to rise and set in the oven. However, there was a limit to the power of xanthan. Yes, it helped to build structure, but the cake was still dense and heavy. We turned to the eggs to solve this problem.

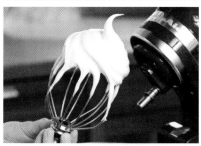

3. WHIP EGG WHITES AND SUGAR: We needed to find another way to add extra lift and support for these wide, flat cake layers. Focusing on the mixing method, we found that separating out the egg whites and whipping them into stiff peaks easily solved this problem. Adding cream of tartar and sugar to the whites as they whipped helped create a stable meringuelike mixture that did not deflate when folded into the cake batter. Whipping the egg yolks with additional sugar also helped to ensure that as much air as possible was trapped in the batter, giving it a light, fluffy texture.

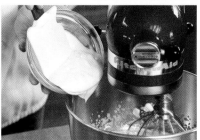

4. USE SOUR CREAM: Buttermilk is often used in traditional yellow cakes for moisture and flavor, but in this cake it made the batter too loose and resulted in layers that were dense and gummy. Instead, we used sour cream, which gave us a thicker batter that baked up taller and fluffier. And the sour cream helped make the crumb especially tender. The tang of the sour cream also helped balance the sweetness of the white chocolate.

Birthday Cupcakes

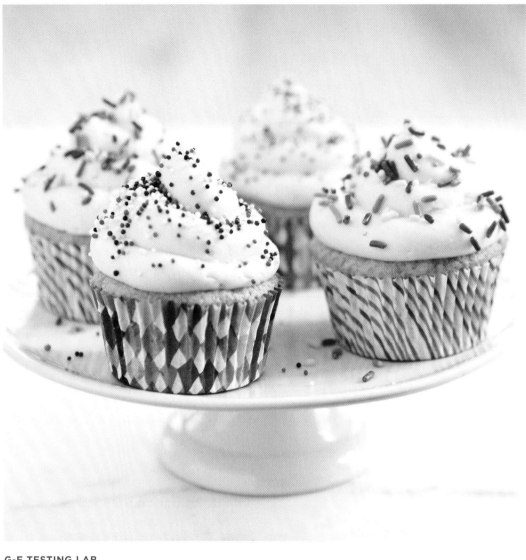

G-F TESTING LAB

FLOUR SUBSTITUTION	King Arthur Gluten-Free Multi-Purpose Flour 6½ ounces = **⅔ cup plus ½ cup**	Bob's Red Mill GF All-Purpose Baking Flour 6½ ounces = **1⅓ cups**
	Note that cupcakes made with King Arthur will not rise as well and will taste slightly pasty, and cupcakes made with Bob's Red Mill will have a coarser crumb and a distinct bean flavor.	
CHOCOLATE	Not all brands of chocolate are processed in a gluten-free facility; make sure to read the label.	
XANTHAN GUM	Do not omit the xanthan gum; it is crucial to the structure of the cupcakes. For more information, see page 16.	

WHY THIS RECIPE WORKS

In our quest for tender cupcakes with a slightly domed top and a light, open crumb, we began with our Yellow Layer Cake (page 282). We immediately found that we didn't need to whip the egg whites. In fact, whipping the eggs was creating a huge dome, which made frosting the cupcakes a challenge. In addition, the cupcakes were so fluffy that they fell apart in our hands. Using the easiest mixing method (combining everything in a bowl) was a step in the right direction—the cupcakes were more compact and less crumbly. Unfortunately, they were still doming too much. We needed the baking soda (it helped with browning and tenderness) but found we could reduce the amount of baking powder substantially. While these adjustments had solved the structural problems in these little cakes, the change in mixing method meant that the butter wasn't getting emulsified into the batter. In the end, we swapped the butter for oil, as we had done in many other gluten-free cakes (see page 306 for more details). Thankfully, the white chocolate and sour cream kept the cupcakes plenty rich, so tasters didn't miss the butter flavor, especially when the cakes were piled high with frosting. Use the scaled-down frosting variations for cupcakes on page 284 or page 290. Once frosted, serve the cupcakes within a few hours.

Birthday Cupcakes
MAKES 12 CUPCAKES

4	ounces white chocolate, chopped
6	tablespoons vegetable oil
6½	ounces (¾ cup plus ⅔ cup) ATK Gluten-Free Flour Blend (page 13)
1	teaspoon baking powder (see page 20)
½	teaspoon xanthan gum
½	teaspoon salt
⅛	teaspoon baking soda
2	large eggs
2	teaspoons vanilla extract
3½	ounces (½ cup) sugar
⅓	cup sour cream
2	cups frosting

1. Adjust oven rack to middle position and heat oven to 325 degrees. Line 12-cup muffin tin with paper or foil liners.

2. Microwave white chocolate and oil together in bowl at 50 percent power, stirring occasionally, until melted, about 2 minutes. Whisk mixture until smooth, then set aside to cool slightly. In separate bowl, whisk flour blend, baking powder, xanthan gum, salt, and baking soda together.

3. In large bowl, whisk eggs and vanilla together. Whisk in sugar until well combined. Whisk in cooled chocolate mixture and sour cream until combined. Whisk in flour blend mixture until batter is thoroughly combined and smooth.

4. Using ice cream scoop or large spoon, portion batter evenly into prepared muffin tin. Bake until cupcakes are set on top and spring back when pressed lightly, 20 to 22 minutes, rotating muffin tin halfway through baking. Let cupcakes cool in muffin tin on wire rack for 10 minutes. Remove cupcakes from tin and let cool completely, about 1 hour. (Unfrosted cupcakes can be stored in airtight container at room temperature for up to 1 day.)

5. Spread or pipe frosting over top of cupcakes and serve.

TEST KITCHEN TIP
Piping Frosting onto Cupcakes

Frosting cupcakes with a small icing spatula or butter knife is certainly easy, but for an extra-special presentation consider using a pastry bag fitted with a large star tip.

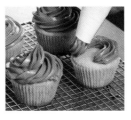

Swirl frosting into tall pile on top of cupcake, starting at outer edge of cupcake and working toward center.

Chocolate Layer Cake

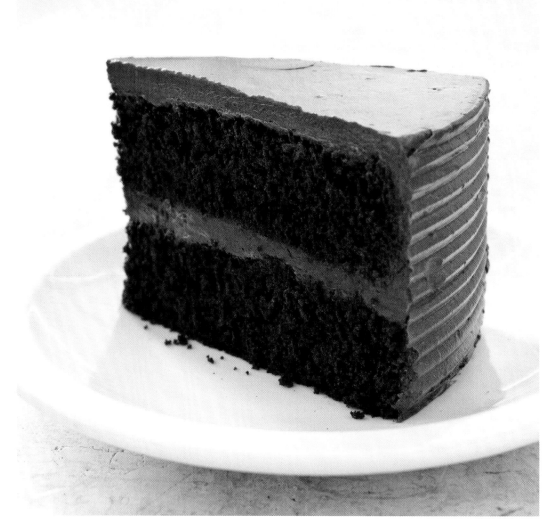

G-F TESTING LAB

FLOUR SUBSTITUTION	King Arthur Gluten-Free Multi-Purpose Flour 7 ounces = 1¼ **cups**	Bob's Red Mill GF All-Purpose Baking Flour 7 ounces = 1¼ **cups plus 2 tablespoons**
	Note that cake made with Bob's Red Mill will have a slightly coarser crumb and an earthy flavor.	
CHOCOLATE AND COCOA	Not all brands of chocolate and cocoa are processed in a gluten-free facility; make sure to read the label.	
XANTHAN GUM	Do not omit the xanthan gum; it is crucial to the structure of the cake. For more information, see page 16.	

WHY THIS RECIPE WORKS

Everyone loves a rich-tasting chocolate cake, but too often the gluten-free translation is less than appealing. Instead of the dense, bricklike versions we turned out in our initial testing, we wanted fluffy, tender, moist layers that baked up tall and sturdy. A combination of cocoa powder and melted bittersweet chocolate provided the best chocolate flavor, but we were afraid the melted chocolate was weighing down our cakes. When we tried a cake made with all cocoa powder, the results were dismal—dry and dense, with a very flat chocolate flavor. Instead, we kept the chocolate and cocoa combination and swapped out the traditional butter for oil, which had proven successful in other gluten-free cakes. This not only gave our cake better texture, but also brought a richer, cleaner chocolate flavor to the forefront. Another combination of ingredients was necessary for leavening our rich layers: baking powder, baking soda, and xanthan gum. The soda helped to keep the cake tender, while the powder gave it lift, and the xanthan gum provided necessary structure. Chocolate cake recipes often call for sour cream to add moisture and richness, but this cake batter was already thick and plenty rich. Switching to whole milk gave us better results. Once frosted, our rich chocolate layer cake was an impressive sight. Use the Creamy Chocolate Frosting on page 284, or any of the easy frostings on page 290. See detailed frosting instructions on page 291. Once frosted, serve the cake within a few hours.

Chocolate Layer Cake
SERVES 10 TO 12

- 1 cup vegetable oil
- 6 ounces bittersweet chocolate, chopped
- 2 ounces (⅔ cup) unsweetened cocoa powder
- 7 ounces (1⅓ cups plus ¼ cup) ATK Gluten-Free Flour Blend (page 13)
- 1½ teaspoons baking powder (see page 20)
- 1 teaspoon baking soda
- 1 teaspoon xanthan gum
- 1 teaspoon salt
- 4 large eggs
- 2 teaspoons vanilla extract
- 10½ ounces (1½ cups) sugar
- 1 cup whole milk
- 4 cups frosting

1. Adjust oven rack to lower-middle position and heat oven to 350 degrees. Grease two 9-inch round cake pans, line bottoms with parchment paper, and grease parchment.

2. Microwave oil, chocolate, and cocoa together in bowl at 50 percent power, stirring occasionally, until melted, about 2 minutes. Whisk mixture until smooth, then set aside to cool slightly. In separate bowl, whisk flour blend, baking powder, baking soda, xanthan gum, and salt together.

3. In large bowl, whisk eggs and vanilla together. Whisk in sugar until well combined. Whisk in cooled chocolate mixture and milk until combined. Whisk in flour blend mixture until batter is thoroughly combined and smooth.

4. Divide batter evenly between prepared pans and smooth tops. Bake until toothpick inserted into center of cake comes out clean, 30 to 32 minutes, switching and rotating pans halfway through baking.

5. Let cakes cool in pans on wire rack for 10 minutes. Run knife around edge of cakes to loosen. Remove cakes from pans, discard parchment, and let cool completely on rack, about 1½ hours. (Cake layers can be wrapped tightly in plastic wrap and stored at room temperature for up to 1 day.)

6. Place 1 cake layer on platter and spread 1½ cups frosting evenly over top using small icing spatula or butter knife. Top with second cake layer, press lightly to adhere, then spread remaining 2½ cups frosting evenly over top and sides. Serve.

VARIATION

Chocolate Sheet Cake

Four cups of frosting is enough to generously frost the top and sides of the cake.

Grease 13 by 9-inch baking pan, line bottom with parchment paper, and grease parchment. Scrape all of batter into prepared pan; baking time will not change. Let cake cool completely in pan on wire rack, about 2 hours. Run knife around edge of cake to loosen. Remove cake from pan, discard parchment, transfer to platter, and frost.

Easy Vanilla Frosting

MAKES 4 CUPS

Even if you omit the added salt, salted butter will ruin this recipe. The heavy cream is a simple refinement that gives this fast frosting a silky quality—don't omit it.

24	tablespoons (3 sticks) unsalted butter, cut into 24 pieces and softened
3	tablespoons heavy cream
2½	teaspoons vanilla extract
¼	teaspoon salt
12	ounces (3 cups) confectioners' sugar

1. Using stand mixer fitted with whisk, whip butter, cream, vanilla, and salt together on medium-high speed until smooth, 1 to 2 minutes. Reduce mixer speed to medium-low, slowly add sugar, and whip until incorporated and smooth, 1 to 2 minutes.

2. Increase speed to medium-high and whip frosting until light and fluffy, 3 to 5 minutes.

VARIATIONS

Easy Vanilla Frosting for Cupcakes

This variation will yield enough for 12 cupcakes.

Cut all ingredient amounts by half; follow procedure as directed.

Coffee Frosting

Add 2 tablespoons instant espresso or instant coffee to butter mixture before beating. (For cupcakes, add just 1 tablespoon instant espresso or instant coffee.)

Almond Frosting

Add 2 teaspoons almond extract to butter mixture before beating. (For cupcakes, add just 1 teaspoon almond extract.)

Coconut Frosting

Add 1 tablespoon coconut extract to butter mixture before beating. (For cupcakes, add just 1½ teaspoons coconut extract.)

TEST KITCHEN TIP **Preparing Cake Pans**

For nearly all gluten-free cakes (except Lemon Pound Cake and Almond Cake), we found it unnecessary to waste our valuable flour blend on pan preparation. We rely on greased parchment instead.

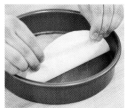

Spray bottom and sides of cake pan with vegetable oil spray, then line bottom of pan with parchment paper (cut to fit), and spray parchment paper.

TEST KITCHEN TIP

Storing Cakes and Cupcakes

In general, we find that gluten-free baked goods really suffer in the refrigerator, and cakes are no exception. Their texture becomes very dry. Most cake layers and cupcakes can be wrapped in plastic and stored on the counter for a day—that is, as long as they are unfrosted. When you're ready to serve, make and apply the frosting. Once frosted, cakes and cupcakes will keep on the counter for a few hours.

TEST KITCHEN TIP Frosting a Layer Cake

The steps below outline the test kitchen's basic method for frosting a layer cake. A rotating cake stand makes this process a bit easier, but any flat platter can be used. The four strips of parchment paper help keep the platter neat and clean. If you notice that the cake layers are covered with loose crumbs, use a pastry brush to gently brush the crumbs away before you start. (If left in place, the crumbs will become embedded in the frosting and mar the appearance of the cake.) We like to use an offset spatula when frosting any cake. The wide, flexible blade lets you spread the icing with minimal pressure. For a particularly smooth finish, dip the spatula in hot water when performing step 6. And for a more homestyle appearance, don't smooth out the frosting as shown in step 6; instead, use a soupspoon to create billowy swirls in the frosting. Simply press the back of the spoon into the frosting, then gently twirl the spoon as you lift it away.

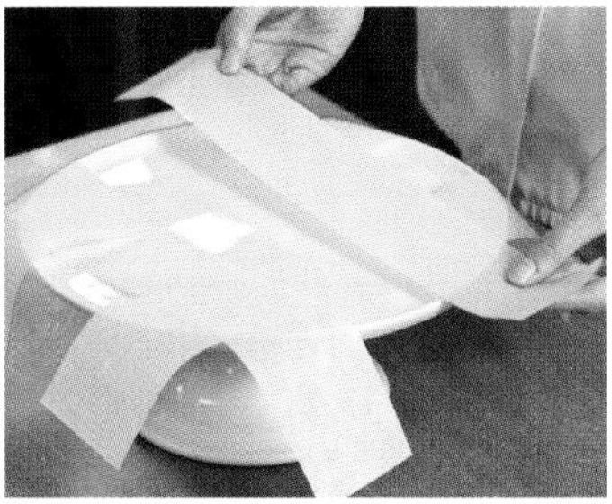

1. Cover edges of cake platter with strips of parchment paper to help keep it clean. Slide pieces of parchment out from under cake once frosting job is done.

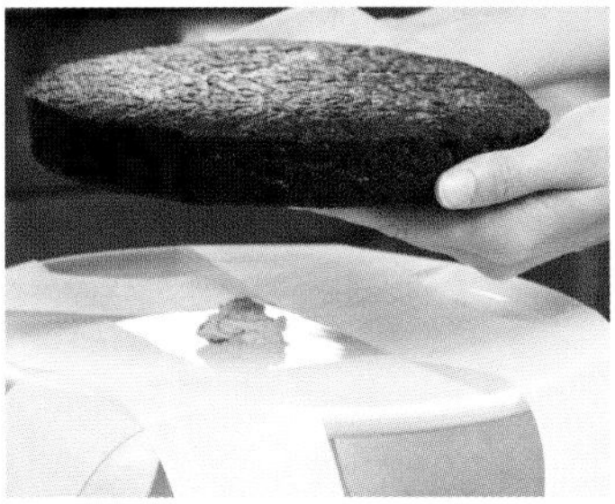

2. Dollop small amount of frosting in center of platter to help anchor bottom cake layer to platter and prevent it from sliding around.

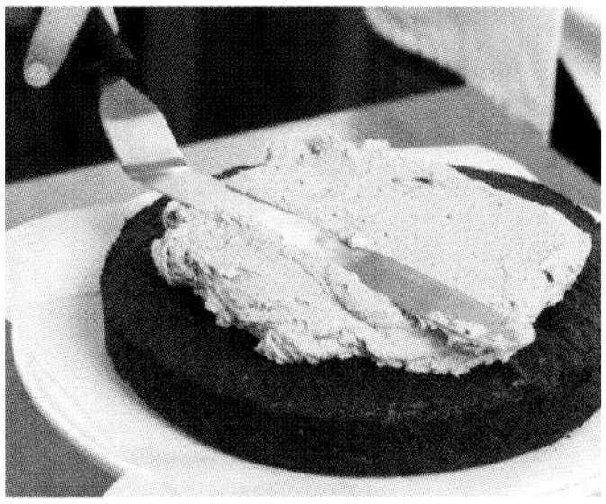

3. Place cake layer on platter, dollop 1½ cups frosting in center, and spread it into even layer right to edge of cake.

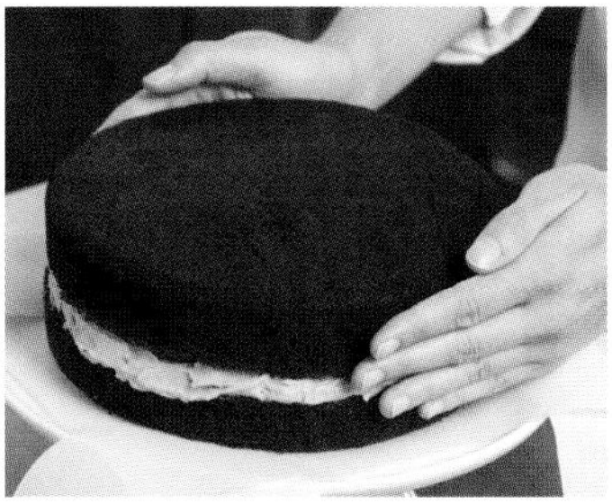

4. Lay second cake layer on top and brush away any large crumbs. Dollop more frosting on top and spread lightly to edge of cake.

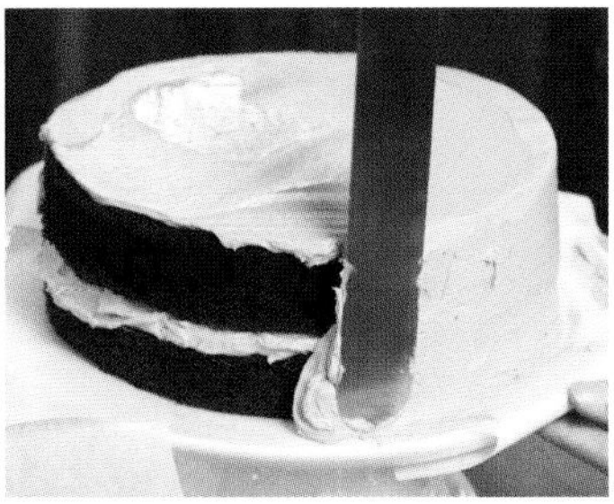

5. Gather several tablespoons frosting on tip of icing spatula, and gently smear onto side of cake. Use gentle motions, don't press too hard on cake, and clean spatula as needed.

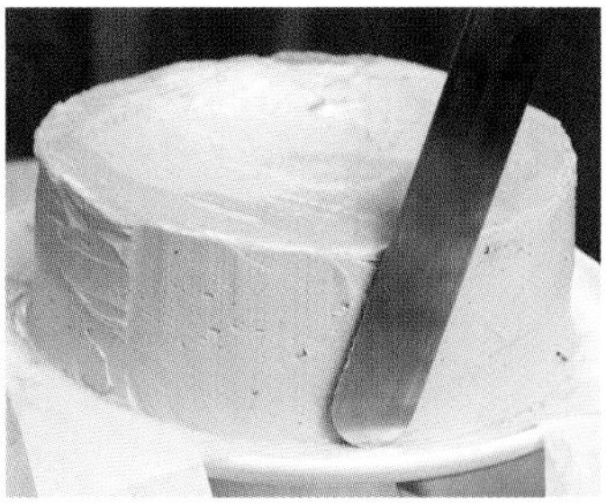

6. Gently run edge of spatula around sides to smooth out bumps and tidy area where top and sides of cake merge.

Dark Chocolate Cupcakes

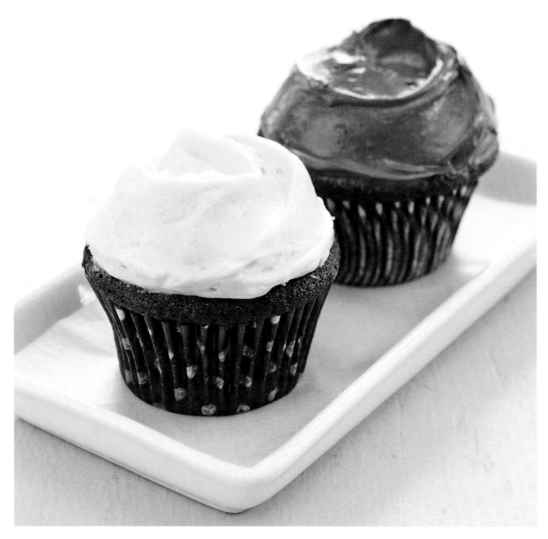

G-F TESTING LAB

FLOUR SUBSTITUTION	King Arthur Gluten-Free Multi-Purpose Flour 3½ ounces = ½ **cup plus 2 tablespoons**	Bob's Red Mill GF All-Purpose Baking Flour 3½ ounces = ⅔ **cup**
	Note that cupcakes made with Bob's Red Mill will have a slightly coarser crumb and an earthy flavor.	
CHOCOLATE AND COCOA	Not all brands of chocolate and cocoa are processed in a gluten-free facility; make sure to read the label.	
XANTHAN GUM	Do not omit the xanthan gum; it is crucial to the structure of the cupcakes. For more information, see page 16.	

WHY THIS RECIPE WORKS

The ultimate chocolate cupcakes are moist and tender with rich chocolate flavor. Taking a cue from the success of our moist and tender Chocolate Layer Cake (page 288), we scaled the recipe to fit in a standard 12-cup muffin tin and simply adjusted the baking time. The combination of rich chocolate flavor and light, fluffy crumb once again fooled tasters into thinking these cupcakes couldn't possibly be gluten-free. Use the scaled-down frosting variations for cupcakes on page 284 or page 290. Once frosted, serve the cupcakes within a few hours.

Dark Chocolate Cupcakes
MAKES 12 CUPCAKES

½	**cup vegetable oil**
3	**ounces bittersweet chocolate, chopped**
1	**ounce (⅓ cup) unsweetened cocoa powder**
3½	**ounces (¾ cup) ATK Gluten-Free Flour Blend (page 13)**
¾	**teaspoon baking powder (see page 20)**
½	**teaspoon baking soda**
½	**teaspoon xanthan gum**
½	**teaspoon salt**
2	**large eggs**
1	**teaspoon vanilla extract**
5¼	**ounces (¾ cup) sugar**
½	**cup whole milk**
2	**cups frosting**

1. Adjust oven rack to lower-middle position and heat oven to 350 degrees. Line 12-cup muffin tin with paper or foil liners.

2. Microwave oil, chocolate, and cocoa together in bowl at 50 percent power, stirring occasionally, until melted, about 2 minutes. Whisk mixture until smooth, then set aside to cool slightly. In separate bowl, whisk flour blend, baking powder, baking soda, xanthan gum, and salt together.

3. In large bowl, whisk eggs and vanilla together. Whisk in sugar until well combined. Whisk in cooled chocolate mixture and milk until combined. Whisk in flour blend mixture until batter is thoroughly combined and smooth.

4. Using ice cream scoop or large spoon, portion batter evenly into prepared muffin tin. Bake until toothpick inserted into center of cupcakes comes out clean, 16 to 18 minutes, rotating muffin tin halfway through baking. Let cupcakes cool in muffin tin on wire rack for 10 minutes. Remove cupcakes from tin and let cool completely, about 1 hour. (Unfrosted cupcakes can be stored in airtight container at room temperature for up to 1 day.)

5. Spread or pipe (see page 287) frosting over top of cupcakes and serve.

SMART SHOPPING **Cocoa Powder**

This potent source of chocolate flavor is nothing more than unsweetened chocolate with much of the fat removed. Cocoa powder comes in natural and Dutched versions. Dutch-processed cocoa has been treated with an alkaline substance to make it less acidic (Dutching also darkens the cocoa's color). In some cases, the type of cocoa can make a noticeable difference, but for the recipes in this book we had good results with both regular (natural) brands as well as Dutched cocoas. Our favorite brand of natural cocoa is Hershey's Natural Unsweetened Cocoa; our favorite Dutch-processed cocoa is Droste Cocoa.

Red Velvet Cupcakes

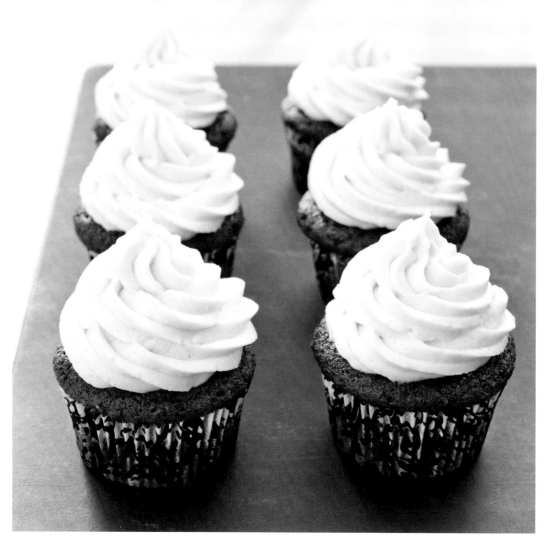

G-F TESTING LAB

FLOUR SUBSTITUTION	King Arthur Gluten-Free Multi-Purpose Flour 6 ounces = ¾ **cup plus** ⅓ **cup**	Bob's Red Mill GF All-Purpose Baking Flour 6 ounces = ⅔ **cup plus** ½ **cup**
	Note that cupcakes made with King Arthur will be slightly pasty, and cupcakes made with Bob's Red Mill will have an earthy flavor.	
COCOA	Not all brands of cocoa are processed in a gluten-free facility; make sure to read the label.	
XANTHAN GUM	Do not omit the xanthan gum; it is crucial to the structure of the cupcakes. For more information, see page 16.	

✓ WHY THIS RECIPE WORKS

Red velvet cupcakes derive their color from food dye mixed with cocoa powder, and their tender texture from the reaction that occurs when buttermilk and vinegar are combined with baking soda. As with our Birthday Cupcakes (page 286), we achieved a moister, more tender crumb with oil instead of butter, especially when we used rich sour cream as the dairy element. The vinegar in the classic recipe didn't work the same way in the gluten-free version, especially with sour cream in the mix instead of buttermilk. We eventually discovered we could make these cupcakes without it. The combination of baking powder and baking soda used in traditional recipes was key, as was adding a little xanthan gum to keep these little cakes from crumbling when you eat them. For a cupcake with more chocolate flavor, we bumped up the cocoa powder from the usual tablespoon or two to a full ¼ cup. Once frosted, serve the cupcakes within a few hours.

Red Velvet Cupcakes
MAKES 12 CUPCAKES

- 6 ounces (1⅓ cups) ATK Gluten-Free Flour Blend (page 13)
- ¾ ounce (¼ cup) unsweetened cocoa powder
- 1 teaspoon baking powder (see page 20)
- ½ teaspoon salt
- ¼ teaspoon xanthan gum
- ⅛ teaspoon baking soda
- 8¾ ounces (1¼ cups) sugar
- ⅔ cup sour cream
- 6 tablespoons vegetable oil
- 2 large eggs
- 1 tablespoon red food coloring
- 1½ teaspoons vanilla extract
- 2 cups Cream Cheese Frosting for Cupcakes

1. Adjust oven rack to middle position and heat oven to 350 degrees. Line 12-cup muffin tin with paper or foil liners. Whisk flour blend, cocoa, baking powder, salt, xanthan gum, and baking soda together in bowl.

2. In large bowl, whisk sugar, sour cream, oil, eggs, food coloring, and vanilla together until combined. Whisk in flour blend mixture until batter is thoroughly combined and smooth.

3. Using ice cream scoop or large spoon, portion batter evenly into prepared muffin tin. Bake until toothpick inserted into center of cupcakes comes out clean, 18 to 20 minutes, rotating muffin tin halfway through baking. Let cupcakes cool in muffin tin on wire rack for 10 minutes. Remove cupcakes from tin and let cool completely, about 1 hour. (Unfrosted cupcakes can be stored in airtight container at room temperature for up to 1 day.)

4. Spread or pipe (see page 287) frosting over top of cupcakes and serve.

Cream Cheese Frosting
MAKES ABOUT 4 CUPS
Low-fat cream cheese will make the frosting soupy. If the frosting becomes soft, refrigerate it until firm.

- 16 ounces cream cheese, softened
- 10 tablespoons unsalted butter, cut into 10 pieces and softened
- 2 tablespoons sour cream
- 1½ teaspoons vanilla extract
- ¼ teaspoon salt
- 8 ounces (2 cups) confectioners' sugar

1. Using stand mixer fitted with whisk, whip cream cheese, butter, sour cream, vanilla, and salt on medium-high speed until smooth, 1 to 2 minutes. Reduce mixer speed to medium-low, slowly add sugar, and whip until smooth, 1 to 2 minutes.

2. Increase speed to medium-high and whip frosting until light and fluffy, 3 to 5 minutes.

VARIATION
Cream Cheese Frosting for Cupcakes
This variation will yield enough for 12 cupcakes.

Cut all ingredient amounts by half; follow procedure as directed.

Carrot Sheet Cake

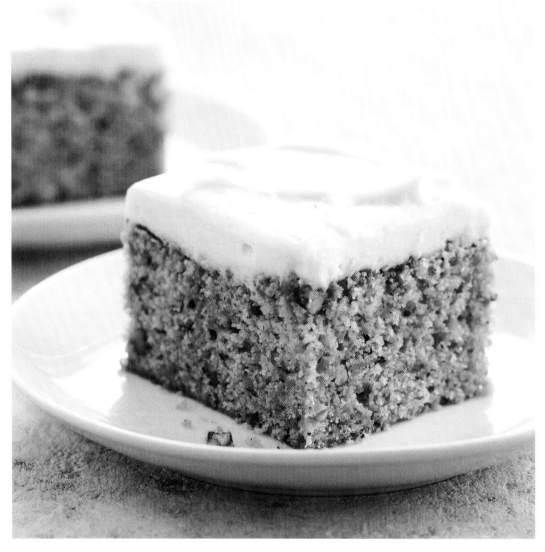

G-F TESTING LAB

FLOUR SUBSTITUTION	King Arthur Gluten-Free Multi-Purpose Flour 12½ ounces = **2¼ cups**	Bob's Red Mill GF All-Purpose Baking Flour 12½ ounces = **2½ cups**

Note that cake made with King Arthur will taste a bit starchy, and cake made with Bob's Red Mill will have a mild bean flavor.

WHY THIS RECIPE WORKS

Carrot cake is typically a bowl cake made with oil rather than butter, and our early testing confirmed that this direction would work. As usual, we needed to go down on oil to account for our flour blend's inability to absorb fat. After many rounds of testing, we landed on ¾ cup of vegetable oil—half as much as we use in the test kitchen's favorite carrot cake recipe with wheat flour. With so little fat, the cake was a bit dry. We solved this problem by using more brown sugar (and less granulated sugar). We not only liked the molasses flavor provided by the brown sugar but also the extra moisture it added. We found that the simplest mixing method was the food processor. We used the processor fitted with the shredding disk to prepare the carrots, then swapped out the blade to combine the eggs, sugars, and oil. The whirring blade of the food processor ensured that the oil and eggs were well emulsified, which helped keep the oil from making the cake heavy or dense. (If you don't own a food processor, shred the carrots on a box grater and use an electric mixer to combine the eggs, sugars, and oil.) Once frosted, serve the cake within a few hours.

Carrot Sheet Cake
SERVES 15

- 12½ ounces (2¾ cups) ATK Gluten-Free Flour Blend (page 13)
- 1¼ teaspoons baking powder (see page 20)
- 1 teaspoon baking soda
- 1¼ teaspoons ground cinnamon
- ½ teaspoon ground nutmeg
- ½ teaspoon salt
- ⅛ teaspoon ground cloves
- 1 pound carrots, peeled
- 7 ounces (1 cup) granulated sugar
- 7 ounces (1 cup packed) light brown sugar
- 4 large eggs
- ¾ cup vegetable oil
- 1 cup pecans or walnuts, toasted and chopped (optional)
- 4 cups Cream Cheese Frosting (page 295)

1. Adjust oven rack to middle position and heat oven to 350 degrees. Grease 13 by 9-inch baking pan, line bottom with parchment paper, and grease parchment. Whisk flour blend, baking powder, baking soda, cinnamon, nutmeg, salt, and cloves together in large bowl.

2. In food processor fitted with large shredding disk, shred carrots; transfer carrots to bowl (you should have about 3 cups). Wipe out food processor bowl and fit with metal blade. Process granulated sugar, brown sugar, and eggs until frothy and thoroughly combined, about 20 seconds. With processor running, add oil in steady stream. Process until egg mixture is light in color and well emulsified, about 20 seconds.

3. Transfer egg mixture to large bowl. Using rubber spatula, stir in shredded carrots, flour blend mixture, and nuts, if using, until thoroughly incorporated. Pour batter into prepared pan. Bake until toothpick inserted into center of cake comes out clean, 35 to 40 minutes, rotating pan halfway through baking.

4. Let cake cool completely in pan on wire rack, about 2 hours. Run knife around edge of cake to loosen. Remove cake from pan, discard parchment, and transfer to platter. (Cake can be wrapped tightly in plastic wrap and stored at room temperature for up to 1 day.)

5. Spread frosting evenly over top, and sides if desired, using small icing spatula. Serve.

VARIATION
Carrot Layer Cake
See page 291 for instructions on frosting a layer cake.

Grease two 9-inch round cake pans, line bottoms with parchment paper, and grease parchment. Divide batter evenly between pans and reduce baking time to 25 to 30 minutes. Let cakes cool in pans on wire rack for 10 minutes. Run knife around edges of cakes to loosen. Remove cakes from pans, discard parchment, and let cool completely on rack, about 1½ hours, before frosting.

Gingerbread Cake

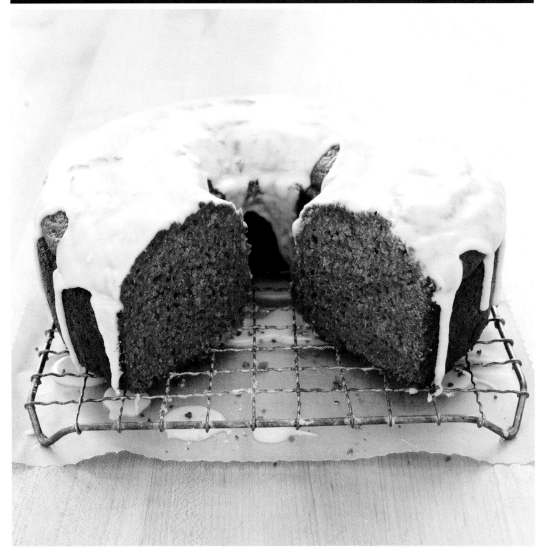

G-F TESTING LAB

FLOUR SUBSTITUTION	King Arthur Gluten-Free Multi-Purpose Flour 13 ounces = **2¼ cups plus 2 tablespoons**	Bob's Red Mill GF All-Purpose Baking Flour 13 ounces = **2½ cups plus 2 tablespoons**

Note that cake made with King Arthur will not rise as well and will be a bit denser, and cake made with Bob's Red Mill will be wetter, will not dome properly, and will have a slight bean flavor.

✅ WHY THIS RECIPE WORKS

Old-fashioned gingerbread cake is rather austere (there's no frosting) but satisfying nonetheless because of the complex ginger and spice flavors. Employing both ground ginger and grated fresh ginger as well as cinnamon and black pepper ensured the cake had sufficient punch. Most recipes rely on molasses as well as brown and granulated sugars, and we saw no reason to depart from tradition. Melted butter imparted a greasy texture, so we switched to vegetable oil supplemented with a significant helping of sour cream (1¼ cups), as we had done in other cake recipes. (See page 306 for more on why gluten-free flours have a hard time absorbing melted butter.) During testing, the center of the cake occasionally collapsed. Up to this point, we had been scraping the batter into a large rectangular baking pan. Would switching to a tube pan (which heats from the outside as well as the center hole) help? As we hoped, the cake rose better (and there was no longer a center that could sink), but the texture was still heavy and dense. Adding more eggs (four in total) upped the protein content and ensured a better rise, as did using a lot of baking powder (4 teaspoons) as well as ¾ teaspoon of baking soda. The switch to the tube pan made us reconsider our original unwillingness to frost this cake. Yes, a dusting of confectioners' sugar would be a sufficient finish, but mixing that sugar with maple syrup (plus a little water and a pinch of salt) was just as easy and so much better. The glaze dribbled down the sides of this statuesque cake, adding both drama and yet another layer of flavor.

Gingerbread Cake
SERVES 12

CAKE
- 1¼ cups sour cream
- 4 large eggs
- ⅔ cup molasses
- 3½ ounces (½ cup packed) light brown sugar
- 3½ ounces (½ cup) granulated sugar
- ⅓ cup vegetable oil
- 1 tablespoon grated fresh ginger
- 13 ounces (2¾ cups plus 2 tablespoons) ATK Gluten-Free Flour Blend (page 13)
- 4 teaspoons baking powder (see page 20)
- 1 tablespoon ground ginger
- ¾ teaspoon baking soda
- ½ teaspoon salt
- ¼ teaspoon ground cinnamon
- ⅛ teaspoon pepper

GLAZE
- 4 ounces (1 cup) confectioners' sugar
- 5 teaspoons water
- 1 tablespoon maple syrup
  Pinch salt

1. FOR THE CAKE: Adjust oven rack to middle position and heat oven to 350 degrees. Grease 16-cup tube pan.

2. Whisk sour cream, eggs, molasses, brown sugar, granulated sugar, oil, and fresh ginger together in bowl until combined. In large bowl, whisk flour blend, baking powder, ground ginger, baking soda, salt, cinnamon, and pepper together. Whisk sour cream mixture into flour blend mixture until batter is thoroughly combined and smooth.

3. Pour batter into prepared pan and smooth top. Bake until top of cake is just firm to touch and skewer inserted into center comes out clean, 45 to 50 minutes, rotating pan halfway through baking. Let cake cool in pan on wire rack, about 1½ hours. Run thin knife around edge of cake to loosen, then remove cake from pan and return it to wire rack.

4. FOR THE GLAZE: Whisk all ingredients together until smooth. Pour glaze evenly over top of cooled cake. Let glaze set for 20 minutes before serving. (Cake can be wrapped in plastic wrap and stored at room temperature for up to 2 days.)

Applesauce Snack Cake

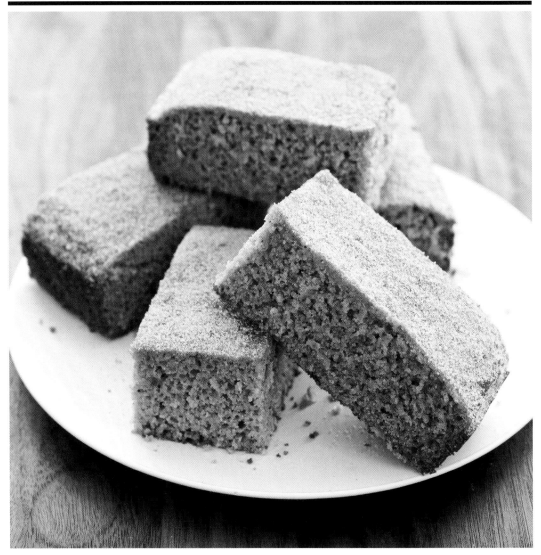

G-F TESTING LAB

FLOUR SUBSTITUTION	King Arthur Gluten-Free Multi-Purpose Flour 7½ ounces = **1¼ cups plus 2 tablespoons**	Bob's Red Mill GF All-Purpose Baking Flour 7½ ounces = **1½ cups**
	Note that cake made with King Arthur will not rise as well and will be denser and slightly pasty, and cake made with Bob's Red Mill will have a coarser crumb, will be slightly drier, and will have a distinct bean flavor.	
XANTHAN GUM	The xanthan gum can be omitted, but the cake will be more crumbly and will not rise quite as well.	

✅ WHY THIS RECIPE WORKS

One of the test kitchen's favorite cakes is a decidedly humble affair—an applesauce snack cake that is permeated with the sweet flavor of apples and infused with warm spice notes. Three-quarters of a cup of applesauce guaranteed robust apple flavor as well as the moistness needed, and small amounts of cinnamon, nutmeg, and cloves offered subtle spice flavor. Tasters preferred a modest of amount of sugar, and a mix of granulated and brown sugar lent more complexity to this simple cake. The biggest problem we faced was greasiness. We tried using oil rather than butter, but we really missed the buttery flavor in this unfrosted cake. Trimming the amount of butter from a whole stick to just half a stick solved the problem and preserved enough of the butter flavor to satisfy our tasters. Adding two extra eggs replaced some of the lost richness (without contributing any greasiness) and introduced more protein to the mix, which meant a sturdier crumb and a better rise. Supplementing the baking soda in the classic recipe with baking powder ensured there was enough leavener (especially in the oven) to create a stable cake with a tender, open crumb. Sprinkling a little cinnamon-sugar over the baked cake while it was still warm produced a crunchy, sweet crust.

Applesauce Snack Cake
SERVES 8

7½ ounces (1⅔ cups) ATK Gluten-Free Flour Blend (page 13)

2 teaspoons baking powder (see page 20)

1 teaspoon baking soda

¼ teaspoon xanthan gum

3 large eggs

3½ ounces (½ cup) plus 1 tablespoon granulated sugar

1¾ ounces (¼ cup packed) light brown sugar

½ teaspoon salt

½ teaspoon plus pinch ground cinnamon

¼ teaspoon ground nutmeg

⅛ teaspoon ground cloves

4 tablespoons unsalted butter, melted and cooled

¾ cup unsweetened applesauce, room temperature

1 teaspoon vanilla extract

1. Adjust oven rack to middle position and heat oven to 325 degrees. Grease 8-inch square cake pan, line bottom with parchment paper, and grease parchment. Whisk flour blend, baking powder, baking soda, and xanthan gum together in bowl to combine.

2. In large bowl, whisk eggs, ½ cup granulated sugar, brown sugar, salt, ½ teaspoon cinnamon, nutmeg, and cloves together until well combined and light-colored, about 20 seconds. Whisk in melted butter until combined. Whisk in applesauce and vanilla to combine. Whisk in flour blend mixture until batter is thoroughly combined and smooth.

3. Pour batter into prepared pan. Bake until toothpick inserted into center of cake comes out clean, 30 to 35 minutes, rotating pan halfway through baking.

4. Mix remaining 1 tablespoon sugar with remaining pinch cinnamon, and sprinkle evenly over warm cake. Let cake cool completely in pan on wire rack, about 2 hours. Run thin knife around edge of cake to loosen. Remove cake from pan, discarding parchment, and transfer to platter. Serve. (Cake can be wrapped tightly in plastic wrap and stored at room temperature for up to 1 day.)

VARIATION

Ginger-Cardamom Applesauce Snack Cake
Substitute ½ teaspoon ground ginger and ¼ teaspoon ground cardamom for cinnamon, nutmeg, and cloves. Substitute 1 tablespoon finely chopped crystallized ginger for cinnamon in step 4.

Rustic Plum Torte

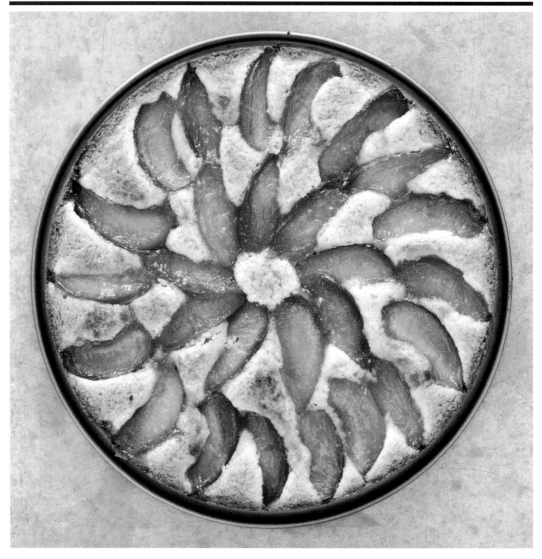

G-F TESTING LAB

FLOUR SUBSTITUTION	King Arthur Gluten-Free Multi-Purpose Flour 4½ ounces = ½ **cup plus** ⅓ **cup**	Bob's Red Mill GF All-Purpose Baking Flour 4½ ounces = ¾ **cup plus 2 tablespoons**
	Note that torte made with Bob's Red Mill will have a slight bean flavor.	
XANTHAN GUM	The xanthan gum can be omitted, but the torte will be more crumbly.	

✓ WHY THIS RECIPE WORKS

Many European cuisines have recipes for dense, single-layer cakes topped with seasonal fruit, and we particularly like the version made in Austria and Germany with summer plums. After an initial round of testing, we settled on a batter in which ground almonds replaced some of the flour. The high protein content of the almonds compensated for the low protein content in our gluten-free flour blend. The ground nuts also made the batter quite thick and thus better able to support the fruit. We also found that a little xanthan gum was necessary to build structure. As for the plums, we poached them in a few tablespoons of jelly and brandy to brighten their flavor. (Don't add this liquid to the cake pan; however, it can be reserved and served with the finished cake, ideally over a scoop of vanilla ice cream.) The cake can be served with ice cream or whipped cream. This cake is best served the day it is made.

Rustic Plum Torte
SERVES 8

- 3 tablespoons brandy
- 2 tablespoons red currant jelly or seedless raspberry jam
- 1 pound red or black plums, halved, pitted, and cut into 8 wedges
- 5¼ ounces (¾ cup) granulated sugar
- ⅓ cup slivered almonds
- 4½ ounces (1 cup) ATK Gluten-Free Flour Blend (page 13)
- ½ teaspoon baking powder (see page 20)
- ¼ teaspoon salt
- ¼ teaspoon xanthan gum
- 6 tablespoons unsalted butter, cut into 6 pieces and softened
- 1 large egg plus 1 large yolk
- 1 teaspoon vanilla extract
- ½ teaspoon almond extract
  Confectioners' sugar

1. Cook brandy and jelly together in 10-inch nonstick skillet over medium heat until thick and syrupy, 2 to 3 minutes. Remove skillet from heat and place plums cut side down in syrup. Return skillet to medium heat and cook, shaking pan to prevent plums from sticking, until plums release their juices and liquid reduces to thick syrup, about 5 minutes. Let plums cool in skillet, about 20 minutes.

2. Adjust oven rack to middle position and heat oven to 350 degrees. Grease 9-inch springform pan, line bottom with parchment, and grease parchment.

3. Process granulated sugar and almonds together in food processor until nuts are finely ground, about 1 minute. Add flour blend, baking powder, salt, and xanthan gum and pulse to combine, about 5 pulses. Add butter and pulse until mixture resembles coarse sand, about 10 pulses. Add egg, yolk, vanilla, and almond extract and process until smooth, about 5 seconds, scraping down bowl if needed (batter will be very thick and heavy).

4. Scrape batter into prepared pan and smooth top. Stir plums to coat with syrup, then arrange wedges in two rings over top of cake. Bake until cake is golden brown, 40 to 50 minutes, rotating pan halfway through baking.

5. Run knife around edge of cake to loosen. Let cake cool in pan on wire rack for at least 30 minutes. Remove cake from pan, discard parchment, and transfer to serving platter. Dust with confectioners' sugar and serve warm or at room temperature.

Lemon Pound Cake

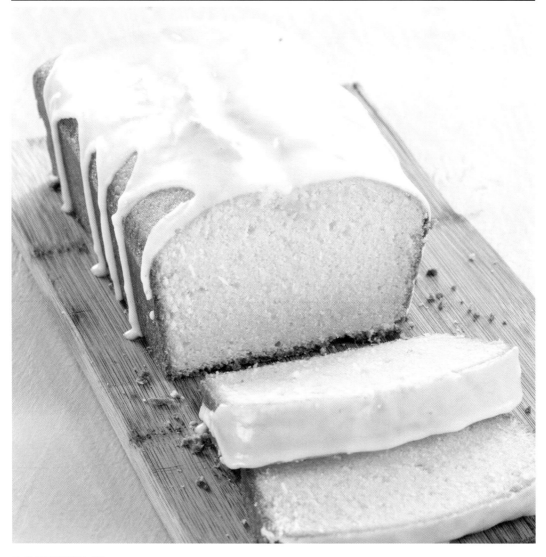

G-F TESTING LAB

FLOUR SUBSTITUTION	King Arthur Gluten-Free Multi-Purpose Flour 7 ounces = 1¼ **cups**	Bob's Red Mill GF All-Purpose Baking Flour 7 ounces = 1¼ **cups plus 2 tablespoons**
	Note that pound cake made with King Arthur will not rise as much and will be denser, and pound cake made with Bob's Red Mill will have a coarser crumb and a distinct bean flavor.	
XANTHAN GUM	Do not omit the xanthan gum; it is crucial to the structure of the cake. For more information, see page 16.	

✓ WHY THIS RECIPE WORKS

Making a superior lemon pound cake (fine-crumbed, rich, moist, and buttery) is not an easy feat. That's because the classic recipe—with just flour, butter, sugar, and eggs—contains no leavener. Using the test kitchen's favorite recipe as our guide, we began our testing by simply subbing in our gluten-free flour blend for all-purpose flour. The resulting cake was overly tender (it crumbled too easily), greasy, and gummy. Adding a bit of xanthan gum improved the structure so the cake didn't crumble. Reducing the amount of butter (the classic recipe contains two sticks) helped with the greasiness, but it also made the cake dry. We tried oil, but tasters rejected this swap—pound cake must taste buttery. We switched gears and looked to replace some of the butter with something else. After several rounds of testing, we ended up swapping out one stick of butter for an equal amount of cream cheese. Unlike butter, which separates into water and fat in the oven, cream cheese—which is much more stable—didn't cause the greasiness problem that plagued our all-butter gluten-free pound cakes. To get the most lemon flavor, we pulsed the zest in the food processor with the sugar. Since we were already using our food processor, we found that we could mix the batter with it as well, as it ensured a perfect emulsification of the eggs, sugar, and melted butter. The crumb was still a tad gummy and heavy, but adding a small amount of baking powder increased lift and produced a consistent crumb with just the right density.

Lemon Pound Cake
SERVES 8

CAKE
- 7 ounces (1⅓ cups plus ¼ cup) ATK Gluten-Free Flour Blend (page 13)
- 1 teaspoon baking powder (see page 20)
- ½ teaspoon salt
- ¼ teaspoon xanthan gum
- 8¾ ounces (1¼ cups) granulated sugar
- 2 tablespoons grated lemon zest plus 1 tablespoon juice (2 lemons)
- 4 large eggs
- 4 ounces cream cheese
- 1½ teaspoons vanilla extract
- 8 tablespoons unsalted butter, melted

GLAZE
- 2 ounces (½ cup) confectioners' sugar, sifted
- 2 teaspoons lemon juice

1. FOR THE CAKE: Adjust oven rack to middle position and heat oven to 350 degrees. Grease and flour 8½ by 4½-inch loaf pan. Whisk flour blend, baking powder, salt, and xanthan gum together in bowl.

2. Pulse sugar and zest together in food processor until combined, about 5 pulses. Add lemon juice, eggs, cream cheese, and vanilla and process until combined, about 15 seconds. With processor running, add melted butter in steady stream until combined, about 20 seconds. Transfer mixture to large bowl. Add flour blend mixture and whisk until batter is thoroughly combined and smooth.

3. Pour batter into prepared pan. Bake 15 minutes. Reduce oven temperature to 325 degrees and continue to bake until cake is golden brown and toothpick inserted into center comes out clean, about 40 minutes, rotating pan halfway through baking. Let cake cool in pan on wire rack for 10 minutes. Run knife around edge of cake to loosen. Remove cake from pan and let cool completely on rack, about 2 hours.

4. FOR THE GLAZE: Whisk sugar and lemon juice together in bowl until smooth. Spread glaze over cake, allowing some to drip down sides. Let glaze set for at least 15 minutes before serving. (Cake can be wrapped in plastic wrap and stored at room temperature for up to 2 days.)

VARIATION
Lemon–Poppy Seed Pound Cake
Add ⅓ cup poppy seeds to batter with flour blend mixture in step 2.

TEST KITCHEN TIP **Making Lemon Pound Cake**

There are three main challenges in creating a great lemon pound cake—getting enough lemon flavor, incorporating the fat to make an emulsified batter, and adding the flour to what's already a thick batter. Grinding the lemon zest with the sugar in a food processor releases a ton of flavor, and the whirring blade of the food processor also does a great job of incorporating the melted butter into the batter. Unfortunately, the food processor doesn't do a very job good of incorporating the flour evenly to produce a smooth batter. Moving operations to a large bowl and using a whisk enables you to incorporate the flour easily and evenly.

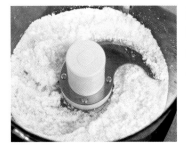

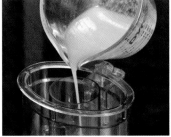

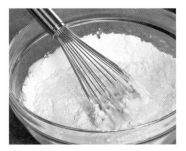

1. Pulse sugar and zest in food processor until combined, about 5 pulses. The sugar breaks down zest so its essential oils are evenly distributed in cake batter.

2. Add lemon juice, eggs, cream cheese, and vanilla and process until combined, about 15 seconds. With machine running, add melted butter through feed tube in steady stream until combined, about 20 seconds.

3. Transfer mixture to large bowl. Add flour blend mixture and whisk until batter is thoroughly combined and smooth.

TEST KITCHEN TIP **Baking with Butter vs. Oil**

In the test kitchen, our preference is to use butter rather than oil in most baked goods, including cakes. In most recipes, butter tastes better. (There are exceptions, such as carrot cake, which is typically made with oil to ensure a very moist, very tender crumb.) But as we developed gluten-free cakes, we found that oil generally worked better, and butter was the "exception."

That's because the butter imparted a greasy texture to many cakes and cupcakes. In some recipes, we simply replaced the butter with oil and added sour cream for some dairy richness. In other recipes, we kept the butter but looked to other solutions to mitigate greasiness. For example, in our Lemon Pound Cake we replaced half the butter with cream cheese.

But the question lingered: Why does butter make baked goods feel and taste greasy when oil doesn't, especially since oil is 100 percent fat and butter is just 80 percent fat (the rest is mostly water)? Shouldn't butter, which has less fat, make baked goods less greasy?

The answer, as we learned, has to do with how butter and oil interact with the proteins in the flour. When oil is mixed with flour, it evenly coats the flour particles, producing baked goods with a consistent crumb. (Oil also tends to make baked goods that are a bit more compact and thus a bit moister.) In contrast, butter coats the flour particles unevenly, and small clumps of fat end up pooling together. It turns out that the water in the butter is actually the problem—it weakens the bonds between the fat in the butter and the protein molecules in the flour. (And the problem is exacerbated in gluten-free recipes because the flour has so little protein to begin with.) It's these unattached pools of butter that end up giving gluten-free baked goods their oily mouthfeel and greasy texture.

Almond Cake

✓ WHY THIS RECIPE WORKS

Almond cake is typically a simple, unfrosted single-layer cake with rich nut flavor. It is both elegant and casual. Despite the bold almond flavor and beautiful appearance, most traditional almond cakes are heavy and dense and come across more as a sweet confection than as a cake. Most recipes are made with almond paste and flour, plus sugar and eggs. By switching out the traditional almond paste for ground almonds, we reduced the sweetness quotient and boosted the nut flavor. This swap also made the cake lighter and less candylike. Traditional recipes don't contain much flour, so using our gluten-free flour blend worked fairly well, although we found it necessary to use an extra egg to boost the protein content and thus improve the structure of the cake. If blanched sliced almonds cannot be found, use 1 cup of slivered almonds in the cake and ⅓ cup of unblanched sliced almonds for the topping. This cake is very sticky, so be sure to grease and flour the cake pan well. Serve with Orange Crème Fraiche or simply dust with confectioners' sugar. Refer to pages 308-309 when making this recipe.

Almond Cake
SERVES 8 TO 10

- 1½ cups plus ⅓ cup blanched sliced almonds, toasted
- 4½ ounces (1 cup) ATK Gluten-Free Flour Blend (page 13)
- ¾ teaspoon salt
- ¼ teaspoon baking powder (see page 20)
- ⅛ teaspoon baking soda
- 4 large eggs
- 7 ounces (1 cup) plus 2 tablespoons sugar
- 1 tablespoon plus ½ teaspoon grated lemon zest (2 lemons)
- 1 teaspoon almond extract
- 4 tablespoons unsalted butter, melted
- 4 tablespoons vegetable oil

1. Adjust oven rack to middle position and heat oven to 300 degrees. Grease and flour 9-inch round cake pan and line bottom with parchment paper. Pulse 1½ cups almonds, flour blend, salt, baking powder, and baking soda in food processor until almonds are finely ground, 10 to 15 pulses; transfer to bowl.

2. Place eggs, 1 cup sugar, 1 tablespoon zest, and almond extract in now-empty food processor and process for 2 minutes. With processor running, add melted butter, followed by oil, in steady stream, until incorporated. Add almond-flour mixture and pulse until fully combined, 4 to 5 pulses.

3. Scrape batter into prepared pan, smooth top, and sprinkle with remaining ⅓ cup almonds. Using fingers, combine remaining 2 tablespoons sugar and remaining ½ teaspoon lemon zest in bowl until fragrant, then sprinkle over top.

4. Bake until center of cake is set and toothpick inserted into center comes out clean, 55 to 65 minutes, rotating pan after 40 minutes. Let cake cool in pan on wire rack for 15 minutes. Run knife around edge of cake to loosen. Remove cake from pan, discard parchment, and let cool completely on rack, about 1½ hours. Serve. (Cake can be wrapped tightly in plastic wrap and stored at room temperature for up to 2 days.)

Orange Crème Fraiche
MAKES ABOUT 2 CUPS

- 2 oranges
- 8 ounces (1 cup) crème fraiche
- 2 tablespoons sugar
- ⅛ teaspoon salt

Grate 1 teaspoon zest from oranges; set aside. Cut away remaining peel and pith from oranges. Over bowl, use paring knife to slice between membranes to release segments. Cut segments into ¼-inch pieces, place in fine-mesh strainer, and let drain. Whisk orange zest, crème fraiche, sugar, and salt together in medium bowl. Fold in strained orange pieces, cover, and refrigerate until chilled, about 1 hour, before serving.

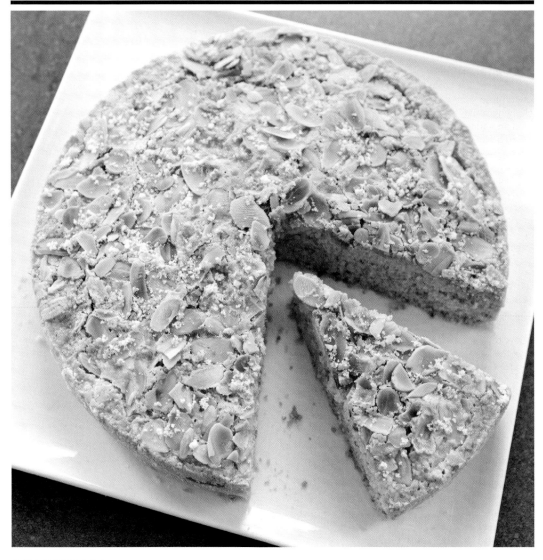

G-F TESTING LAB

FLOUR SUBSTITUTION	King Arthur Gluten-Free Multi-Purpose Flour 4½ ounces = **½ cup plus ⅓ cup**	Bob's Red Mill GF All-Purpose Baking Flour 4½ ounces = **¾ cup plus 2 tablespoons**

Note that cake made with Bob's Red Mill will be crumbly and have a distinct bean flavor.

Rebuilding an Italian Classic

THE PROBLEM This Italian favorite, typically made with almond paste or ground almonds plus sugar, a little flour, butter, and eggs, is a sweet, dense, almost pound cake–like cake. We set our sights on developing a gluten-free version, thinking it would be an easy task given how little flour it typically requires. Using the test kitchen's most recent almond cake recipe as a starting point, we simply replaced the all-purpose wheat flour with an equal amount of our gluten-free flour blend. The result? A very dense, flat, and greasy cake. Developing a gluten-free version of this cake was not going to be a simple fix. Here's what we learned.

TOAST AND GRIND ALMONDS A key factor in this recipe is infusing the cake with deep almond flavor. Marzipan, ground almonds, almond extract, and almond paste are often used either alone or in combination. Taking a hard look at almond paste, we zeroed in on the fact that it is made of 50 percent almonds and 50 percent sugar. Given that our flour blend is already on the sweet side as a result of its two rice flours, the addition of almond paste made the cake cloyingly sweet. Grinding sliced almonds seemed like a much better route and would help us control the sweetness. Toasting the almonds deepened their flavor and made them easier to grind, plus the ground almonds helped give the cake a nice texture. We still needed to reduce the amount of sugar to 1 cup (most recipes call for 1¼ to 1½ cups).

THE CREAMING ISSUE Traditional almond cakes cream butter and sugar before incorporating the eggs and dry ingredients. This method relies on the flour to produce gluten and create structure. Obviously we needed a different approach. We first turned to the egg foam method, which requires whipping the eggs and sugar for a full 2 minutes before incorporating melted butter and flour; beating the eggs like this not only incorporated lots of air but unraveled their protein strands so they could hold on to that air. This created the lift and structure that would normally come from gluten. But it was actually a bit too much lift for this particular cake, which is not supposed to be tall and fluffy. Was there a middle ground?

USE THE FOOD PROCESSOR We wanted to stay true to the dense, rich texture that is the hallmark of this cake. Since we were already grinding the almonds in the food processor, we tried using it to whip and aerate the sugar and eggs, wondering if it would make a difference. Not only could we successfully whip the eggs and sugar in the food processor, but, unlike the mixer, its sharp blade damaged some of the protein strands of the eggs, resulting in less overall lift. Now we had the moist interior we were looking for without all the unintended fluffiness.

A MIX OF BUTTER AND OIL Now that we were making the cake batter in the food processor, we needed to switch from softened butter to melted butter. We have found that our flour blend does not absorb fat in the same way that all-purpose flour does. To combat greasiness, we ended up using less butter, but that also made the cake a bit dry. Vegetable oil actually does a better job than butter of creating a moist crumb. (Oil-based carrot cakes are a good example of this phenomenon.) Replacing half the butter with oil helped keep the cake moist while still providing the flavor benefits associated with butter.

Flourless Chocolate Cake

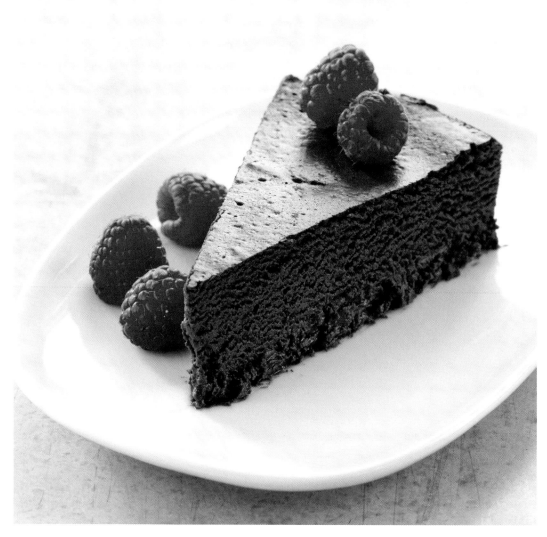

G-F TESTING LAB

CHOCOLATE   Not all brands of chocolate are processed in a gluten-free facility; make sure to read the label.

WHY THIS RECIPE WORKS

Flourless chocolate cake should serve as an ultimate expression of pure chocolate flavor, with a rich, dense texture that still retains some delicacy. Unfortunately, many versions are too heavy, while others are gritty. Yes, this cake should be rich, but it shouldn't be leaden, and it must be smooth and creamy. We found it imperative to whip the eggs in order to lighten the batter. Baking the cake in a water bath created a gentle moist-heat environment that ensured a smooth, creamy result. It's also important to remove the cake from the oven while it is still a little underdone. The cake will continue to cook and firm up as it cools. Good-quality chocolate is very important to the flavor and texture of this cake. You can substitute ¼ cup warm water mixed with 1 teaspoon instant espresso or instant coffee for the strong coffee. If substituting an 8-inch springform pan, increase the baking time to 22 to 25 minutes. This cake is very rich, so small slices are best. For neat, professional-looking slices, clean the knife thoroughly after each cut.

Flourless Chocolate Cake
SERVES 12 TO 14

1	**pound bittersweet chocolate, chopped**
16	**tablespoons unsalted butter, cut into 16 pieces**
¼	**cup strong coffee**
8	**large eggs, room temperature**
	Confectioners' sugar
10	**ounces (2 cups) raspberries**

1. Adjust oven rack to lower-middle position and heat oven to 325 degrees. Grease 9-inch springform pan, then line bottom with parchment paper. Wrap outside of pan with two 18-inch square pieces heavy-duty aluminum foil. Lay dish towel in bottom of roasting pan and place wrapped cake pan on towel. Bring kettle of water to boil.

2. Microwave chocolate, butter, and coffee in large bowl at 50 percent, stirring often, until melted, 1 to 3 minutes; set aside to cool slightly.

3. Using stand mixer fitted with whisk, whip eggs on medium-low speed until frothy, about 1 minute. Increase speed to high and whip until eggs are very thick and pale yellow, 5 to 10 minutes. Gently fold one-third of whipped eggs into chocolate mixture with rubber spatula until few streaks remain. Repeat twice more with remaining whipped eggs and continue to fold batter until no streaks remain.

4. Scrape batter into prepared pan and smooth top. Set roasting pan on oven rack and pour boiling water into roasting pan until it reaches about halfway up sides of springform pan. Bake cake until edges are just beginning to set, a thin crust has formed over top, and cake registers 140 degrees about 1 inch from edge, 18 to 20 minutes. (Do not overbake.)

5. Let cake cool in roasting pan for 45 minutes, then transfer to wire rack and let cool until barely warm, 2½ to 3 hours, running knife around edge of cake every hour or so. Wrap pan tightly in plastic wrap and refrigerate until set, at least 12 hours and up to 2 days.

6. About 30 minutes before serving, run knife around edge of cake and remove sides of pan. Carefully slide cake, still on parchment, onto serving platter. Before serving, dust with confectioners' sugar and garnish with raspberries.

TEST KITCHEN TIP **Setting Up a Water Bath**

Some cakes are baked in a "water bath," which means that the cake pan is partially immersed in water to ensure gentle heating. A water bath reduces the risk of overcooking cheesecakes and other delicate flourless cakes. Wrap the springform pan with two pieces of foil to prevent leaking.

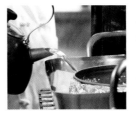

Line roasting pan with dish towel. Place springform pan in roasting pan, fill, place pan in oven, and carefully add boiling water until it reaches halfway up sides of springform pan.

Conversions & Equivalencies

The recipes in this book were developed using standard U.S. measures following U.S. government guidelines. The charts below offer equivalents for U.S., metric, and imperial (U.K.) measures. All conversions are approximate and have been rounded up or down to the nearest whole number.

EXAMPLE:

1 teaspoon = 4.9292 milliliters, rounded up to 5 milliliters
1 ounce = 28.3495 grams, rounded down to 28 grams

VOLUME CONVERSIONS

U.S.	METRIC
1 teaspoon	5 milliliters
2 teaspoons	10 milliliters
1 tablespoon	15 milliliters
2 tablespoons	30 milliliters
¼ cup	59 milliliters
⅓ cup	79 milliliters
½ cup	118 milliliters
¾ cup	177 milliliters
1 cup	237 milliliters
1¼ cups	296 milliliters
1½ cups	355 milliliters
2 cups (1 pint)	473 milliliters
2½ cups	591 milliliters
3 cups	710 milliliters
4 cups (1 quart)	0.946 liter
1.06 quarts	1 liter
4 quarts (1 gallon)	3.8 liters

WEIGHT CONVERSIONS

OUNCES	GRAMS
½	14
¾	21
1	28
1½	43
2	57
2½	71
3	85
3½	99
4	113
4½	128
5	142
6	170
7	198
8	227
9	255
10	283
12	340
16 (1 pound)	454

CONVERSIONS FOR INGREDIENTS COMMONLY USED IN BAKING

Baking is an exacting science. Because measuring by weight is far more accurate than measuring by volume, and thus more likely to achieve reliable results, in our recipes we provide ounce measures in addition to cup measures for many ingredients. Refer to the chart below to convert these measures into grams.

INGREDIENT	OUNCES	GRAMS
1 cup granulated (white) sugar	7	198
1 cup packed brown sugar (light or dark)	7	198
1 cup confectioners' sugar	4	113
1 cup cocoa powder	3	85
4 tablespoons butter* (½ stick, or ¼ cup)	2	57
8 tablespoons butter* (1 stick, or ½ cup)	4	113
16 tablespoons butter* (2 sticks, or 1 cup)	8	227

* In the United States, butter is sold both salted and unsalted. We generally recommend unsalted butter. If you are using salted butter, take this into consideration before adding salt to a recipe.

OVEN TEMPERATURES

FAHRENHEIT	CELSIUS	GAS MARK (IMPERIAL)
225	105	¼
250	120	½
275	135	1
300	150	2
325	165	3
350	180	4
375	190	5
400	200	6
425	220	7
450	230	8
475	245	9

CONVERTING TEMPERATURES FROM AN INSTANT-READ THERMOMETER

We include doneness temperatures in many of the recipes in this book. We recommend an instant-read thermometer for the job. Refer to the above table to convert Fahrenheit degrees to Celsius. Or, for temperatures not represented in the chart, use this simple formula:

Subtract 32 degrees from the Fahrenheit reading, then divide the result by 1.8 to find the Celsius reading.

EXAMPLE:
"Roast chicken until thighs register 175 degrees."
To convert:
175°F − 32 = 143°
143° ÷ 1.8 = 79.44°C, rounded down to 79°C

Weight-to-Volume Equivalencies for GF Flours

Different brands of wheat flour all contain the same ingredients so they measure out the same. However, different gluten-free flour brands contain different ingredients, which will pack differently. For this reason, weight-to-volume equivalencies vary from brand to brand, as you can see from the information below.

You can easily avoid this problem (and never look at this chart again), if you simply weigh your flour (this is how our recipes are written). Ten ounces of gluten-free flour blend is the same, no matter the brand. If you decide to measure flour by volume, the G-F Testing Lab feature will give you the relevant conversion information.

This chart will be helpful if you're trying to rework another recipe (not in this book) and you're using either our homemade blend or flours made by King Arthur or Bob's Red Mill. See page 14 for more details on why we recommend these two brands if you decide not to make our homemade blend.

OUNCES	ATK GLUTEN-FREE FLOUR BLEND	BOB'S RED MILL GF ALL-PURPOSE BAKING FLOUR	KING ARTHUR GLUTEN-FREE MULTI-PURPOSE FLOUR
1	3½ tablespoons	3 tablespoons	3 tablespoons
1.5	⅓ cup	5 tablespoons	¼ cup
2	7 tablespoons	6 tablespoons	6 tablespoons
2.5	⅓ cup plus ¼ cup	½ cup	7 tablespoons
3	⅔ cup	½ cup plus 2 tablespoons	⅓ cup plus ¼ cup
3.5	¾ cup	⅔ cup	½ cup plus 2 tablespoons
4	¾ cup plus 2 tablespoons	½ cup plus ⅓ cup	¾ cup
4.5	**1 cup**	¾ cup plus 2 tablespoons	½ cup plus ⅓ cup
5	1 cup plus 2 tablespoons	**1 cup**	⅔ cup plus ¼ cup
5.5	1¼ cups	1 cup plus 2 tablespoons	**1 cup**
6	1⅓ cups	⅔ cup plus ½ cup	¾ cup plus ⅓ cup
6.5	¾ cup plus ⅔ cup	1⅓ cups	⅔ cup plus ½ cup
7	1⅓ cups plus ¼ cup	1¼ cups plus 2 tablespoons	1¼ cups
7.5	1⅔ cups	1½ cups	1¼ cups plus 2 tablespoons
8	1¾ cups	1½ cups plus 2 tablespoons	¾ cup plus ⅔ cup
8.5	1¾ cups plus 2 tablespoons	1⅔ cups	1⅓ cup plus ¼ cup
9	**2 cups**	1½ cups plus ⅓ cup	1½ cups plus 2 tablespoons
9.5	2 cups plus 2 tablespoons	1¾ cups plus 2 tablespoons	1¾ cups
10	2¼ cups	**2 cups**	1½ cups plus ⅓ cup
10.5	2⅓ cups	2 cups plus 2 tablespoons	1⅔ cups plus ¼ cup
11	1¾ cups plus ⅔ cup	1⅔ cups plus ½ cup	**2 cups**
11.5	2⅓ cups plus ¼ cup	2⅓ cups	1¾ cups plus ⅓ cup
12	2⅔ cups	2¼ cups plus 2 tablespoons	1⅔ cups plus ½ cup
12.5	2¾ cups	2½ cups	2¼ cups
13	2¾ cups plus 2 tablespoons	2½ cups plus 2 tablespoons	2¼ cups plus 2 tablespoons
13.5	**3 cups**	2⅔ cups	1¾ cups plus ⅔ cup
14	3 cups plus 2 tablespoons	2½ cups plus ⅓ cup	2⅓ cups plus ¼ cup
14.5	3¼ cups	2¾ cups plus 2 tablespoons	2½ cups plus 2 tablespoons
15	3⅓ cups	**3 cups**	2¾ cups
15.5	2¾ cups plus ⅔ cup	3 cups plus 2 tablespoons	2½ cups plus ⅓ cup
16	3⅓ cups plus ¼ cup	2⅔ cups plus ½ cup	2⅔ cups plus ¼ cup
16.5	3⅔ cups	3⅓ cups	**3 cups**

Index

E

Easy Stovetop Macaroni and Cheese, *140,* 141

Easy Vanilla Frosting, 290

Easy Vanilla Frosting for Cupcakes, 290

Edamame, Shiitakes, and Ginger, Quinoa Pilaf
with, 81

Eggplant

Parmesan, *136,* 137–39

Roasted, and Sesame, Soba Noodles with, *120,* 121

Eggs, 17

English Muffins

freezing, 209

recipe for, *186,* 187

Evaporated milk, shopping for, 141

F

Fish. *See* Anchovy(ies)

Fish sauce, shopping for, 127

Flame tamers, 79

Flaxseeds

Hearty Country Flax Bread, 179–81, *180*

shopping for, 181

Florentine Lace Cookies, 231–33, *232*

Flour

almond, about, 18

buckwheat, about, 18

chickpea, about, 18

masa harina, about, 18

masarepa, about, 204

oat, about, 18

rice, about, 19

wheat, about, 5–7

see also Gluten-Free Flour Blend

Flourless Chocolate Cake, *310,* 311

Foil sling, creating, 237

Fresh Fruit Tart, *278,* 279

Fresh Pasta, *98,* 99–101

Alfredo, 103

al Limone, 102

sauces for, 102–3

shaped, preparing, 103

with Tomato–Brown Butter Sauce, 102

Fresh Strawberry Pie, *256,* 257

Fried Chicken, 147–49, *148*

Frostings

Almond, 290

applying to layer cake, 291

Chocolate, Creamy, 284

Chocolate, Creamy, for Cupcakes, 284

Coconut, 290

Coffee, 290

Cream Cheese, 295

Cream Cheese, for Cupcakes, 295

piping onto cupcakes, 287

Vanilla, Easy, 290

Vanilla, Easy, for Cupcakes, 290

Fruit

Dried, Almond Granola with, *60,* 61

Fresh, Tart, *278,* 279

Tropical, Individual Pavlovas with, *262,* 263

see also Berry(ies); *specific fruits*

Fudgy Brownies, *236,* 237

Fusilli

with Basil Pesto, *106,* 107

with Kale–Sunflower Seed Pesto, 107

with Roasted Red Pepper Pesto, 107

with Spring Vegetable Cream Sauce, *108,* 109

G

Ginger

-Cardamom Applesauce Snack Cake, 301

Gingerbread Cake, *298,* 299

Gingerbread Cake, *298,* 299

Gluten

defined, 5

development of, 5

-free diet, key challenges, 7

science of, 5

Gluten-Free Flour Blend

America's Test Kitchen, 13

binders in, 16

buying vs. homemade, 14

homemade, developing, 12–13

measuring, 15